Health Research

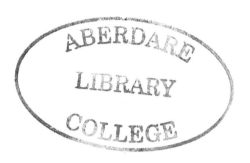

Health Research

Catherine Anne Berglund

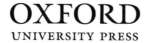

OXFORD
UNIVERSITY PRESS

OXFORD
UNIVERSITY PRESS

253 Normanby Road, South Melbourne, Victoria, Australia 3205

Oxford University Press is a department of the University of Oxford.
It furthers the University's objective of excellence in research, scholarship,
and education by publishing worldwide in

Oxford New York

Athens Auckland Bangkok Bogotá Buenos Aires Calcutta
Cape Town Chennai Dar es Salaam Delhi Florence Hong Kong Istanbul
Karachi Kuala Lumpur Madrid Melbourne Mexico City Mumbai Nairobi
Paris Port Moresby São Paulo Singapore Taipei Tokyo Toronto Warsaw

with associated companies in Berlin Ibadan

OXFORD is a registered trade mark of Oxford University Press
in the UK and certain other countries

National Library of Australia
Cataloguing-in-Publication data:

Health Research.

Bibliography.
Includes index.
ISBN 0 19 551218 9.

1. Health—Research. I. Berglund, Catherine Anne.

362.1/072

Indexed by Ross Gilham
Illustrations by Richard Dall
Cover design by MAPG
Typeset by Desktop Concepts P/L, Melbourne
Printed through Bookpac Production Services, Singapore

Editor's Dedication

For two friends and colleagues: Julie Walters, the first person to suggest that I write a research book, and Phillip Godwin, who encouraged me to embark on this project.

Both friends are sadly missed and fondly remembered.

Contents

Figures

Tables

Abbreviations

ADL	activities of daily living
AIDS	acquired immune deficiency syndrome
AIHW	Australian Institute of Health and Welfare
ANOVA	analysis of variance
CDC	Center for Disease Control (USA)
CQI	continuous quality improvement
Cwlth	Commonwealth
H0	null hypothesis
H1	alternative hypothesis
HIV	human immunodeficiency virus
HREC	human research ethics committee
IEC	institutional ethics committee
IMRAD	introduction, method, results and discussion
KS	Kaposi's sarcoma
MRC	Medical Research Council (United Kingdom)
NHMRC	National Health & Medical Research Council, Australia
NHL	non-Hodgkin's lymphoma
p-value	probability of incorrect rejection of null hypothesis
PAR	participatory action research
RCT	randomised controlled trial
Type I error	error of rejection of true null hypothesis
Type II error	error of rejection of true alternative hypothesis
Type III error	error of correct inference for wrong reasons
WHO	World Health Organization (United Nations)
WWW	world wide web

Contributors

Catherine A. Berglund BSc(Psychol) PhD (Community Med)
Catherine Berglund is the editor of this book, and a contributing author of chapter 1, 'Beginning the quest', chapter 12, 'Ethics as part of research', and chapter 14, 'Writing and publishing'. The breadth of this text is influenced by her interest in increasingly diverse methodologies in health research. Her PhD thesis, on the ethics of research with human participants, spanned the disciplines of research methods and ethics. Catherine lectures in ethics and research at the University of New South Wales. Her first book, *Ethics for Health Care*, published by Oxford University Press in 1998, could be used as a companion to *Health Research*.

Deborah Black BSc Dip Ed M Stats PhD
Deborah Black, an experienced statistician and Senior Lecturer in the School of Community Medicine, University of New South Wales, has for some years worked on health projects, and taught researchers and students how to use statistical tools sensibly. She has explained the process of statistical application to data in a straightforward way in her contribution, chapter 5, 'Numbers and more'. Deborah has also combined with a clinician, Sue Irvine, to present an informed enquiry process which makes use of statistics, in chapter 8, 'So, how is the treatment going?'

John A. Devereux BA LLB DPhil
John Devereux is a Professor in law at the University of Queensland. His text, *Medical Law: Text, Cases and Materials*, is published by Cavendish. John has served as a Law Reform Commissioner, and has taken an academic interest in children and medical treatment decision-making. He has contributed chapter 13, 'Disciplines and boundaries', which alerts researchers to legal boundaries in the conduct of their health research.

†Phillip Godwin RN Dip NrEd BHA BM MHPEd
Phillip Godwin had a unique combination of training and experience in nursing, medicine, health administration, and health personnel education. He brought this experience to bear in his contribution, chapter 2, 'Using research in practice'. Phillip was the Senior Health Education Officer (Medical Education) with the Australasian Society for HIV Medicine Inc.

Andrew Grulich MBBS MSc PhD FAFPHM
Andrew Grulich is a Senior Lecturer in epidemiology at the National Centre in HIV Epidemiology and Clinical Research, Sydney. His PhD concerned the epidemiology of cancer in people with AIDS, and he presents an enquiry on this topic in his chapter 6, 'How is our health?', as an example of epidemiological analysis. He has ten years experience in teaching epidemiology to medical students and postgraduate students in public health.

Dusan Hadzi-Pavlovic BSc(Psychol) MPsychol
Dusan Hadzi-Pavlovic is a Senior Hospital Scientist, with the South Eastern Sydney Area Health Service, and Adjunct Senior Lecturer, School of Psychiatry, University of New South Wales. He is a research psychologist who is well known for his capability of explaining complex statistical issues in simple terms. He works with clinicians, and with applied health data. He has co-contributed chapter 7, 'Meaningful categories', and concentrates on ordinal statistics.

Ben Haneman MBBS FRACP
Ben Haneman is a consultant physician with an interest in the history of medicine. He has been awarded an AM in Australia, and a Cruz de Caballero de la Orden de Merito Civil in Spain. He is well known for his writings in medicine and history of medicine. His contribution to chapter 3, 'Great expectations', includes a case study of an early Australian public health concern.

C. D'Arcy J. Holman MBBS MPH PhD FAFPHM
D'Arcy Holman is Professor in Public Health and Director, Centre for Health Services Research, Department of Public Health, the University of Western Australia. He has worked with Jeanette Ward to co-contribute chapter 4, 'Who needs to plan?'.

Susan Irvine MB ChB SM MPH MPM FRACMA FAFPHM
Susan is active in general practice as well as postgraduate teaching, and is a Senior Lecturer in the School of Community Medicine, University of New South Wales. Her academic interests are in behaviour change for health, and health policy. She has co-contributed chapter 8, 'So, how is the treatment going?', to illustrate the partnership of clinical and statistical inquiry in the research process.

Alix G. Magney BA(Sociology)
Alix Magney has co-contributed chapter 11, 'Assistants and mentors'. Alix's background is in sociological research. She is currently undertaking a PhD in the School of Sociology, University of New South Wales, with an interest in negotiation of health issues.

Elizabeth O'Brien Cert Nursing BN MPH
Elizabeth O'Brien has worked for many years in both the hospital system and the community as a nurse. In recent years, she has brought her clinical experience to public health-related research. She has co-authored chapter 11, 'Assistants and mentors'.

Natalie O'Dea BEc (Soc Sci)
From a background in humanities and social sciences research, Natalie is now a private consultant, and contributes to health education. Working with Deborah Saltman, she has brought her understanding of education practice and training to health professional education, and regularly evaluates training programs. Natalie has co-contributed chapter 10, 'Quality and quantity'.

Lisa Parker BMed Sc MBBS(Hons)
Lisa Parker is a medical practitioner, who has worked in clinical practice and pathology. Lisa is completing her Masters on the history of autopsy and the human body, and presents part of her research as a case study in chapter 3, 'Great expectations'. Lisa is a recently appointed Registrar in Palliative Care at the Sacred Heart Hospice, St Vincent's Hospital, Sydney.

Mary Phipps MSc
As an experienced statistician, Mary Phipps has been involved on a large number of clinical and health related research projects. She has co-authored chapter 7, 'Meaningful categories', which highlights the use of categorical statistics with health data. She publishes on mathematical and applied aspects of statistics, and is a Senior Lecturer in the School of Mathematics and Statistics at the University of Sydney.

Jan Ritchie Dip Phty MHPEd PhD
Jan Ritchie is an experienced qualitative researcher and Senior Lecturer in the School of Medical Education, University of New South Wales. She has published widely on her own, and with others, on health issues and interventions. Jan largely works in context, with rich material from community participants. Her doctorate work was a participatory process on health issues with steel workers. Her contribution, chapter 9, 'Not everything can be reduced to numbers', gives an overview of qualitative methods and uses examples from her research experience.

Deborah C. Saltman MBBS MD FRACGP FAFPHM

Deborah Saltman is Professor of General Practice at the University of Sydney, and an experienced researcher. Her research interests range from clinical to professional development issues, and she is active in the continuing medical education of general practice colleagues. Deborah has contributed chapter 10, 'Quality and quantity', which illustrates a range of methods in health research practice.

Vanessa Traynor BA

Originally from a history and philosophy of science background, Vanessa Traynor has had experience working on health projects as diverse as medical records in general practice, policy evaluation, and ethics in the general practice setting. Vanessa has a working understanding of both qualitative and quantitative methods. She is completing a Masters of Community Health, and has co-authored chapter 11, 'Assistants and mentors'. Vanessa is currently a Research Officer with the Discipline of General Practice, Newcastle University.

Jeanette E. Ward MBBS MHPEd PhD FAFPHM

With training in medicine, and health education, Jeanette Ward is well placed to comment on research design choices which are useful and rigorous. Jeanette Ward is Associate Professor and Director of the Needs Assessment and Health Outcomes Unit, in the Central Sydney Area Health Service, and Honorary Fellow, School of Medical Education, University of New South Wales, and brings her broad understanding of research and clinical contexts to bear in her research. She has published widely, and is well known for her attention to detail in the conduct of research. She has contributed chapter 4, 'Who needs to plan?'

Preface

Health research should not be a daunting discipline to understand, nor to undertake. This text, *Health Research*, makes the subject of research approachable and understandable. It is aimed at health care workers who need to understand research so that they can bring the best knowledge to their practice of health care. It is also aimed at researchers, particularly beginning researchers, who need a reference text handy as they design and conduct their projects. The text is also useful for undergraduate and postgraduate students who are learning about research and beginning to develop some critical analysis skills. The text starts with the quest to learn and understand, and follows examples of what may be learned through various methods.

Health Research is a text which can be used as a manual. The main objective of the text is to offer reasoned choices in inquiry processes in health.

Health research, while traditionally quantitative, is increasingly using qualitative methods. Such methods were once confined to the social and behavioural sciences. Conversely, social health researchers are increasingly using some form of quantitative methods. The modern-day health researcher needs to be skilled in both qualitative and quantitative methods. The health researcher can be from any discipline, from medical to nursing to psychology, epidemiology, through to the social sciences. The contributors in this text range across those disciplines.

In *Health Research*, qualitative and quantitative methods are explained, and many examples are included, so that the reader can see how researchers implemented their own research choices, and how they interpreted research in their context.

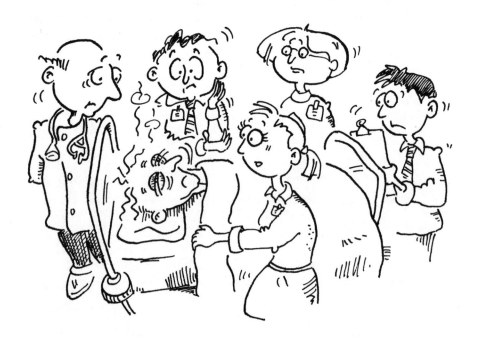

1

Beginning the quest

CATHERINE BERGLUND

This chapter looks at the drive to learn about health and the quest for new knowledge and understanding of influences on our health. The importance for health of this continuing process in training, skill development, clinical practice, and health services planning and delivery is discussed. The range of possible methods of gathering information or acquiring knowledge is broached.

Critical analysis of information which is already available is described as a skill which can be learnt, and some easy-to-follow steps are given to start readers on this path. Pointers are given to critical analysis skills that are followed up in other chapters, and in particular, those analysis skills that relate to qualitative and quantitative methods. The issue of inherent bias, even in 'objective' methods, is discussed. A preference for inductive or deductive research frameworks is presented as the readers' and the researchers' choice. Research methods that may suit individuals' preferences in positivism and relativism are canvassed.

Your interest in health and research

As readers of this text, you probably have a variety of reasons for being intrigued by health and research. The pursuit of health, and the pursuit of an explanation for illness, is both universal and elusive. Fables dating back to the first recordings of human endeavour feature tales of sickness and restoration of health, and of the value of maintaining health in the face of adversity. Vast plagues and threats to populations, and their consequences, are incorporated into stories in all cultures. The puzzle of the cause of illness appears as a thread in those stories. In stories about the cholera epidemic of the nineteenth century, a common theme was that people who succumbed had weakened themselves spiritually, in a form of sin, such as drinking, overeating, or sexual excess. Ministers of religion of that time also suggested that the cumulation of sin had weakened the community's resistance against disease.[1] In stories of illness from China, health was thought to depend on the harmony of nature. Natural forces of light, dark, heat and cold, and so on, needed to be balanced for people to remain healthy. The two main forces were termed yin and yang, and these were thought to be in a constant state of change. Xings (chings) were thought to be connected with control over certain body parts—for instance, the xing of fire with heart, small intestines and tongue; and that of water, with kidneys and ears; wood with gall bladder and eyes; metal with lungs, large intestines and nose; and earth with stomach, spleen and mouth. Protective compounds were made, both herbal and metal based, and artificially made gold was thought to be the much sought-after elixir of immortality.[2] In ancient India, broken bones and such were attributed to everyday causes, but deities were thought to bring other diseases, and incantation rites and herbs were used to try to expel those. Animal and human sacrifices were made to appease the deities.[3] Ludwig Edelstein, a scholar of medicine in ancient times, suggests that physicians in ancient Greece opposed theories that demons caused illnesses. Those demonic theories suggested that illnesses were in the domain of the magician to try and heal, rather than the physician. So Greek physicians understood illnesses to be caused by sun, air, winds, or the nature of man, but many laypeople then assumed that these forces were expressions of the gods. The god Asclepius, a rational god, was the god of physicians and patients according to Greek legend. Edelstein conceded though that the lay theory of illness as the wrath of the gods persisted in ancient times. It is noted in Galen's writings, Galen arguing against the use of incantations by proper physicians.[4]

Regardless of the assumed cause of illness in those stories, there is a sense of timelessness of the drive to understand what protects a state of health, and to understand what threatens our health. The stories describe how, by virtue of the human condition, we are mortal, and prone to illness. They also relate how we depend on supportive environments and nutrition for optimal existence. There is a sense of collective endeavour to ensure the best possible health for the people in our own communities.

Community expressions of the importance of certain goals in modern times are available. For instance, the World Health Organization's aim for the world community to take responsibility for the health of all peoples in all nations is an ambition that extends not only to the physical, but also to the psychological, social and environmental features of health. It is a goal that extends beyond absence of disability.[5] It is up to each of us to decide how we can best contribute to collective endeavours, given the skills and responsibilities that we possess. Health professions are entrusted with certain skills to be used in the pursuit of health as a collective endeavour.

Taking stock of how our health is, and how the health of others in our community is, is the first step. Deciding what could be done to maintain, restore, or improve health status is the next step. Examining how effective intervention has been informs the next cycle of assessing health and deciding what to do to maintain, restore or improve the human condition. Each of these steps of setting goals, assessment of status, and pursuit of the goals, is hotly contested in health research.

You need to understand the health and medical research that goes on around you, and you need to understand the results of that research. Your interest may be to understand enough about research so that you can critically assess whether the research is to be relied on, and then interpret the results in a way that is meaningful for your clinical practice, or for the management of your own health. Some of you will also be generators of research. You need to be able to plan and carry out data collection and analysis, and to let others know of what you have found. Both of those pursuits require a certain understanding of the research process. This text should equip you with that understanding.

Professional goals

Health professionals need all sorts of information just to get their job done. They need to know how their patient is, and has been. They need to know what useful management or treatment they could offer, and they need information on what might be the best options for each individual patient. The information that they use is a mixture of fact, observation, perception, intuitive experience and judgment. The knowledge that they seek is geared for use in practical contexts.

As health care students undergo training, they wade through textbooks and attend countless lectures to learn how the human body functions, and the characteristics of certain human conditions. They become used to looking for up-to-date information on health status, and treatment regimens. They learn directly from their supervisors and clinical teachers, and amass a working base of information, facts and supervised clinical experience, so that they too can start to assess patients and plan courses of treatment.

Health care professionals rely on their own factual base, and on their experience, so that they can recognise the health issues in their patients, and so that they know what might be reasonable to do to restore health, or at least improve comfort, for their patients. They also rely on the experiences of others. They talk in tea rooms and corridors with their colleagues to learn how their peers approached clinical issues in other patients. They attend conferences and read journals so that the experiences of others' patients, as told by the patients and/or interpreted by their health care professionals, are known to them. They also look to see if any more formal research is relevant to their patient population. Research, in large part, is the summary of the experience of patients and other health care professionals, often gathered systematically. The collective professional knowledge assumes importance because it represents such close observation of patients with particular health conditions, or experience with so many more patients than any one health care professional could hope to achieve single-handed. It aims to be reliable, in the sense that contextual features are teased out, or even controlled for, when interpreting clinical data.

Responsibility to research

That collective knowledge continues to be generated, as increased understanding of the human body and our living environments is attained, as new conditions are identified, and as new (hopefully improved) treatments or management plans are tried. A key professional aim is to bring about improvement in the health status of people, and communities, and improvement in health care for those people. Improvement in health care service delivery is a shared professional and community aim. Health research plays a central part in the evaluation of any progress in health status, health care, or service delivery.

Different professions' codes of ethics emphasise the responsibility to be up to date so as to provide optimal care and to contribute to the generation of new knowledge. All codes feature continuing education for the professional, even when 'trained', so that the standard of care improves.[6] To take part actively in research is seen as a responsibility as well. For instance, the New Zealand Medical Association *Code of Ethics* states: 'Recognise that medical progress is based on research which ultimately must rest on experimentation and systematic observations involving human subjects. Accept a responsibility to medicine to participate in such studies where possible.'[7] The Australian Medical Association's *Code of Ethics* states: 'Where possible, accept a responsibility to advance medical progress by participating in properly developed research involving human subjects.'[8] For nurses, the responsibility is expressed as: 'Research is necessary to the development of the profession of nursing. Research should be conducted in a manner that is ethically defensible.' This explanatory statement appears under the value statement that 'Nurses promote and uphold the provision of quality nursing care for all people.'[9] In their codes of ethics, other health care professions express similar positive responsibilities: to be aware of latest practice and research, and to be part of research.[10] Acceptance of these responsibilities means they continue to enquire into professional practice possibilities, and to search for improvement of care for individuals.

Values that were agreed to be essential to the practice of medicine, and that formed an integral part of the profession of medicine, have been listed by the British Medical Association. A spirit of inquiry was one of those values. The other core values were: respect, commitment, caring, compassion, integrity, competence, responsibility, confidentiality and advocacy.[11]

This spirit of inquiry crosses the boundaries of institutions, professions, and nations, but remains culturally influenced. Consultation with communities about their health issues has become a feature of health care, and health research. Information about values and assumptions which communities hold about their health, and certain treatment options, is necessary, and gathering that information is now a recognised part of the process of health research. It is discussed in some detail by Jan Ritchie, in her chapter 'Not everything can be reduced to numbers' and is prominent in the historical chapter 'Great expectations' by Lisa Parker and Ben Haneman. The setting of goals of health research and health care is a value-laden exercise. That process is discussed in a number of chapters in this text, particularly in relation to the planning stages of research, and is summarised in the chapter on ethics.

Context and values

The value and pursuit and desire for a certain good has characterised philosophical discussion of science for centuries. In a modern and famous essay entitled 'Science and ethics', Bertrand Russell asserts that the very pursuit of a good is a matter for personal opinion and for debate.

> Whatever our definition of the 'Good', and whether we believe it to be subjective or objective, those who do not desire the happiness of mankind will not endeavour to further it, while those who do desire it will do what they can to bring it about. I conclude that, while it is true that science cannot decide questions of value, that is because they cannot be intellectually decided at all, and lie outside the realm of truth and falsehood. Whatever knowledge is attainable, must be attained by scientific methods; and what science cannot discover, mankind cannot know.[12]

Setting the course for research is necessarily value laden. Even the process of being alert to identifying an issue, in among all the noise of context and other health issues, as being worthy of note, is affected by our biases. Classifying the issue as a problem, and one which is worth pursuing, and then deciding how to pursue it is value laden. Max Charlesworth has pointed to the social influence on science, as well as the myth of objectivity in individual application of research methods, to caution researchers to acknowledge their biases and subjectivity in their pursuits.[13] In brief, our assumptions and values and beliefs in relation to health may prove to be a source of fascination for future generations, just as we are fascinated by those of ancient times. That does not necessarily mean that we should not proceed with research, but that we should proceed with caution. This value-laden and contextual aspect of the research endeavour has been a topic of study for social scientists for many decades. While their studies may not be popular with their contemporary scientific and medical research counterparts, comments from the more famous commentators like Karl Popper and Ian Mitroff serve as reminders on bias which are well heard by future researchers.

The goals of medicine, and the treatment goals for individual conditions, are value laden, and not always supported by 'scientific research'. For instance, the goal of medicine of enabling longer life can be queried. It can be asked whether certain treatments have even been proved to have been effective or necessary in that pursuit, and also, whether the goal is worth pursuing at the cost of disfigurement, or other debilitating symptoms. In other words, the goal may be acceptable to some, but not others, and may be assessed in relation to the burden that it leaves for patients to bear.[14]

Cases, stories and inquiry

Health professionals push for better knowledge, and search for information actively. They let others know of their experiences. They are frequently part of a process of gathering information, or even formally testing a new treatment process. In chapter 2, 'Using research in practice', Phillip Godwin explains the interactive nature of health care professions and research. He argues that health carers, by their pursuit of better health status for their patients, and better health care, are at the very least, informal participants in the process of health research.

Clinical wisdom is based on experience with individuals, not just the application of theory and fact in disease processes. The experiences and stories of individuals become part of the process of clinical care. In recent years, more emphasis has been given to the narrative, or story, told by patients, or by clinicians, in understanding the process of health, illness, and restoration of health.

The way the health care professional tells a clinical story has an expected format. The age, background, 'history', and medical features of a patient are described. The medical developments are told like a story line. As outlined by Kathryn Montgomery Hunter, stories can be used to describe the predictability of progress of a patient, in response to certain treatment, or to highlight oddities, puzzles which colleagues may be able to help solve, the patient who does not 'fit' into routine experience. AIDS (acquired immunodeficiency syndrome) related conditions were reportedly identified, in part, from anecdotes in tea rooms, told by clinicians who were seeing strange combinations of conditions, and talking about them as stories on their breaks.[15] At a similar time, unusual summaries of treatment regimens were identified in larger data gathering exercises. Deborah

Black, in her statistics chapter, notes that routine analysis of patterns of prescription revealed an odd quantity of rarely used drugs for highly unusual conditions in a relatively small geographical area in the United States. The conditions for which the drugs were prescribed would later become known as AIDS-related conditions. The analysis of prescriptions was just one way of summarising what was happening in treatment with a large number of patients, not really any different to hearing the clinicians tell their stories of what they were doing in treatment settings, but with large numbers of clinicians at one time.

Howard Brody, also intrigued by storytelling of cases by clinicians, views clinical stories as part narration of the uniqueness of the individual, and part science, in the drive to 'explain the patient's illness by means of generally applicable laws'.[16]

Some commentators have noted that this emphasis by clinicians on individual case stories is really a casuistry type process. The clinicians observe fact and context in individual cases, and try to apply that evolving wisdom when they encounter new clinical cases.[17] This is a pragmatic process, rather than rigid application of theory.

The systematic analysis of stories of health and illness, as told by patients and by health care professionals, is an emerging discipline in health research. It is particularly prominent in ethics research, in examining stories which contain decisions that have explicit or implicit value or moral features and, in that context, is termed narrative ethics.[18]

A variety of methods

The history of health research is marked by an ongoing debate about appropriate methodology. This debate has in part been due to a historical debate about the form of reasoning that is appropriate for medicine and health. The following precis of the change in scientific reasoning more than three hundred years ago is drawn from a chapter in a recent book on the tasks facing medicine.[19]

In a scientific leap in the seventeenth century, Descartes penned the Cartesian thinking process, in which a deductive process leads from a certain foundation to conclusions. This process was the opposite to that suggested by Francis Bacon, in which an inductive process started with less general relations, and then moved to the derivation of general laws. Descartes emphasised rational thought and direct observation, particularly as a way of testing theory, and also a purposeful distinction between facts and values. Miles Little suggests that the medical 'conviction that objective tests are better than subjective impressions, even when the impression seems to tell us something important',[20] is a lasting influence of Cartesian thinking.

Generally, the deductive form of reasoning corresponds to positivism. The form of reasoning which corresponds to inductive reasoning is more compatible with relativism. If you choose to see positivism and relativism as being on a continuum, the drive to search for facts or experiences would vary, and the certainty of relying on 'facts' would change by degrees.

Wesley Salmon has charted different types of understanding as including: meanings, empathy, purposes, and natural phenomena. Conceptual understanding would be pursued under 'meanings', and empirical sciences would be pursued under 'natural phenomena'. The different types may simply contribute facets of understanding, but the tradition attached to each can vary considerably. According to Salmon, 'We come to understand a meaning when we can say what something means; we come to understand a phenomenon when we can explain why it occurred.'[21] While Salmon argues for the 'scientific' form of understanding, and emphasises knowledge of basic mechanisms and objective evidence in achieving that, he also acknowledges the pursuit of understanding in the psychological or experiential sense.

The key question in the modern debate on health research methods is how to capture and summarise the rich and diverse information about the health of individuals and their communities, and how to capture any change that may occur in individuals, or in those people as a group. The challenge is partly about individual examination, and partly about inquiry into factors which impact on whole groups of people. In chapter 3, 'Great expectations', Lisa Parker explores the history of wondering about the human body and inquiring into causes of death by examination of the body, and Ben Haneman tells a story of early protective health measures championed by a clinician in charge of the welfare of people en route to the new colony of Australia.

For most of the twentieth century, health research relied on observation of individuals, with accurate measurement of properties in those individuals, and then on statistical manipulation of the results of that measurement. This is termed quantitative research. It quantifies meaningful properties, in number quantities, and provides number measurements to summarise each person, or groups of people. The number measurements can also be relied on to examine differences between groups of people. Statistics, a mathematical process of number summary and comparison, is used in that process. The history of quantitative research methods lies in the physical sciences, and is, broadly speaking, used in a deductive approach.

Research that relies on conceptual exploration, and sorting of themes and understandings for individuals, or groups of people, has emerged as an alternative discipline in health research. Termed qualitative research, this method emphasises meaningful issues, rather than measurement. The history of qualitative research methods lies in the humanities, in the social sciences, and is, again broadly speaking, used in an inductive approach.

The debate regarding methods ranges right across the process of research, from who or what should be part of the investigation process, to what sort of information should be collected, to what type of summary and comparison process should be used. Editorials are frequently written on the issue of different method processes being appropriate, and in fact necessary, under qualitative and quantitative frameworks. One editorial, written by Janice Morse, the editor of the journal *Qualitative Health Research*, concentrates on why samples (people under investigation in a research study) are chosen in different ways in qualitative and quantitative research. Essentially, Janice Morse explains that qualitative research methods focus on experiences and issues, rather than general characteristics of numbers of people. In qualitative research, having rich data means having people in a study who are prepared to talk in depth about their experiences with a researcher. Great numbers, or even representative numbers from a group, will not necessarily result in a better understanding of the topic issue or experience. People are included in the research sample until 'saturation' is reached, that is, until themes, which emerge when people talk about their experiences, become repetitive and no new issues seem to be being raised.[22]

Whereas quantitative research is geared towards explaining the normal or average experience, qualitative research is aimed at explaining the range of experiences. The very use of 'normative' statistics relies on having some confidence in the sample being reasonably representative of a group, and in the numbers being large enough to have confidence in being able to approximate the 'normal' experience. Each of the later chapters on quantitative and qualitative methods explains how to decide on a sample of people for study, and how to gather information about those people. Issues of sampling are noted by Jeanette Ward and D'Arcy Holman in chapter 4, 'Who needs to plan?', and by Jan Ritchie in chapter 9, 'Not everything can be reduced to numbers'. The assumptions of statistical tests, in summarising information about a sample of people and in comparing measurement information across time, or between groups of people, receive considerable attention in the detailed statistics chapters. The assumptions vary for different types of number measurements and manipulations.

Measurements

The types of number measurements in common use in quantitative health research are continuous, or parametric, interval, ordinal and categorical measures. These are different because of the meaning of their units of measurement. Consider the following simple examples to think about the different choices in measurement units.

If you were in hospital, you would have your temperature taken regularly, usually by nursing staff. This is because temperature is thought to be one indication of how the body is working. If the temperature is elevated, we say someone has a fever, or simply, someone has a temperature. So, how is that decided? A rough guide is to place a hand on your forehead, to see if it 'feels' hot. But if you want a bit more accuracy, a thermometer is used (often orally). The thermometer has a recording of temperature on it, and the reading of temperature is the unit of measurement of body temperature, say in units of heat, Celsius or Fahrenheit. The units of heat are really on a continuous scale. You could draw a line from the lowest temperature imaginable, even negative temperatures, and continue that line to the highest temperature imaginable. People could, theoretically, be measured as having a temperature at any point on your continuous line, provided the appropriate instruments to measure it were available. Your temperature, all going well, will be like most people's and will be measured at about the same 'normal' or 'average' temperature (about 37°Celsius, or 98.4°Fahrenheit). Your temperature can be plotted on a graph too, to demonstrate part of the picture of your health and recovery process. Because it is on a scale that is like a continuous line, and one which is the same increase or decrease in temperature between units of measurement, it is interval, parametric data.

Now, imagine that a nurse asks you to give him an idea of how much pain you are in. He says, 'Thinking of all the numbers from 1 to 5, can you describe what you are feeling? Tell me 1, if you have no pain at all, and 5 if you are in severe pain, or pick one of the numbers in between for slight, or significant pain that is in between.' That sort of measurement is an ordinal measure. The numbers have a sense of increase or decrease, because we understand them in that way, but there is no guarantee that the difference between 1 and 2 is the same as the difference between 2 and 3, and so on. The possible responses are simply ordered, like lining up a group of kids by height. One child might be one and a half years old, and really only knee high. The next might be two, and marginally taller. The next might be a six year old, and up to your waist height. The next might be fifteen, and as tall, or taller than you. You can order the children by lining them up from smallest to tallest, but you will not claim that the differences in height between each of them is the same. For convenience, you could say that they were 'very short', 'short', 'medium' and 'tall', meaning their heights in relation to your own concept of height (which needs to be checked with different raters to ensure reliable categorisation). The alternative of course, is to measure their height, and note in parametric measures what their exact heights are (i.e. 65 cm, 67 cm, 130 cm, 170 cm, etc.).

Now, back to the hospital. Next, imagine that a medical student comes by and asks what sort of operation you had. She says she has a few options in mind: did you for instance, have a hip replacement, or cardiac surgery? She also makes a note of whether you are female or male. These are discrete categories. There is no relationship between them. They cannot be pictured on a spectrum or continuum, or in terms of increase or decrease of properties. They explain the existence, or not, of a property or experience in a dichotomous fashion. These are examples of categorical measures.

When all of this information about you is summarised and collected, it is termed 'data'. It may be that this information tells something about your state of health, and it might be that we would like to analyse it further, pooling the number summaries of how you are with similar measurements of other people.

Statistics will help, but only if the appropriate statistical tools are used. The emphasis in this text is for you to understand when tests are appropriate for given sets of data.

You can read about parametric statistics tests in Deborah Black's chapter 5, 'Numbers and more', and Deborah Black and Sue Irvine's chapter 8, 'How is the treatment going?'. Tests that are used to understand the health of whole populations, in epidemiological research, are outlined by Andrew Grulich in chapter 6, 'How is our health?'. Mary Phipps and Dusan Hadzi-Pavlovic's chapter 7, 'Meaningful categories', is on categorical and ordinal statistics.

Collecting qualitative data

The exploration of issues and the drawing of concepts into themes for further consideration is at the heart of qualitative analysis. The first step is the 'raw' exposition of issues from an individual's perspective.

Thinking back to the hospital example, you could even be asked to tell your story of how you feel. Your story could be about your physical symptoms, and it could also be about how you feel being ill, and how being in hospital is affecting you and those close to you. Qualitative investigation is characterised by open-ended questions, and opportunities to talk and explain perceptions about oneself, one's social context and life context.

Combining methods

In recent years, perhaps over the last ten years or so, a maturity has emerged in health research. It is now possible to conduct research that makes use of both methodologies; to explore health issues using the tools available in both qualitative and quantitative methods. The challenge for health professionals in the twenty-first century is to have a working knowledge of both types of methods, so that they can understand the experience of others in health care. That experience may be expressed by patients or modern-day health care professionals in terms of number measurements, or thematic concepts, or both. The challenge for health researchers is to have sufficient understanding to decide when each method may be useful, and plan appropriate research. This text includes relevant detail on quantitative research processes and qualitative research processes, and illustrates how both are used in partnership, in Deborah Saltman and Natalie O'Dea's chapter 10, entitled 'Quality and quantity'.

One way of thinking about combining qualitative and quantitative research methods, despite the often-noted conflict in combining different paradigms, is that each can be used in different stages of the same research. For example, preliminary qualitative study can generate ideas and hypotheses to test, to see if concerns or themes that are noticed when talking to some people in depth are in fact generalisable to a larger population sample. Alternatively, preliminary quantitative research can be helpful in establishing range of variation, so that 'purposive sampling' can be achieved more efficiently. That is, a small group of people can be selected for intensive and detailed investigation. Once a purposive sample is derived, an issue can be explored in more detail with a few people.[23]

Increasingly, studies have parallel arms, which explore a topic of interest using both methods. Researchers are being encouraged to use the methods as complementary, rather than antithetical. In one briefing article on the benefits of qualitative methods in health and health research, three main roles of qualitative research are suggested. The first is, as a preliminary process in research, to describe a situation or behaviour and so provide better understanding of it. The second is to supplement quantitative research in a triangulation type validation process, where results are compared for similarities and 'conversion'. The third is to explore complex phenomena, or areas that are not amenable to quantitative research.[24]

Critical analysis skills are essential in all methodologies. Critical thought about the issues to explore, useful ways to summarise those issues, and the meaning or interpretation of information pervade research. You can practise simple search, summary and interpretation exercises to aid in this process.

Try exercise 1.1 in pairs.

Exercise 1.1

You want to learn something about one of the following 'injury risk' topics:

- parental perception of children's risk of injury in the home
- community perception of hazards in everyday life
- young men's perception of road rules and risk of motor vehicle accident

First, decide where to find a piece of information on your topic. Bear in mind you are searching for perception, not 'fact'. You may like to look in newspapers, or magazines, or even talk to people about their perception directly.

Collect the information, and keep it in full as your 'data'. It may be your transcribed conversation or the article you found. Either way, it is your raw information. To practise summary, take a paragraph and condense it into a short written piece on the key issues. The issues should be the ones that your informants think are key, not what you think should be key! Show a friend your summary, then let him/her see the original data and ask whether you captured all the key issues as portrayed in the original data, and whether you captured them faithfully (or accurately).

In health research, once issues of what information to collect have been decided, the problem becomes how to collect, summarise, and make that information available to practising clinicians. The importance of disseminating research findings, of writing and publishing research ideas and pursuits, is emphasised in the chapter on writing and publishing.

The enormous task of keeping up to date with all literature has posed a challenge to health care professionals. The availability of masses of 'evidence' has spawned creative approaches to collecting, summarising and disseminating key findings. The evidence-based medicine (EBM) movement is one of those new approaches. It assumes that clinical practice, and clinical decision-making, should be conducted taking into account the documented experiences of many professionals with patients with similar conditions, and also taking into account systematic reviews or actual research data on treatment options for patients with particular conditions. EBM is becoming a feature in health research, driving the collection of researched clinical data. The founders of EBM continue to ponder whether clinicians will avail themselves of such detailed clinical research data, even though it is conveniently collected in libraries, such as the Cochrane Library, and is becoming routinely available on-line in computerised form.[25] Evidence-based medicine, and its preference for types of data, is discussed by Phillip Godwin, in chapter 2, 'Using research in practice'; and by Jan Ritchie, in chapter 9, 'Not everything can be reduced to numbers', and is noted by Jeanette Ward and D'Arcy Holman, in chapter 4, 'Who needs to plan?'.

Deciding how to pursue an issue will also depend on your training and skill. Try exercise 1.2 sometime with a group. This works well as a brainstorming session with research students too. The exercise highlights how the same issue can lead to different research questions, and different research plans, depending on the skills and resources that are available. A research tip: Learn to identify research issues and then pose research questions and form research plans. Having a number of options is key before designing a study.

The health issue is the natural starting point, and the health context is the natural place to begin, as in chapter 2.

Exercise 1.2

Take a letter to an editor from one of your own profession's journals to use as a starting point for group discussion.

As you read the letter, brainstorm what the health issues are that need to be investigated.

Then, put different 'skill' hats on. Make some people administrators of health institutions, some nurses, some doctors, some social workers, and some from one other health profession. Make other people health policy-makers (i.e. from the government), epidemiologists, occupational health and safety officers, and laboratory scientists (either benchtop scientists or pathology workers, etc.). Ensure that there is a group representing your own health profession.

In those small skill groups, write a 'question' that you would like to answer to help understand one of the health issues which the group has identified from the letter. This is your research question.

You could take the exercise further and plan a research design to get an answer to your question.

2
Using research in practice

PHILLIP GODWIN

This chapter looks at what research means in a practice setting. It explores the history of health professions from the viewpoint of past experience, cumulative data in the real sense, structured research, and communication with other practitioners. With the explosion of health-related information, there exists a real difficulty for busy practitioners. They need to identify what information they require to make informed clinical decisions, and they need to identify where that information can be readily accessed. The possession of critical analysis skills to use in that process is imperative.

The need to broadly identify the paradigms that exist in clinical settings is inherent in using research in practice. Health care delivery is both an art and a science. Kernick suggests that the basis of modern science is uncertain, and that we live in a chaotic system.[1] Clinical practice is experimental in the sense that it is reflected on throughout the process of treatment and management. Practice is altered for groups and individuals. Clinical research can itself also remain experimental, in the sense of being flexible, utilising both quantitative and qualitative methodologies, and being altered so that it is appropriate to context. It is much more than the randomised controlled trial. The importance of reflecting on history is also illustrated in detail in chapter 3, 'Great expectations'.

In attempting to explain the discipline of research in clinical settings, this chapter will consider a number of issues—searching for information on outcomes; summing up of evidence; the quality of clinical trials and meta-analyses; overuse and underuse of medical procedures—and draw on various

sources—the *National Statement on Ethical Conduct*; a conceptual framework for evidence-based practice; databases and evidence-based medicine in
general practice; evidence-based surgery and general practitioners' use of evidence databases. Additionally, the issue of research going drastically wrong
cannot be excluded from this discussion.

Have we learnt from past experience?

At face value, we could assume that we have learnt from past experience. However,
this is not always borne out in fact. In 1850, Dr Ignaz Semmelweis advocated hand-
washing to prevent the spread of puerperal fever.[2] He observed, in the absence of
any rigorous research methodology, that there was a higher incidence of puerperal
fever in women during childbirth attended by physicians, compared with women
attended by midwives. He concluded that this occurred as a result of physicians
failing to wash their hands between undertaking autopsies and examining their
patients. It should be noted that the practice of hand-washing by midwives indeed
was best practice, yet was not recognised as such by their professional medical colleagues. At that time, Semmelweiss was regarded by his peers as being of unsound
mind for making this observation. The conclusion of his peers may also be a comment on the fact that nurses were of lesser status, and had less power to influence
their medical colleagues at that time. Semmelweiss was ostracised by his profession, and relegated to a mental asylum. In 1865, following his incarceration, he pur-
posely slashed his hand with a scalpel during an autopsy, and died three days later.
The story is as much a lesson in visionary nursing practice and the importance of
that health care role as of practice informed by adequate research.

There are now numerous studies which suggest that hand-washing by health
professionals is still not universally practised. Semmelweis stated that 'frequently
we, as physicians, are blinded by our narrow views and dogma'. Semmelweis was
also a lone practitioner who noticed something, and tried to convince others of
what he saw. Our research history is full of examples of discomfort with lone cam-
paigners. We tend to operate more by group consensus, and well-accepted research
is usually peer-reviewed and conducted research. Yet, even with peer-reviewed
research and policies on universal infection control, procedures such as hand-washing between patients continues to be a problem in some clinical settings. The fact
that such an obvious and routine practice of hand-washing remains underrecog-
nised points to our ability to underestimate the lessons of the past. On balance
however, we have heeded many lessons gleaned from collective experience.

Kernick suggested that a momentous event occurred in 1948: the first medical
randomised controlled trial. It was a move to large numbers of identical clinical

interventions, and correspondingly large numbers of observations, collected in a systematic fashion. 'The experiment was quite straightforward. Patients with tuberculosis, unaware they were taking part in a clinical study, were randomized to receive streptomycin or nothing. With a plunge of the syringe, 3000 years of medical treatment based on experience and perceived effectiveness were at an end.'[3]

The issue of the relationship between truth, honesty and evidence remains vexed. The robust nature of information collected in specific settings, and the use of that information for guidance in other settings, is debated. That of informed consent and individual agreement to take part in research trials is discussed in some length in chapter 12, 'Ethics as part of research'.

Kernick further suggests that:

> decisions in life are based on a cognitive continuum. Wired to the cardiological bed, the heart disease succumbs to inferential statistics. But patients come and go: to the real world where attempts to impose a spurious rationality on an irrational process may not always succeed; where structures are highly complex and disease thresholds may not be met; where decisions are based on past experience, future expectations, and complex human interrelationships; where doctors and patients have their own narratives; where time scales exceed those of the longest trial; and where the mechanisms of poverty are the greatest cause of dys-ease.[4]

Kernick has, like many others, highlighted the need to question the validity and reliability of evidence, and has acknowledged the relevant place of uncertainty in research. This is to acknowledge an uncertainty of factors involved in disease and disease progression. It is also an uncertainty in the many measures that we have available to us to measure health and health progress in research settings. In a practical manner, the statistics chapters in this text give prominence to the uncertainty of statistical test results. Statistical tests are just reasoned assessments and summaries of complex situations, and should be cautiously interpreted with continual reference to the situation to which they are applied. To continue to question and ponder the meaning of a situation is a key part of the clinical and research process.

Coupled with this uncertainty is a reasoned assessment of the levels and quality of evidence provided by any research project. For any practice to become mainstream, and perhaps be contained in clinical practice guidelines, the health profession would need to define and have considerable confidence in the evidence for applying that practice within certain well-defined clinical conditions. Confidence, to the clinician, is validity, reliability and consistency in research terms. These are discussed further in chapters 4 and 9. The range of bias within research studies is a concern of bodies such as the NHMRC.[5] Bias is an inherent problem, even in randomised controlled trials. There are other contextual biases, as noted earlier in this chapter and also elsewhere in this book. Put simply, all confounding variables cannot be eliminated in clinical research and health care. Who assesses the available evidence from clinical work, and then constructs the clinical practice guidelines is a matter of debate. The assessors, the research constructs, and the research findings, and the health care professionals, which are all open to inherent bias, together form what comes to be known as the 'evidence'.

Exercise 2.1

As a small group exercise, think of an area of your clinical practice which seems to lack concrete evidence.

Try to stay with an example from your own professional practice.

Just as the Semmelweiss story raises nursing and medical practice issues in relation to routine hand-washing, there may be other everyday practices which impact on more than one profession.

Look for evidence in the literature supporting the practice, and evidence which suggests that the practice should not be continued.

In pursuing your topic, ask:

- How common is this practice?
- What are the levels of evidence which support this practice?
- What evidence do you have that the practice is helpful to your clients?
- What evidence do you have that it poses risks for your clients?
- Would you recommend that this practice be re-examined, continued without change, or ceased? Give your reasons for your conclusion.

Searching for information

Health care professionals want to know what the best practice is for each of their patients or clients. They learn to search for up-to-date and relevant information. There seems to have been a shift in where and how that information is accessed. Previously, health carers would search for information in textbooks and professional journals in medical libraries, and they would ask their fellow professionals for information. Now, there is an additional increasing reliance on direct access to information by clinicians and other health service providers.

The appropriate search is crucial, and haphazard searches can mean poor information for the clinician to act on. Brettle, Long, Grant and Greenhalgh have suggested that two common problems exist in searching for information via abstract type indexes: missing relevant papers; and accessing too many irrelevant studies.[6] Either problem can result in misleading conclusions and, potentially, inappropriate clinical management.

The solution therefore lies in developing effective search strategies. These strategies have been well enunciated in the literature on evidence-based medicine. While search strategies appear initially complex, their application is more user-friendly. Brettle et al. conclude that 'when improving health care quality, decisions should be made on the basis of sound research evidence while using appropriate outcome criteria and measures (effects). Finding this evidence is problematic'.[7]

This is not to suggest that busy clinicians should regard information seeking as an onerous task, even given obvious time constraints. Practical strategies such as journal clubs, grand rounds, medical record audits and special interest groups can prove invaluable in clinical settings. Patients are often useful, as partners, in searching for information. They can present to their primary carer with the research data themselves.

In searching for information, the critical question of interpreting data has to be considered. Indeed, limiting clinical errors is paramount. Wright, Jensen and Wyatt argue there are three main criteria for interpreting data, namely: perception, attention, and memory. Clinical errors in interpretation of data can arise from 'illegible handwriting, or type on computer screens or printouts. These perceptual difficulties can lead to confusion over drug names'. Loss of detail can also result from the inefficient reading so caused.

Another confounding variable is the clinician's memory processes, including such factors as pattern recognition, substitution, misunderstanding, distortion of facts, and transposition errors. It should be acknowledged that memory lapses by clinicians are not infrequent, and can be directly associated with issues such as time of day, and workload. Wright et al. suggest that a solution is 'to format records so that all information can be recorded as soon as it is elicited'.[8]

Further, it is useful to recognise the impact of visual factors (e.g. headings and columns), and clarity of language (e.g. succinct medical notation avoiding ambiguity), in aiding the accurate interpretation of textual data. The role of computers today in facilitating data interpretation is obvious, however the authors point out that 'the use of a computer is not a substitute for good design'.[9]

Any discussion on using research in clinical settings cannot ignore the assertion that 'one answer is not always enough'. Lau et al. propose that meta-analysis, which quantitatively combines evidence from diverse studies, is increasingly useful in clinical practice.[10] It should be noted that meta-analysis does, however, have its critics, who raise questions of heterogeneity of variables, and the ability to generalise results. The authors conclude, 'given the problems, it is perhaps surprising that meta-analyses have agreed quite well with large trials addressing a similar "homogeneous" question. Clinical trials and meta-analyses mostly have addressed the question of how well a treatment works overall. Both of these approaches, while useful in estimating a population effect, do not show how to treat individuals'.[11]

Any summing up of evidence requires explicit criteria and transparent methodology. That evidence must be integrated appropriately into the clinical context, including to patients who are different from those in the trials, by virtue of confounders. The clinical practitioner, when undertaking research, needs to be cognisant of variables such as individual values, co-morbidity (patients having more than one defined condition or disease), and other confounding variables.

To test or not to test

In an age requiring cost containment and increased accountability, the issue of overuse and underuse of medical procedures is inescapable in clinical practice. It is also an issue when new treatment possibilities are being explored, informed by recent clinical research. Put simply, new research results can prompt different exploration of each patient's condition, leading to an assessment of whether a particular treatment process should be tried. Both routine and innovative testing of a patient can be challenged on grounds of appropriateness.

The different ways of deciding if a test is appropriate have a common feature: they rely on access to previous research on the application and usefulness of the test being considered. The methods, or assessment processes have themselves been scrutinised.

A parallel three-way replication of the Rand-University of California at Los Angeles 'appropriateness method' was examined to see if it was useful when applied to two medical procedures.[12] The authors conclude that the appropriateness method of identifying overuse is considerably lacking in accuracy. The authors do however note that their results for identifying underuse of procedures are far more accurate. Other methods such as meta-analysis, decision-analysis, and cost-effectiveness analysis, are also subject to variable interpretation. This study highlights the need for further research to identify which procedures would benefit from appropriateness method analysis.

Further empirical evidence on usefulness of tests and their use in different contexts would enhance the debate on appropriate decision-making in relation to the efficacy of ordering tests. There is an obvious dilemma for busy interns, residents and registrars ordering tests. They face inherent challenges of understanding the health conditions that people have, and of using the resources available to them in a reasoned and efficient way. The use of 'appropriateness methods' to make decisions on testing can be combined with the experienced reasoning of their supervisors and colleagues, which represents the cumulative experience of appropriate and inappropriate testing as well. Sometimes, Health Insurance Commission (HIC) counsellors perform an educative role for the young practitioners, helping them to identify overuse of pathology tests, when available information combined with a confidence in their own clinical reasoning would have given them an equivalent result.

Evidence-based practice: Valid science or a flash in the pan?

A fierce debate currently rages over the merits of evidence-based practice. There can be no argument that such lively discourse is useful and should be strongly encouraged.

As a starting point, it is important to consider a conceptual framework. This framework centres upon implementing research into practice; clinical effectiveness; evidence-based practice; facilitation and change-management. According to Kitson, Harvey and McKormack, the 'successful implementation of research into practice is a function of the interplay of three core elements—the level and nature of the evidence, the context or environment into which the research is to be placed, and the method or way in which the process is facilitated'.[13]

Approaching research from this perspective requires a shift from the traditional randomised clinical controlled trial to a qualitative approach. Kitson et al. highlight such issues as the role of focus-group facilitation in implementing research. Facilitation in this context is coupled with change. This represents quite a significant departure from previously held values on sound research. It should be noted, however, that issues of construct and face validity require further analysis and debate. Kitson et al. conclude that 'the framework has limited construct and face validity and has been set out to stimulate debate in this important but complex area'.[14]

O'Flynn and Irving state that 'the concept of an evidence-based approach to surgical practice has a sound historical basis through the founder of scientific surgery, John Hunter, and the first advocate of surgical outcomes research... While embracing the concepts, however, neither used the term evidence-based'.[15]

These authors raise some compelling questions in relation to the lack of randomised controlled trials in the surgical literature. They assert that a number of challenges face surgeons in adapting to this imperative.

> First, an urgent need exists for pragmatic trials to test the acceptability and effectiveness of new interventions against established surgical procedures. Second, the quality of the surgical literature needs to be improved with less reliance on case series and reviews with unsound methods. Third, critical appraisal skills need to be a part of every surgeon's armamentarium. The wide variations that exist in surgical practice are undeniable and embarrassing, but the increasing publication of surgery-related systematic reviews and evidence-based practice guidelines points to a change in surgical culture. The biggest challenge will be the implementation of high-quality evidence into routine clinical practice.[16]

Even though this represents a British perspective, the Australian surgical fraternity should be commended in their collaboration with the Commonwealth government to develop an Australian Safety and Efficacy Register of New Interventional Procedures-Surgical (ASERNIP-S) through the Royal Australasian College of Surgeons (RACS).

An editorial in the *Medical Journal of Australia* outlines that 'external clinical evidence can be ranked in a hierarchical framework with the randomized controlled trial at the top, meta-analysis or systematic reviews in the middle, and clinical experience at the bottom. From this framework of information, clinical practice guidelines are currently evolving'.[17]

Solomon and McLeod reinforce this approach to randomised controlled trials in surgery, adding that 'if RCTs can be performed, other strategies to increase the number and quality of RCTs may be needed: Education of surgeons in clinical research methods; Improved funding of surgical RCTs; Compulsory evaluation of new techniques and technology before their general adoption is permitted'. The same authors commendably cite Hippocrates' assertion that 'one must attend in medical practice not primarily to plausible theories, but to experience combined with reason'.[18]

It is difficult to conclude with any degree of certainty the direction which evidence-based medicine will follow into the new millennium. It is, however, fair to say that this scientific approach is in essence not new.

Databases and evidence-based medicine use in general practice

It would be an omission for this chapter not to mention the specialised sources on evidence-based medicine. Van Der Weyden comprehensively cites the following: 'specialized extract journals such as Evidence Based Medicine, Evidence Based Mental Health, and Evidence Based Nursing and the inception and growth of the Cochrane Collaboration and the Cochrane Library. The latter includes the Database of Systematic Reviews and the Database of Abstracts of Reviews of Effectiveness, available either online or on CD-ROM'.[19] Van Der Weyden goes on further to state that, according to previous reports in the *Medical Journal of Australia*, '72% of Australian neonatologists and 44% of obstetricians regularly used evidence databases to guide their care of patients'.

In the same editorial, Van Der Weyden refers to an outstanding report by Young and Ward on Australian general practitioners' use of the Cochrane library.[20] Young and Ward found that 'although 43% of GPs (14% at work) had access to the Internet and 22% were aware of the Cochrane Library, only 6% had access to it and 4% had ever used it. These findings are mirrored in the United Kingdom, where the Cochrane Library Database of Reviews has a higher recognition rate among GPs (40%) but the rate of use (4%) is remarkably similar'.[21]

This evidence adds weight to the argument that we need to consider both quantitative and qualitative data in ensuring best practice in clinical practice. The rapid expansion of computerisation in general practices should be acknowledged.

Looking for guidance

Clinicians are increasingly becoming involved in organised research, which goes beyond the individual clinical experience. There is ample guidance available for clinicians should they wish to be involved in research.

The *National Statement on Ethical Conduct in Research involving Humans* represents a significant national initiative for research in Australia.[22] This chapter will not examine in detail each section of the *National Statement*, which should be referred to separately by all readers of this text. The general ethics issues are explored in chapter 12, 'Ethics as part of research'. However, the section on clinical trials does require specific clarification.

The *National Statement* provides a definition of clinical trials. In essence, a number of criteria (not an exhaustive list) must be included in a detailed protocol, so that the protocol can be considered prior to its conduct:

- an explicit statement of the aims of the trial
- the credentials of the researchers
- the design of the clinical trial (such as specific question/s; validity of hypothesis; effectiveness of intervention; risk/benefit analysis)[23]

Interestingly, the clinical objective and nature of the clinical process is open to discussion. For instance, natural and complementary therapies can also be tested within the paradigm of a clinical trial. The key issue is that an agreed and explained methodology is followed within each trial.

There are a number of methodological provisions, which need to be applied and which are listed within the *National Statement*. Before a clinical trial is approved, the protocol must conform to a number of directives including:

(a) this Statement;
(b) the World Medical Association Declaration of Helsinki;
(c) where relevant, the CPMP/ICH Note for Guidance on Good Clinical Practice (CPMP/ICH-135/95) and the ISO 14155 Clinical Investigations of Medical Devices and the requirements of the TGA; and
(d) any requirements of relevant Commonwealth or State/Territory laws.[24]

Other issues addressed in the approval process are: the use of placebos; conflict of interest; budgetary implications; and compensation for injury suffered as a consequence of participation in the trial. A rigorous reporting and review mechanism is in place. In addition, provisions for the termination of a trial are explicitly described.

Every other section of the *National Statement* remains relevant and applicable to research in clinical settings, and should be read and discussed among your colleagues.

Research gone horribly wrong

While it is not my intention to conclude this chapter on a pessimistic note, it is imperative to acknowledge that, on occasion, research performed with the most altruistic intentions can inadvertently result in tragic consequences. Tragic consequences are even more stark when there was previously no danger to the participant. This can occur when healthy volunteers are called for as part of a research program, either as a control type group, or as a way of understanding what the normal body would do in certain situations.

The ethical principles of beneficence and non-maleficence, namely to care and to do no harm, can fail in not only the research methodology, but also in its implementation. Day, Chalmers, Williams, and Campbell cite the following example: 'A healthy 19-year-old United States college student volunteer in a clinical research program underwent a bronchoscopy and died as a result of acute lignocaine toxicity. The major contributing factor in the tragedy was that the research failed to specify an upper dose limit for lignocaine spray, although previous versions of the protocol had done so'.[25]

It is almost inconceivable that, with rigorous research protocols and procedures that we now have, such an event could occur as recently as 1996, and possibly even to date. It highlights the inherent risk that any intervention in the health of research subjects carries. It also highlights the immense responsibility that researchers undertake when they conduct health research.

In some instances, simply knowing, or being deemed to have known, that greater risks were posed to patients in certain situations can attract harsh peer criticism if harm occurs. This means that health care professionals must be aware of the latest information on treatment, and also on the success of that treatment when it is delivered by their own team. This is exemplified by the Bristol case, in which a cardiac surgery team was challenged over its continuing practice with poor outcomes for some of the children under their care. Bolsin, one of the former medical professionals with the team, became concerned, and his concern eventually prompted a full investigation into the responsibilities of the medical practitioners concerned. Bolsin summarised the outcome of the investigation and professional hearing on the matter:

> in June 1998, the Professional Conduct Committee of the General Medical Council of the United Kingdom (the body which regulates British doctors) concluded the longest-running case it has considered this century. Three medical practitioners were accused of serious professional misconduct relating to 29 deaths (and four survivors with brain damage) in 53 paediatric cardiac operations undertaken at the British Royal Infirmary between 1988 and 1995. All three denied the charges but, after 65 days of evidence over eight months (costing £2.2 million), all were found guilty.[26]

This tragic series of treatment episodes was of particular concern as the surgery suggested for the children allegedly had a lower chance of success with the Bristol team than at other centres, but parents were allegedly not informed of this.

Moving forward

These cases beg the question that we started with earlier in this chapter: have we learnt from our mistakes? As Kernick rightly points out, 'Only a fool would deny the importance of evidence, but it may be wise at times of rapid change to proceed with circumspection—to adopt a pragmatic approach accepting the few things we know for certain, and learning to live with the uncertainty of most of the grey zones in medicine. Best perhaps to seek honesty, not truth. Caution rules OK'.[27]

In summing up, it is clear that research in practice is far from exact, either as an art or a science. The challenge that all practitioners face is to ask the right questions; seek accurate information; and make informed decisions to the best of their own ability at any given time.[28]

3

Great Expectations

LISA PARKER AND BEN HANEMAN

This chapter, by two clinicians with interests in the history of medicine, offers an insight into how society can determine our understanding of the human body and of dangers to our health. The first section of the chapter, by Lisa Parker, gives a historical account of different methods of researching the physical body, from ancient to modern times, and comments on social and religious contexts of the developing knowledge. The reader is left with a distinct impression that we, in our modern age, may also have an understanding of the human body that is historically and culturally determined. The second section of the chapter, by Ben Haneman, tells a story of a clinician's concern for the welfare of all passengers during the course of their journeys by boat from England to the colony of New South Wales. An inquiring process is described, as the clinician strives to identify what causes illness, and then advocates changes to the passengers' living conditions, with the aim of reducing the risks to their health during the journey. This is an early public health research story.

The human body
LISA PARKER

The internal human body has been a source of fascination and curiosity since the beginning of civilisation, possibly even before. The body is a key focus of modern health care and health care research. How we conceptualise the human body is dependent on contemporary medical philosophies. What we seek to 'know' depends on what health professionals and researchers already believe about the way the body behaves in sickness and in health. When we had a supernatural theory of medicine, there was little investigation into the physical properties of the body. When humoral medicine was prominent, practitioners' predominant interest was in the physical properties of blood, bile and phlegm. In our own times, we may well come to realise that our contemporary visions of the body are constrained by modern assumptions and dominant theories. As such, our research methods are similarly culturally and temporally defined.

This chapter uses historical methods of research. As you read, you will notice a reliance on historical documents which record events and views, and a reliance on secondary analysis of historical interpretations. A useful reference for historical research in medicine is that by Osborne and Mandle.[1]

Dissection of the human body has always been restricted by the great respect and fear of the dead body that is an inherent part of human culture. The first part of this chapter follows the historical story of the resulting conflict between the desire to examine and dissect the corpse and social demands to preserve the dignity and physical integrity of the body. It also explores the variable interpretations of the dissected body, which have depended upon the result of this conflict, as well as upon contemporary scientific theories. Interest in the dead body has historically been promulgated by the scientific, medical and judicial communities. These communities have been keen to explore human internal structure in order to better understand anatomy, and to search for the cause of death.

Human anatomy is of interest to people, both for its own sake, and for the information that it might give regarding man's identity, *raison d'être*, or the Christian soul. It has also been used to examine internal human bodily function, or physiology, and to explore the concepts of life and death. The physical body is a constant focus in the search for longevity and the secrets of eternal life.

The cause of death is also of interest. Those responsible for the medical care of a community seek to learn from death by exploring the internal corpse for physical or spiritual signs as to the cause of death. It is hoped that this will enable future deaths to be anticipated and if possible prevented. Such an examination is called an *autopsy*. Those responsible for the legal structure of a community search the corpse for the cause and circumstances of suspicious deaths, in order to inflict the appropriate retribution upon a possible perpetrator. Both the internal and external appearances of the body are relevant in this regard. The internal examination is called a *medico-legal* or *forensic autopsy*.

Respect for the dead is a universal phenomenon in human society. The act of disturbing the body is surrounded by strong cultural taboos and dissection tends to be seen as an unwelcome act of desecration. This is exemplified by the frequent use of criminals for dissection throughout history, and the not uncommon practice of using dissection as a method of punishment itself.

The strength of such taboos is dependent upon changing social attitudes towards death, the body and ideas regarding the medical and legal professions. The strongly religious societies of the ancient world tended to live very much with the dead spirits in their midst, and fear and respect for such spirits made dissection almost unthinkable. During the equally religious Dark Ages, interference with the corpse was seen as abhorrent because of its suggestion of interest in the physical body, which was mortal and sinful, and therefore not worthy of investigation.

Religion in itself has not always prevented dissection, particularly during the early Calvinist years when exploration of the physical body was seen as a way of reaching out towards and understanding God, but in general, highly religious societies have been loath to condone dissection. Most religions have strong central tenets, focusing on the afterlife and the importance of respect for the physical remains of the dead. Such tenets are not negotiable, and produce a society with a uniform attitude towards dissection of the human body.

During the Renaissance when the pervasive power of the Church waned, and interest in academia was high, dissection became much more socially acceptable. Attendance at a scientific dissection became, in fact, a popular social pastime, frequented by the lay community as well as the more academic members of society. For the first time in human history, it was possible to explore internal human bodies on a large scale.

Constantly changing dissecting practices are the result of what has generally been a truce, albeit uneasy, between the variably inquisitive medical and legal communities, and labile social attitudes. The truce has been sporadically disrupted, and events such as the widespread grave robbing of the eighteenth and early nineteenth centuries in England resulted in pervasive social distrust of human dissection. As the modern era unfolded, the desire for knowledge of the body took precedence over the social abhorrence of interfering with the dead. During the mid twentieth century, human dissection occurred on a scale never before attempted.

What follows is a presentation of this fascinating and ever changing story of human dissection within its historical context. Historical events are gleaned from medical and social writings, including actual reports of dissection and autopsy. Some of these reports have been included in the text, to indicate the level of medical understanding, and prevalent social attitudes.

Later in this chapter, you will be prompted to explore the history of an issue which interests you. As you read about some of the earliest recordings of exploration of the human body, notice the way historical sources are relied on, and analysis of interpretations of events in history are culturally based as well.

Ancient Egypt

Modern understanding of ancient Egyptian medicine is gleaned from the writings of Greek and Roman commentators (including Homer, Herodotus, Hippocrates, and Pliny) and more recently from several medical *papyri*,[2] which were discovered in the nineteenth century.[3] Egyptian medical practices were heavily borrowed from the Babylonians, and were dominated by supernatural forces. Unlike the embalmers, the Egyptian physicians had little need for knowledge of internal human anatomy.

Despite the relative lack of interest from the medical profession, the regular practice of embalming meant that the anatomical knowledge of the Egyptian culture was significantly better than that of previous cultures or other contemporary societies. The Egyptians named many internal organs including the heart, brain, liver, lung, spleen, bladder and stomach.[4] There was occasional medical commentary on organ appearance, as described in the Edwin Smith Papyrus:

> If you examine a man [having] a gaping wound in his head, reaching the bone, smashing his skull and breaking open his brain, you should feel his wound. You find that smash which is in his skull [like] the corrugations which appear on [molten] copper ... and something therein throbs and flutters under your fingers like the weak place in the crown of the head of a child when it has not become whole.[5]

The 'corrugations' felt through the shattered bone undoubtedly represent the gyri and sulci of the human brain, which 'throbs and flutters' under cardio-respiratory influence. There was also some appreciation of the localisation of disease, and the Smith Papyrus discusses the physical effects of brain injury, noting that the results depend upon which side of the brain is injured.[6] According to the Roman medical historian, Pliny, the Egyptians even performed autopsies of sorts, 'for to search out the maladies whereof men died.'[7] Indeed Pliny went on to say that such a practice proved that radishes were successful in curing *phthysicke*, pulmonary ulceration.

There is no record of bodies being opened for forensic purposes, despite the legendary existence of Imhotep, supposedly the first medico-legal expert in the Western world, revered as a God in the latter centuries of the ancient Egyptian civilisation. According to Egyptian legend, Imhotep was the physician to the pharaohs c. 3000 BC. He was also trained in the legal profession, thus combining the two sciences of medicine and law.[8] There are, however, no records or legends of Imhotep using dissection as part of his investigation for medico-legal cases.

Despite its relative sophistication, there were significant limitations to Egyptian human anatomy. The hieroglyphs used to represent human internal organs are recognisably animal in origin, unlike the hieroglyphs for external structures, which are more obviously human.[9] In addition, there are few Egyptian words for non-organ based anatomical structures such as bones, compared with the well-named visceral organs.

These limitations have several explanations. First, the amount of anatomical detail known to the embalmers might in fact have been quite limited. The abdominal incision was small, and unlikely to reveal much about the position and relationship of the internal organs. The brain was removed piecemeal, destroying its structure, and the heart was left *in situ*, and therefore rarely seen. Organs that were visualised *in toto* were not dissected, and thus only their external appearance was known. Bones, muscles, vessels, nerves and certain abdomino-pelvic organs were not viewed at all by the embalmers.[10]

Second, the embalmers had little reason to exploit the academic potential of their job. Aside from being able to localise the organs with limited visual assistance, and identify the different entities, they were not expected or required to understand complicated details of internal human structure. Why or even how should they note that the human uterus contained a single cavity only, rather than a bicornute cavity as in the ox?

Discourse between the physicians and the embalmers was probably very limited. Medical practitioners had significant religious importance, and a high social status. It is unlikely that there was much regular exchange of ideas and knowledge between these lofty priest-like doctors and the socially unacceptable embalmers.[11]

Finally, doctors had minimal interest in the internal physical structure of the human body, since their medical system was based on spiritual rather than anatomical foundations. There was little stimulus for the medical accumulation of anatomical knowledge.

In combination, these factors meant that the Egyptian understanding of the internal human body was less detailed than might have been expected, given the unique opportunities available. The Egyptians left a significant contribution to early human anatomy that was used and enlarged by later cultures.

Ancient Greece

One of the greatest civilisations of the ancient world undoubtedly belonged to the Greeks. The first people to settle in the lands of modern day Greece were the Minoans, who flourished on the island of Crete, c. 2000 BC – 1450 BC. They were invaded c. 1450 BC by the Mycenaeans, from the city of Mycenae on the

Peleponnese peninsula. The Homeric tales, such as the siege of Troy, probably date from this Mycenaean civilisation, c. 1650 BC – 1100 BC.

In such an exciting age one would expect that the Greek body as defined by the medical gaze would be significantly different from that created by the other ancient cultures, as in fact it was. The permissive nature of the polytheistic Greek religion played an important part in this.

Supernatural forces were prominent in early theories of medicine, notably that produced by the cult of Aesclepius, the principal God of healing, who rose to prominence c. 700 BC.[12] Unlike the Indians however, later Greeks had no dominant religious philosophy attached to their medical theories, and the scholars of the Golden Age were free to explore different ideas in medical science. 'Schools' of medicine developed in Sicily, Ionia, Southern Italy and Cos, where philosophers, medical teachers, practitioners and students gathered to discuss, learn, experiment and contemplate the mysteries of the human body.

There was great interest in the subject of anatomy, and the Greeks routinely dissected animals for this purpose. Alcmaeon (c. fifth century BC) studied in the Crotona School in southern Italy and was a pioneer in this field. From his dissections Alcmaeon noted the physical connections between the brain and the organs of sense, such as the eye. He concluded from this that the brain was the seat of thought and memory.[13] He also recognised that sperm did not come from the spinal cord as was previously believed and he named many nerves, although often confused nerves with ligaments. His contemporary, Diogenes, described blood vessels, but did not distinguish between arteries and veins.[14] Aristotle (fourth century BC) also dissected many animals and described a hierarchy of internal organs.

Due to their animal dissection and scientific interest, the anatomical detail known to the Greeks progressed significantly from the naming of organs and other major structures to the naming of *parts* of organs and their relationship to each other and to vessels, nerves, muscles and bones. The heart, dealt with at length in the Hippocratic writings, was discussed in terms of the pericardium, ventricles, valves and great vessels.[15]

Hippocratic medicine

It was in this time of burning scientific curiosity and improved anatomical knowledge provided by detailed animal dissection that a radical new medical philosophy was created. Hippocrates was educated in Cos, an Ionian island off the coast of Asia Minor, c. 370 BC, and was thus conversant with the anatomical discoveries and philosophical debates mentioned above. His medical principles and practices are inferred from the many ancient Greek texts known as the Hippocratic writings.

Hippocrates' great legacy was to create a medical system devoid of supernatural influences, based entirely upon sensate observations and treatments of natural origin. Other medical cultures had included simple physical treatments in their medical armaments, but, without exception, basic theories of disease had been supernatural. Hippocrates challenged this tradition, arguing that bodily ills resulted entirely from natural causes, and that the body could be treated by supportive physical therapy, allowing it to use its own innate healing mechanisms. Magic, superstition and prayer were useless as treatment modalities in Hippocratic philosophy.

Central to Hippocrates' theory of medicine was a physiological system based on four humors: black bile, yellow bile, phlegm and blood. The humors existed in harmony in the healthy body, but, as in the ancient Chinese and Ayurvedic theories, imbalances caused disease. Significantly different, however, was Hippocrates' rejection of the belief that supernatural forces were the fundamental cause behind this imbalance.

By 800 BC city-states such as Athens and Sparta were developing and as populations expanded, the Greeks settled in other areas around the Mediterranean, including modern France, Spain, southern Italy, and northern Africa. By the 'Golden Age' (c. 500 BC – 350 BC) the Greeks were producing great art, making significant scientific advances and developing a democratic political system.

The humoral theory was partly based on real anatomy in that physical correlates for the four humors existed. In addition each organ was assigned a specific and unique balance of humors, and each humor supposedly derived from a specific bodily source, assumptions that might well have been linked with physical observations. Ultimately, however, the humoral philosophy of medicine was based on theoretical assumptions rather than empirical observation.

A contemporary physiological concept was that air is taken into the body via the lungs. The Greeks believed that air was contained within the body in vessels, a theory possibly arising from the fact that elastic arteries, which constrict after death, will expand again once incised, thus giving the appearance of containing air. This internal air or *pneuma* was thought to be the source of the body's innate heat.[16]

The physical, anatomical body was extremely important to the Hippocratic doctors. An important tenet of Hippocrates' medical system was the emphasis on personal observation as a method of diagnosis. Supernatural portents and astrological signs were rejected in favour of simple inspection, palpation and smell. Porter commented that Hippocrates' unique legacy was his recognition of the fact that, 'medicine [is] expertise in the body.'[17] Ultimately however, the Greeks were limited by their inability to directly view the internal aspects of the dead human body. The detailed case histories in the Hippocratic collection are notable for their complete absence of autopsy findings. Despite this, Greek interest in anatomy and their careful documentation of animal dissection made a significant contribution to medicine, laying the foundation for a new medical system, and providing an important background for later anatomical discoveries.

The Roman Empire

The Ptolemic rule over Egypt and Alexandria came to an end when the last of the dynastic rulers, Cleopatra VII, was conquered in battle by the Romans in 32 BC.

She suicided in legendary fashion and Egypt was absorbed into the rapidly expanding Roman Empire. Starting from humble beginnings on the banks of the River Tiber, c. 750 BC, the Roman Empire grew to include, at its height (c. 117 AD), most of modern-day Europe, Britain, northern Africa and parts of the Middle East.[18] In 286 AD the Roman Empire divided into East and West, with the Eastern capital at Byzantium, later renamed Constantinople after Emperor Constantine the Great. The Western Empire declined from 400 BC, but the Byzantine Empire continued in strength through the Middle Ages.

The Romans were much more superstitious than the Greeks whose Empire they had conquered, but the Romans adopted the Greek polytheistic religion, converting it to their own unique style. The dead Roman body was honoured but also greatly feared and was quickly cremated after death. It is probable that it was the Roman occupation of Alexandria that led to the gradual decline in human dissection in that city. By 150 AD regular, open dissection had ceased at Alexandria and elsewhere in the known world.[19]

Despite this, the Romans actively pursued the science of anatomy. Like many other aspects of Roman life, medicine was based on Greek ideas. Roman physicians inherited all existing medical theories and anatomical knowledge and also a strong drive for further investigation. The Roman taboo against dissecting the human was dealt with by using man-like mammals. The primates were similar in both visceral and muscular appearances. Apes and monkeys were available in greater numbers than humans had ever been, and slow, careful and detailed dissections gave rise to significant advances in anatomy. Vivisection was also widely practised, and enabled a new understanding of physiology, particularly of the nerves and muscles.[20]

One of the greatest names in Roman anatomy, or indeed in the entire history of human anatomy, is Claudius Galen. Galen (130 AD – 200 AD) was born in the Holy Roman Empire at Pergamum in Asia Minor. Pergamum was a great medical centre, with a famous medical school and there Galen was able to study the latest medical knowledge and philosophy. He later travelled to Alexandria to continue his medical education. Human dissection was no longer practised but the city was still regarded as the centre of excellence for medical study. Galen returned to Pergamum to practise medicine, and also spent many years in Rome, where he achieved considerable distinction among his peers for his clinical expertise.[21]

Galen's personal contribution to the internal body picture was greater and more persistent than any other individual influence in the Western world either before or since. Despite never dissecting the human body himself, Galen was accepted as a complete authority on human anatomy, and his anatomical and physiological descriptions were adopted by the whole of the Western world for over a thousand years. The internal human body created by Galen remained in use far beyond the life of the Roman Empire, persisting through the Dark Ages until the European Renaissance.

Galen spent his entire professional life combining a successful clinical practice with extensive research and voluminous writing. He was constantly dissecting and vivisecting animals (particularly the ape and the pig) to explore their anatomy and physiology. Duckworth wrote of his 'insistence upon the endless pursuit of dissection, and the study of things seen, and not of words whether spoken or written.'[22] In Rome, many of Galen's animal dissections were public events, attended by the fashionable nobility.

Such persistent work enabled Galen to make many original discoveries in medical science. By severing the recurrent laryngeal nerve and noting its effect on the voice, he discovered its function. Similarly he noted paraplegia after cutting the spinal cord, and cessation of respiration following the severing of the brainstem at the level of the medulla. He proved that arteries contain blood not air, by tying the femoral arteries in dogs and then incising them. Likewise he proved that urine originates in the kidney and arrives in the bladder via the ureters. He left detailed descriptions of the cranial nerves, and disputed the contemporary belief that nerves originate in the heart.[23] This detailed description of liver dissection is typical of Galen's writing:

> [The liver] ... receives from the mesenterium the veins which extend to its most concave part. The place where all these (veins) gather is called 'portae hepatis.' Now here you will find in all red-blooded animals the very large orifice of a vein. Having inserted into this orifice one of the prepared probes ... and pushing it gently forward along each lobe you should cut the above lying substance with a scalpel ... When you have laid the vein bare without making an incision, remove the surrounding flesh of the viscus ... You will find that one large vein reaches from the 'portae' into each lobe, however many there may be, that it divides up into many small veins like the trunk of a tree into branches, that these again divide into twigs, so to say, that these end in thin offshoots, as it were, and that the space between the vessels is all filled up with the flesh of the viscus ...
>
> Now if the animal is of considerable size, you will be able to preserve, together with the veins, the biliary ducts and the arteries ... For the arterial vessel is somewhat whiter than the vein.
>
> Galen (130 AD – 200 AD)[24]

Just like Alexandrian anatomy, Galen's anatomy contained many details that were incorrect, and reflect his familiarity with the animal rather than the human body. His descriptions include a five-lobed liver (seen in the pig), a bicornuate uterus (ox), a segmented sternum (ape) and flared hip bones (dog).[25] It was a great disappointment to Galen that he never had the opportunity to dissect the human form. He took full opportunity of his time in Alexandria to examine the two remaining skeletons on display, and encouraged fellow physicians to do the same.

Galen's greatest shortcoming was not his lack of opportunity, but his inability to accept the limitations of his material, and his unsubstantiated extrapolation of animal anatomy to the human form. He described human anatomy definitively but inaccurately, unwilling to accept that it might differ from the animal anatomy that he studied so carefully. An understanding of the body led to the use of that anatomical knowledge in research like processes of deduction.

Traditional Chinese forensic medicine

Forensic medicine was relatively far advanced in China compared with Europe. The formal investigation of homicide and suicide was introduced during the Ch'in dynasty (221 BC – 207 BC).[26] In 995 AD a decree was issued specifying the details of the forensic investigation system such that all unusual deaths must be investigated by government/police officials with any cases raising the possibility of foul play receiving a more formal 'inquest'.[27]

In 1247 the judicial official Sung Tz'u released a script titled, *Hsi yuan lu (The Washing away of Wrongs)*.[28] It was intended as an instruction manual for the government officials who had the task of investigating suspicious deaths and was used extensively until 1927 when the Chinese established a new system of inquiry into suspicious deaths with the Chinese National Health Service.[29] According to the *Hsi yuan lu*, all cases proceeding to inquest required a detailed forensic examination of the corpse. This was performed in the open by a lowly man called a *wu-tso* (often an undertaker) for male corpses and by an elderly woman, probably a midwife, for female corpses. The inquest official supervised from a short distance away, often accompanied by government clerks, the accused, the chief village service men and relatives of the deceased. There were no medical personnel present.

Due to the general ban on dissecting the human body, the forensic examination was external only, but it was extremely thorough. Where necessary it included all orifices and visible internal cavities, including the mouth, nose, anus, urethra and vagina. Certainly the inability to dissect did not prevent the Chinese from developing an elaborate system of practical forensic medicine, and this included searches for evidence of invisible internal injuries:

> If on the body there are several blue-black marks, take water and drop it on these marks. If they are injuries, then they will be hard and the water will not flow away. If they are not injuries, they will be soft and the dripped water will run off.
>
> In holding inquests, when any bones have been injured, if the traces are not visible, sprinkle lees and vinegar over the body. In the open air hold newly oiled silk or a translucent oiled silk umbrella between the parts you wish to examine and the sun. The wounds will become visible ...
>
> In very hot months, when the corpse has been covered with mats, the skin of the injured parts will often be white, but uninjured parts will be livid or blackish.
>
> Again, during the hot months, if maggots have not yet appeared at the nine orifices, but they have appeared at the temples, hairline, ribcage, or belly, then these parts have been injured.[30]

Europe in the Middle Ages

As the influence of the Christian Church over daily life declined, secular physicians began to emerge together with secular educational bodies, along the lines of the modern university. Monastic medicine further declined with an edict from the Council of Clermont in 1130, restricting the practice of medicine by monks due to its disruption to religious life.[31]

In those times, academic discourse and experimentation returned to medical education. A thriving medical community in Salerno, in southern Italy, established the first well-known centre for medical education in the medieval period. The school was initially practical in orientation, but by 1080 theoretical teaching and speculation were included in the course and by 1250 the study of anatomy by animal dissection had been introduced.[32] Human dissection remained abhorrent due to religious taboos, with the physicians declaring that it was 'horrible ... especially among us Catholics.'[33] Gradually, other universities around Europe began to offer courses in medicine, including institutions in Paris (1110), Bologna (1113), and Montpellier (1181). These latter two schools, together with the School of Salerno, were the major centres of medical education in medieval Europe.[34]

The only available medical texts were Arabian in origin, as the Christians had not produced or preserved any written medical works during the Dark Ages. Corrupt translations of Hippocrates, Aristotle and Galen were accompanied by original works by the Arabian physicians themselves. Texts by Avicenna, Hali and Rhazes were popular, but relied completely upon Galen's body as their reference point for medical discourse. The early medieval physicians thus continued to promulgate Galen's view of human anatomy.

The division of surgery and medicine

As the Middle Ages progressed, medical practice underwent significant changes. During the Dark Ages medical treatment was largely supportive, although the monks had occasionally practised basic therapeutic surgery. In 1163 however, Pope Calistas passed an edict, *Ecclsia abhorret a sanguine*, forbidding all religious practitioners to perform any surgery.[35] Possibly this was to prevent attempts at crude and generally fatal operations or perhaps it was a reflection of a growing sense of unease at cutting the impure human body. Surgery thus began to attract social stigma, and even the secular physicians started to consider it beneath their dignity. The barbers, who regularly shaved the heads of the priests and other religious people, began to add minor surgical procedures to their repertoire, and gradually these *barber-surgeons* developed considerable expertise in surgical medicine.[36]

A split between the two therapeutic disciplines emerged. University-educated physicians treated their patients with drugs and poultices, in accordance with humoral theories of disease. Apprentice-trained barber-surgeons focused less on theory and more on invasive (minor) surgical treatment. Although not regarded as professionals in the same ways as the physicians were, the barber-surgeons began to form local guilds, which protected their standards and instituted educational requirements. The Fraternity of Barbers in London formed in 1308.[37]

Human dissection and exploration into the Renaissance

Once bodies of the deceased were regularly opened for social and religious reasons, it became possible to conceive of dissecting the dead body for the express purpose of studying its interior. Certainly the medical profession had reached a new level of sophistication and was eager to find new sources of knowledge about the human body. The law was also interested in the human body as part of its search for information in cases of suspicious death. It is likely that medieval human dissection began in the city of Bologna,[38] but it is unclear whether it was first introduced for medical or legal purposes.

Legal systems around Europe had been using medical evidence at murder trials since the Dark Ages, with physicians giving their opinions based upon the external appearance of the dead body. Bologna University was renowned throughout the known Western world for its expertise in law, and the town housed many important and influential legal academics. Given that the Bologna was famous for its law rather than its medicine, Singer suggested that the innovation of human dissection is more likely to have been introduced by the lawyers, rather than the anatomists. 'It seems probable that the earliest reason for examining the human body was simply the gathering of evidence for legal processes. This is a reason, and the only reason, that would have appealed to an official of Bologna University of the 13th century. As time went on post-mortem examination passed into anatomical study.'[39]

The first recorded forensic autopsy in Bologna was performed in 1302, although according to Singer, they were probably occurring for several decades before this.[40] The case was a deceased nobleman, Azzolino, who died under the suspicion of poisoning. Two physicians and three surgeons participated in the autopsy, and concluded that poison was unlikely to have been the cause of death.

The performance of forensic autopsies slowly spread throughout Europe, particularly as many Italian physicians travelled to Paris in the late thirteenth and early fourteenth centuries, seeking to escape civil war in their homelands.[41] The Catholic authorities, far from distancing themselves from the practice, used the autopsy in their own forensic investigations. The Church specifically ordered an autopsy on Pope Alexander V after his suspicious death in 1410.[42]

The new, sophisticated legal system of the Renaissance demanded greater access to a range of evidence and expertise, including medical evidence. The Germanic act *Cado Bamberger* (1507) and the more extensive *Constituito Criminalis Carolina* (1532–33) officially sanctioned the use of medical evidence in legal trials.[43] They insisted upon its use for the investigation of all cases of suspected murder, and all deaths involving violent wounds, poison, hanging, drowning, infanticide or abortion. Charles V enforced the Carolina Code throughout the entire Holy Roman Empire, and similar practices spread to neighbouring countries.[44]

On the continent, it became commonplace for medical practitioners to examine the body in cases of suspicious death, and give their opinions as to the cause of death. Apart from obviously violent deaths, such cases included death by poisoning which was suspected on the basis of circumstantial evidence, such as sudden, unexpected death or rapid putrefaction of the body.[45] The practitioners involved in the examination might be the treating physicians/surgeons or dedicated forensic experts. In 1606 Henry IV of France nominated two surgeons for every large city to examine and report on all cases of wounding and murder.[46]

In England the forensic system was less advanced. Unlike the continental systems for investigating suspicious death, the English coronial system was separate from the police force. The English coroner was usually not formally trained in any profession, his only necessary qualifications being sufficient wealth to enable him to ignore the inherent temptations of the job.[47] Early coroners were unpaid, and therefore naturally loath to pay for expert evidence in their investigations. In 1487 official legislation (3 Hen. 7, c.1) held that coroners should be paid, but only for investigations that resulted in a conviction.[48] The number and extent of investigations and the use of medical evidence therefore remained lower in England than on the European continent.

The extent of the medical examinations in medico-legal cases was variable. Often an external examination alone was considered sufficient, and this might be quite detailed as the following excerpt from the works of the innovative French surgeon, Ambroise Pare (1510–90), indicates:

> Whosoever is found dead in the waters, you shall know whether they were thrown into the water alive or dead. For all the belly of him that was thrown in alive will be swollen, and puffed up by reason of the water that is contained therein. Certain clammy excrements come out at his mouth and nose thrills, the ends of his fingers will be worn and excoriated, because that he dyed striving and digging or scraping in the sand or bottom of the river, seeking somewhat whereon he might take hold to save himself from drowning.[49]

Internal examinations were less common but are certainly recorded. During the sixteenth century the bodies of Popes Leo X and Adrian VI were examined internally because of suspected poisoning, implied by local rumours and the sudden putrefaction of the corpses.[50] There are records of internal examinations in Scotland in the same century. For example Darnley, the husband of Mary Queen of Scots, was allegedly murdered in 1567, and a full autopsy was performed upon his body.[51] Ambroise Pare was a leader in the field of forensic medicine, and is known to have performed a number of forensic autopsies in France during his lifetime.[52]

The medical autopsy

The regular practice of performing autopsies on patients to determine the cause of death purely for medical reasons began in Italy in the fifteenth century. Pietro de Montagna, writing in 1444, claimed to have seen fourteen post-mortems in Padua during his lifetime, but the details are not recorded.[53] The Florentine physician Benivieni (1440–1502) is credited with being one of the first physicians to regularly perform private medical autopsies. He kept notes of his most important clinical cases, and these were published posthumously by his brother in 1507 under the title *De Abditis Causis Morborum*. The text includes 111 case histories and post-mortem reports, the latter performed for the express purpose of finding the cause of death.[54]

By the middle of the sixteenth century, the medical autopsy was being performed more frequently and a number of influential physicians were actively encouraging its use. Girolamo Cardano (1501–76), the Professor of Medicine at Padua and later at Bologna, and Jean Fernal (1506–88), one of the greatest French physicians of the Renaissance, both suggested that autopsies should be used by the astute physician as a check on diagnosis and a form of self-education.[55]

Outside the main educational centres, autopsies were less common, but were still performed in desperate situations. In 1536, Jacques Cartier led an expedition up the St Lawrence River in the New World. After disease (probably scurvy according to Saphir[56]) had affected all but ten and had caused eight deaths out of over one hundred men on board ship, Cartier, in a move reminiscent of the plague times of the Middle Ages, requested a post-mortem on one of the victims. Richard Hakluyt reported on the expedition:

> Some did lose all their strength, and could not stand on their feet, then did their legs swell, their sinnows shrink as black as any coal. Others also had all their skins spotted with spots of blood of a purple colour: then did it ascend up to their ankles, knees, thighs, shoulders, arms and neck; their mouth became stinking, their gums so rotten that all the flesh did fall off ...
>
> Philip Rougement ... died, being 22 years old, and because the sickness was to us unknown, our Captain caused him to be ripped to see if by any means possible we might know what it was, and so seek means to save and to preserve the rest of the company; he was found to have his heart white but rotten, and more than a quart of red blood about it; his liver was indifferent fair, but his lungs black and mortified. His blood was altogether shrunk about the heart, so that when he was opened a great quantity of rotten blood issued out from about his heart ... because one of his thighs was very black without, it was opened, but within it was whole and sound. That done, as well as we could he was buried. In such sort did the sickness continue and increase ...
>
> *Richard Hakluyt, 1536*[57]

The medical autopsy was gradually becoming more frequent and more sophisticated. The interpretation of findings was initially beset with errors resulting from unfamiliarity with the normal dead body. With cumulated experience, medical practitioners were able to make better informed and more accurate observations, and often were able to identify the pathological lesion likely to have been the cause of death.

The forces that led to the scientific use of the autopsy and its sequelae were multiple. Importantly, the academic interest in solid organ and tissue pathology was present, promulgated by such original thinkers as Giovanni Morgagni and Mathew Baille. Simultaneously, and equally importantly, the industrial revolution and subsequent urbanisation of Europe and the United Kingdom resulted in the development of large public hospitals in major cities. This gave medical practitioners unprecedented access to large numbers of diseased individuals, most of whom had no money and therefore, in nineteenth century Europe, no rights. They were, in effect, a giant source of material for experimentation and investigation by the medical profession.

Paris was the centre of medical advancement in the early nineteenth century, this role being facilitated by recent political events. After the French Revolution in 1789 the control of the main public charitable hospital in Paris, the Hotel Dieu, was transferred from the Church to the new government. The paupers at the hospital, previously protected by charitable philanthropists and the Church, were left to the mercy of a government that was happy to allow them to be used as instruments for teaching, both before and after death.[58] In large public hospitals throughout France and also in many Germanic countries autopsies were performed routinely upon all deaths. The Germanic hospitals began to appoint dedicated *autopsists*, and great pathologists such as Carl Rokitansky (1804–78) and Rudolf Virchow (1821–1902) began their careers in this way.[59] The use of public patients for autopsy was not quite so common in England, where the hospitals were still dependent upon charitable donations, and therefore public opinion and sensibilities.

According to the twentieth-century philosopher Michel Foucault, the rise of the public hospital meant that the patient became de-individualised.[60] Medical practitioners viewed patients as recognisable disease entities, rather than individual people with holistic and idiosyncratic illnesses. Because of this new clinical 'gaze' and because of the advancement in morbid anatomy, doctors began to look at the diseased internal human body as a collection of predictable morbid anatomies.

More recently, the Western world has become increasingly secular and scientifically orientated, and attitudes towards dissection have altered once again. Today, the value of scientific experiment is high, and the medical and judicial professions enjoy considerable status and power. Offsetting this is an increased anxiety about mortality and death, fostered by the lack of community faith. There is a general desire to avoid contact with the dead body, and to avoid any discussion or thought that might bring death into the social consciousness. A society that fears and avoids death to this extent finds it hard to discuss or accept a need for dissection of the human body. At the same time, individual rights have become increasingly important, and individuals in society are beginning to demand absolute control over their own bodies in death as in life. Similarly the voice of minority groups within discohesive populations have become increasingly powerful, and it is now necessary to consider the differing demands of separate cultural groups within one general society.

The modern community may have once more moved away from acceptance of dissection, and the access of the medical community to the human cadaver continues to decrease year by year. The use of the dead body has decreased in almost all aspects of scientific life, including education, medical practice and anthropological research. The use of human dissection remains steady only in the investigation of forensic deaths.

Even in times of widespread social acceptance of dissection, the body does not reveal its secrets easily and the interpretation of the internal body is constantly changing. In line with Kuhn's theory of scientific paradigms,[61] the meaning of the internal body appearance is heavily dependent upon prevailing scientific theories. Just as Foucault declared that the 'patient' is created by contemporary medical concepts, so 'the body' has been variably created over different centuries by local theories of physiology and of disease. This concept is emphasised by Armstrong, who declared that, 'what the student sees is not the [anatomy] atlas as a representation of the body but the body as a representation of the atlas.'[62] In the same way, morbid anatomy can be regarded as a representation of contemporary theories of disease.

Try exercise 3.1, either by yourself, or with a small group of fellow students or colleagues.

Exercise 3.1

Identify an historical issue of interest to·you, and begin your own investigation of the issue.

The historical methods book by Osborne and Mandle may be useful.[63]

You may choose to look at:

- methods in health care
- professional practices
- biographical stories of key figures in nursing and medicine
- institutional roles
- social attitudes towards practices and context of health care.

One of the following sources may be a useful starting point in your investigation:

- A 1994 issue of the *Medical Journal of Australia* includes a selection of medical history writings.[64]

- Articles of historical health care interest are routinely investigated and presented to conferences held by the Australian Society of the History of Medicine, and published in their proceedings.[65]
- Texts such as Ackernecht are relied on in this chapter, and provide a concise history of a wide variety of medical issues.[66]

A clinician's concern
BEN HANEMAN

My challenge was to look into the early history of health research in Australia. I have chosen to tell a story of clinical concern for the welfare of passengers en route from England to New South Wales. Some of the passengers were prisoners, some were paying passengers and some were crew. The clinician's concern extended to them all. In constructing this story, I have relied on a number of references that verify the clinician's contribution to early public health, combining clinical reasoning, research and advocacy.[67]

The first well-recognised study on health done in Australia was by Dr William Redfern. He was one of the patriarchs of Australian medicine, indeed of Australian society. In an age when medical science was remarkably ineffective therapeutically, doctors were more concerned and, for their time, more knowledgeable in preventive and public health issues. Perhaps this was a natural compensation. At the beginning of the nineteenth century, the major health problems confronting Australia centred on life in the special circumstances of the new colony and the health of those being shipped to Australia, many of them against their will and with all the implications of being a convict. Sea travel, quite apart from natural hazards, still carried the threat of scurvy and of course contagious diseases.

It is customary to quote Sir Edward Ford who wrote extensively on Dr William Redfern. Redfern's own report on the conditions on convict ships, which were transporting a very special type of new Australians to this continent, was important in this historical account as well. Redfern made one of the major Australian contributions to public health as well as one the earliest. The nature of Redfern's report and the circumstances around the necessity for such a report are both interesting and instructive. The chronicle of Redfern's life, too, is fascinating if not exciting. Both facets of the Redfern story will be detailed in this chapter.

On first consideration, one might argue the place for a brief historical vignette in a serious scientific book on health research in Australia, such as the publication which the reader is now holding. Such questioning is valid and indeed welcomed. Yet in truth, science has no call to be ever proud, nor history always humble. Both disciplines deal with facts. Perhaps, the way those facts appear to be manipulated may reveal differences. History has the great benefit that it throws light on ourselves and the lives we are living. It has been asserted correctly that all history is, in the last analysis, contemporary history. All history, of necessity, is seen with today's eyes. History reveals us to ourselves today as much as it reveals the past and our past. History gives us the rare opportunity—indeed permission—to reflect on the present and perhaps even suggests an agenda for the future.

William Redfern (1775–1833) was born in Canada, though this detail is not certain. His family was connected with Ireland and he studied medicine in London. He passed the examination of the Company of Surgeons, a precursor of the College of Surgeons, in 1797, and within a few days was Surgeon First Mate on HMS *Standard*, a ship with some five hundred souls on board.

Although part of Great Britain's North Sea fleet, it was to carry young Redfern to Sydney Cove. There was much unrest in the British fleet in general, with shocking conditions on board, very poor pay, often no pay, and certainly minimal wages compared with wages that could be commanded ashore. The sailors' living quarters were abysmally bad, the sailors resented fellow crew members who had been press-ganged on board, and were often the dregs of the society at the time. There had been a mutiny at Spithead. Two months later, the mutiny spread to the North Sea fleet and to HMS *Standard* then stationed at Nore.

The mutiny was put down and young Redfern was arrested as a mutineer. He was the most educated, he had been sympathetic to the mutineers and their grievances, had advised them on strategy—for instance, that they should remain united if they were to have any chance of success. Redfern was in court to hear the death sentence announced, but immediately there was a recommendation for mercy. Grounds given were his professional obligation to mix with the mutineers and his concern for their lives and limbs. There was also the matter of his youth, with uncertainty to this day if he was 19 or 22 at the time.

He spent a miserable four years in prison, an experience which cannot have failed to have an influence on him and formed his ideas about justice, about personal interrelationships and about fate. When he was offered transportation to Botany Bay, it was seen as an act of mercy and an offer of a fresh start. He travelled to Sydney on the *Minorca* and was listed as mutineer. In May 1802 he commenced medical duties on Norfolk Island. Within a year he had a conditional pardon and soon after, a full pardon. He acquitted himself very well on Norfolk, doctoring there for some five years, and subsequently moved to Sydney where he worked initially at the old dilapidated hospital at Dawes Point.

It is a point of academic interest that because he had no papers or written evidence of his medical qualifications, he was obliged to sit for an examination administered by Surgeons Thomas Jamison, John Harris and William Bohan. He was judged 'qualified to exercise the Profession of a Surgeon' which made him the first Australian medical graduate and also set a pattern for recognising overseas qualifications.

Redfern was a popular doctor and a successful doctor. He treated members of Governor Macquarie's family, indeed, attended the birth of Macquarie's son. Redfern had also successfully treated John Macarthur's daughter. Dr Redfern also had his enemies, principally the royal commisioner John Thomas Bigge who had such great influence in the colony and whose report is so well and widely known. Bigge found it incomprehensible that a mutineer, someone so manifestly disloyal, could ever find a place, still less a place of responsibility in decent society. He disliked and distrusted Redfern. Some of his enquiries about Redfern were frankly offensive. The prejudice shown against the so-called emancipists, those who had achieved pardon, was a fact of early colonial life and on several occasions Redfern was refused preferment, which he might otherwise merited. He took no pains to ingratiate himself, had a rough manner, had a reputation for bad temper. On one occasion, by way of remonstrance to his apprentice, the young Mr Cowper, he struck a blow that broke his teeth. Not too much should be made of this one incident, though it is on the record.

Redfern, among his duties, had to supervise punishments at the jail but more important was obliged to visit the ships when they berthed. He was in particular concerned with transports which arrived with notably high level of mortality and morbidity. He was requested to make a report to Governor Macquarie and it is on the basis of that report that Redfern gained the credit for his pioneer report on health issues in the transporting of prisoners to Australia.

The event which precipitated Macquarie's request for a report was the arrival of the Male Convict Ship *Surry* on 28 June 1814. Part of the crew and the convicts were found to be 'in a wretched and deplorable State of Disease'. Redfern's report is dated 30 September 1814. It is couched in respectful and circumspect terms, which, today, makes curious if not charming reading:

> Some days since, in a Conversation with your Excellency on the Subject of the Calamitous state of disease, in which the Convicts on the Transports General Hewit, Three Bees, and Surry, Arrived in this country, your Excellency expressed a wish that I should Communicate to you my Sentiments on the possible causes of the diseases, which appeared Among the Convicts on these Transports, on the means of preventing similar Occurences in future, or of counteracting their effects. In obedience to this wish, I have now the honour of Submitting the following detailed observations to your Excellency's Consideration.

Somewhere in his report, Redfern had made note of his heavy involvement in other medical matters. The rules governing Redfern's choice of capitals are quite different from our present rules, and the effect is disconcerting, but lends a certain vigour to his writing.

The report to Governor Macquarie gives painstaking accounts of the conditions found on the three ships and also enquires as to the voyage, the victualling, how much access the prisoners had to time on the deck; the state of cleanliness was particularly focused on. He observed that women, being regarded as posing less threat to security, even potential uprising, were allowed on the deck for significantly greater lengths of time and this was reflected in better (lower) mortality figures.

He complained, for instance, about the reliability of the medical certificates stating that a prisoner was fit to travel. It has been shown independently that some prisoners were so anxious to escape from the hulks where they were incarcerated that they hid their illness and pretended good health. Is there an antonym to malingering?

The quality of the accompanying surgeons was criticised. They were either fresh from medical school, full of book learning but otherwise grassy green, or bad, doctors who had failed in medical professional life, often alcoholics. The circumstances of their work, their subservience to the captain who often made no attempt to hide his scorn, encouraged drunkenness in the ships' doctors.

The ship's officers often stole the convicts' food and later sold it at a profit on reaching their Australian destination. Or for instance, soap was not distributed, and opportunities for keeping themselves clean were denied the prisoners. Particularly noisome were the 'mattrasses' that had been allowed to become soaked without opportunity of drying. In fairness, when the weather was bad, it was difficult to allow the prisoners time on the deck. Moreover, the ventilation was very poor, and fumigation, which was believed to be important, was not practised. The distribution of the anti-scorbutic prophylactic was often omitted.

One focus of attention was clothing, evidently unsuitable. If the transport left in the English summer, it was less of a problem but those leaving in the winter experienced increased illness. A measure as simple as providing an extra blanket was most helpful. His suggestions went into details of types of material and cuts of clothing. Redfern's paragraph introducing his suggestions makes one wonder where his tongue was in relation to his cheek because this is what he wrote :

> Far, very far, from Arrogantly wishing to propose useless innovations in a System already as nearly perfect as possible, Yet with the importance of the Subject pressing on my mind, and urged too by a strong sense of duty, I shall take the liberty most respectfully to submit to Your Excellency's consideration the propriety of suggesting and recommending to his Majesty's Government the following trifling changes and addition in the present Clothing for the Winter Voyage.

Witness now the value of history: have I not demonstrated that reading historic texts could restore the art of making a CEO positively purr as he is stroked?

Suggestions as to clothing led naturally to consideration of cleanliness and an insistence on the distribution of sufficient water to make washing possible. Redfern was much in favour of 'wholesome ablutions'.

The recommendations came under eleven headings. These encompassed warm clothing, cleanliness, the desirability of cold affusions, that masters of transports be better supervised in their custody of the victuals, that more wine for convicts be available, that water allowance not be reduced, that articles of comfort should not be surreptitiously or fraudulently withheld, that each day each convict and his mattrass should be brought up on deck, that the prison be regularly cleaned and fumigated, that better medical officers should be found; the last recommendation, one that perhaps took in all points, was that the medical officer should have control of all matters pertaining to the convicts—indeed, the surgeon superintendent should have at least as much power as the captain of the ship.

These suggestions were put into effect, were very beneficial and a measurable improvement occurred in the morbidity and mortality of subsequent transports. The rates fell to a quarter of what they had previously been. Redfern's great contribution, apart from emphasising what was already known, was the innovative but very logical administrative structure of having the doctor also agent for transport, carrying both the responsibility and the administrative clout.

His recommendations found a strong and useful ally in the Society of Apothecaries, London, which prided itself on the quality of drugs and equipment which it supplied to ships. The society was pressing also for the employment of fully qualified medical practitioners and, naturally, was promoting its own degrees, the MRCS and LSA. The society, with its initiative in teaching and raising the general standards of medical practice, was also having a favourable effect on the health of transported convicts.

William Redfern had many attributes which made him peculiarly suitable for the work he undertook. He was immensely experienced in the field, not only as a theoretician, but also as a practical man. His own life and his personal ups and downs provided him with much sympathy for the subjects of his study. His work was on a real problem, one of great practical and actual concern. He had a powerful patron: Macquarie had taken a liking to him, respected his work and integrity, and when Redfern was attacked, Macquarie took it as a personal affront that his judgment in men should be questioned. Redfern did his work thoroughly, collecting facts and figures. Note too, that it was a study that had been requested, not a gratuitous piece of research. The style of his report was calculated to best gain acceptance and support. In public health matters in particular, the researcher's work is only half done if the research does not become an advocate—better still, an effective advocate—for the cause.

In the beginning, when our white Australian world was being created, Redfern stands out like a biblical figure, by no means perfect, but a righteous man for his generation, both in the field of medicine and in the wider Australian community. He has earned himself a niche in Australian public health.[68]

4

Who needs to plan?

JEANETTE WARD AND D'ARCY HOLMAN

This chapter was written by two researchers who assess health, illness, process and outcomes of health care by applying scientific methods to contemporary health questions. Both observational measures of physical health and perceptual measures of health and treatment decisions and processes can be used in such research. In their explanation of planning issues in this chapter, they present a positivistic approach. This represents a mainstream view on research planning. Qualitative research is noted in this chapter, with helpful tips on how to explore qualitative concepts in essentially quantitative studies. The chapter can be read in conjunction with other chapters which have a different approach, most notably Jan Ritchie's chapter on qualitative methods in health research, in which qualitative paradigms can take the lead in the research design.

The benefits of planning show up in results. This chapter briefly revisits the tenets of scientific method and its centrality in health research. It is the pursuit of 'truth' which informs specification of a research question and selection of an appropriate research design. Experimental and other quantitative designs are best for seeking evidence of attribution, while qualitative methods are best for understanding meaning, especially when contextual insights are needed. This chapter provides a practical overview of issues commonly encountered when planning quantitative research, such as sampling, statistical power, error, bias and probability of proof. In this chapter, multidisciplinary approaches to researchable questions about health, the efficacy of treatments and interventions, as well as the evaluation of health care delivery and the system in which it takes place, are recommended.

Involving representatives of potential users of research results in its initial planning also will enhance the researcher's 'duty of care' to disseminate results and get research into practice. This chapter promotes an iterative process when planning research, particularly as research protocols cannot be modified once the research is under way. At the end of this chapter, readers will be able to develop a researchable question and incorporate various methodological and practical considerations when selecting research designs.

The authors emphasise there is no need to solve the whole puzzle all at once. It will suffice to join the many first-rate scientists at work, adding small but true pieces of knowledge, one at a time.[1]

Scientific tenets of health research

The word 'science' comes from the Latin word *scientia*, which means 'knowledge'. The purpose of scientific inquiry is to create knowledge that clarifies the world around us. Health research shares with other branches of science four major characteristics of scientific inquiry, namely: positivism, theory, empiricism and objectivity.

Positivism

Positivism is the leading principle of a system of encyclopaedic classification of the findings of scientific enquiry, named by the philosopher, Comte. It is the view that all true knowledge is based on a fundamental assumption that the world is not totally chaotic. Rather, it has logical and persistent patterns of regularity, which can be observed, studied and reported. Positivism is a dominant philosophy in the biomedical sciences. However, positivism is sometimes challenged, especially with respect to social phenomena, which are arguably the product of both social laws and human volitional action. Although, in general, social phenomena cannot be predicted with complete accuracy, in part because existing theories, methods of data collection and analysis are insufficiently developed to explain them, there are nevertheless important patterns of regularity in social phenomena to justify adopting a positivist approach to research data collection and analysis.

Theory

A theory is a statement that seeks to explain or predict a particular phenomenon. Scientific theories are used to derive research hypotheses, plan research, make observations and explain the patterns of regularity that are observed. Alternative theories may exist and scientific inquiry is directed towards testing and choosing from these. The strength of a theory can be judged by the extent to which it is *efficient* (i.e., involves few statements and assumptions), *comprehensive* (i.e., explains a broad range of phenomena) and *accurate* (i.e., predicts reliably the results of causal actions or factors). One theory is judged superior to another if it is more efficient, more comprehensive or more accurate in its predictions. A theory is a statement that seeks to encapsulate an explanation or prediction of particular phenomena.

There is an intimate connection between theory and research. When researchers critically examine an existing theory to see if observed phenomena are consistent with what the theory predicts, they are using a *deductive* approach. Researchers who take particular observations to inform the development or confirmation of a general theory are using an *inductive* approach. *Grounded theory* exemplifies the latter. In grounded theory studies, researchers hypothesise inductively from data, most particularly using the subjects' own categories, concepts and even notions of causality. In searching for theories, scientists do not start with a clean slate, but are influenced by a range of general perspectives about what is important, legitimate and reasonable. These perspectives are known as *paradigms* and they typically represent the general perspective adopted by a particular discipline. Sometimes a major new set of theories is introduced that challenges existing perspectives and becomes generally accepted as providing a superior model to explain the world. This is the *paradigm shift*.

Empiricism

Another dominant characteristic of modern scientific inquiry is an acceptance of empiricism, namely that evidence collected from the observation of experience in the world can be used legitimately to corroborate, modify or construct theories.

Objectivity

Empirical evidence is assumed to exist independently of researchers and should ideally be reported and interpreted in a similar manner by different researchers. In practice, perfect objectivity is impossible to achieve in health research, due to the complex nature of the subject matter and the many value-based decisions that are made by researchers with respect to design, data collection, analysis, reporting and interpretation. Research methods, properly used however, strengthen the objectivity of the observational aspects of research. In planning health research (whether qualitative or quantitative), you must be comfortable in working within these principles. It is both causal association and an acceptance that we can alter future health outcomes by applying treatments found to be effective in clinical trials that characterises modern health care from unscientific therapies. It is this expectation that generalisable insights are generated through research that justifies any research effort.

Inference in scientific research

By conducting research, we seek to infer a versatile 'truth' about the universe with which we hope ultimately to inform and improve future health care practice. Therefore, researchers themselves, and users of research, place considerable importance on the validity of research and, consequently, also consider threats to validity.

A useful distinction is that between the validity of measurement and the validity of a research study overall. Measurement validity is concerned with the extent to which a measurement corresponds to the theoretical concept under study (*construct validity*); the extent to which the measurement embraces all important aspects of phenomena that are part of the theory (*content validity*); and the extent to which the measurement stands up to external criteria such as a comparison with a 'gold standard' or the ability to predict an expected outcome (*criterion validity*).

The validity of a research study is the degree to which inferences drawn from the results are warranted when account is taken of the study methods, including sampling methods, and the nature of the study population. *Internal validity* is met when inferences made about the study results are 'true' for the study population. In other words, internal validity is the degree to which the researchers draw valid conclusions about how the results of the study came about within the study itself. Internal validity is concerned with keeping systematic error in a study to a minimal, but it has nothing to do with random error in research; i.e., the role of chance variation. *External validity* is met when inferences made on the basis of study results are correct for the reference population. In other words, the degree to which the insights concluded by the researchers represent a 'truth' for other similar circumstances. External validity is also sometimes known as *generalisability*.

Reliability refers to the 'stability' of research methods and instruments. If the same method described in a scientific article was followed identically by another group, then a reliable study conducted in the same context ought generate virtually the same results. This explains in part why health researchers must be clear and concise when reporting methods used in their studies, such that replication by others is possible. When using specific instruments, obtain psychometric studies that report aspects of reliability such as the test-retest reliability. If your method or instrument is unreliable, then your findings cannot be interpreted. Researchers also need to consider the possibility of differences between users of research instruments. For example, if you plan to measure quality of care by auditing records, then you should confirm the reliability of your audit by having two people independently review records using your protocol. A statistic known as *kappa* will demonstrate *inter-rater reliability*. A high kappa value confirms to others the stability of your protocol in different hands.

Decisions made in planning research ought to be guided by the inferences you can make about the universal 'truth' you seek to understand. By minimising random and systematic errors, researchers maximise validity. To conduct health research, we must be confident and comfortable in accepting that science is a valid activity leading to generalisable insights.

Clarifying your research question

While these global sentiments about 'truth' and validity are fundamental, it is crucial that, as health researchers, you clarify and progressively refine the question you seek to answer in your research.

Hulley and Cummings proposed the acronym FINER as a guide to those new to research when developing a research question:[2]

Feasible
    Adequate number of subjects
    Adequate technical capacity among the research team
    Affordable and manageable in scope
Interesting to the researcher
Novel
Ethical
Relevant
    To scientific knowledge
    To clinical or health policy
    To future research directions

You could practise applying these to the research question that you developed in chapter 1. You may even wish to alter your question after considering the FINER criteria.

Researchers have an ethical as well as scientific responsibility to justify the place of their intended research by appraising the pre-existing backdrop of knowledge and responding to gaps in that knowledge base. Systematic literature reviews and, if appropriate, meta-analyses, will synthesise the extant evidence and identify strategic directions for new enquiry. If no such synthesis exist, researchers are encouraged to consult colleagues, leaders in the field and potential end-users of the research to elicit key issues and contemporary questions. Clearly, the process of peer review typically undertaken by research grant funding bodies such as the National Institutes of Health in the US or the Medical Research Council in the UK provides scrutiny of these aspects of any proposed research idea. Consultation with others active in your research field also ensures your research has relevance, credibility and meaning.

Choosing an appropriate design

If you seek to determine whether a new treatment for a chronic disease significantly improves outcomes over and above current 'best practice', you need to compare outcomes by using a quantitative method. If you seek to determine whether application of multidisciplinary quality improvement processes significantly increase the likelihood of better patient outcomes than medical peer review processes alone, a quantitative method will determine the quantitative changes but qualitative methods will elicit barriers to implementation or incidents critical to success. If you seek to understand what factors influence patients in making a decision about health care treatments, you need qualitative methods to reveal their underlying values, cognitive processes and discourse about treatment effectiveness for example. Quantitative methods are unlikely to provide valid insights in this case.

Quantitative designs

If your question seeks to study the impact of a new treatment of program, then it is important to establish the prevailing level of evidence already available to support your program and, as appropriate, advance knowledge by selecting a rigorous research design. It also is important to be very clear about the variables to study and, in turn, prescriptive about ways to measure these variables.

What are variables?

A concept with a single never-changing value is known as a *constant*. These are rare in health research. By contrast, a concept that has more than one measurable value is a *variable*. A variable capable of effecting change in other variables is an *independent* or *study* variable. A variable whose value is dependent upon one or more other variables is a *dependent* or *outcome* variable. Relationships between study and outcome variables may be direct (positive) or inverse (negative), symmetric or asymmetric (if change in one variable is accompanied by change in the other, but not vice versa); linear or non-linear; spurious or causal. When planning your quantitative research, be explicit about the outcome variables you seek to understand and the hypothesised nature of their association with study variables.

When the association between two variables has been caused by a third or extraneous variable, the relationship is *spurious*. The variable that causes a spurious relationship is called an *antecedent variable* or, in the field of epidemiology, a *confounder*. Another form of confounder is a *suppressor variable*, which conceals the relationship between two variables because it directly affects one and inversely affects the other. A relationship between two variables may also be caused by an *intervening variable*, which is caused by the independent variable and affects the dependent variable. An intervening variable is not a confounder.

If a change in the independent variable does indeed cause an effect in the dependent variable, there is a *causal relationship*. There are three basic requisites to a causal relationship: statistical association, rational sequence of influence, and non-spuriousness. Establishing that these conditions exist is known as the process of *causal inference*. Ruling out alternative explanations other than cause, such as chance variation, confounding and other bias (selection or information bias), is an important part of causal inference. As described above, judicious selection of an increasingly more rigorous design such as moving from observational studies to an experimental design will add to the body of knowledge.

Types of quantitative designs

When a researcher is able to assign the independent or exposure variables to a number of subjects and withhold it from others (who become controls), an experimental design is the one of choice. Randomisation is the cornerstone of true experimental designs such as clinical controlled trials. However, when a researcher is able only to compare people with and without exposure (to an aetiological agent, treatment or health service) and to analyse the results, s/he is conducting a non-experimental analytic study of which there are many types,[3] including: case-control studies, prospective cohort studies, historical (retrospective) cohort studies, prognostic cohort studies, and analytical (hypothesis-driven) cross-sectional studies.

Hypothesis testing remains the cornerstone of analytic designs although they are 'observational' rather than 'experimental'. By contrast, quantitative description of a phenomenon or current outcomes without intervention or prior hypotheses is known as descriptive research. These designs are quantitative. Types of descriptive studies include: case series, community needs assessment, cross-sectional community or professional studies, and population surveillance. Each of these is defined in further detail below, and worked examples of them are included in subsequent chapters. It is worth spending some time on understanding the differences between these types of studies. The designs will naturally lead to different data collection, analysis and interpretation.

More on experimental design

In an experiment, the investigator intentionally alters one or more factors under controlled conditions in order to study the effects of doing so. The most important form of experiment in health research is the clinical trial, which is used to assess the efficacy or effectiveness of treatment in quantitative terms. A distinction can be made between explanatory trials, which assess the effect of the active component of treatment under ideal conditions, and pragmatic trials, which assess the effect of the treatment in practice.

The clinical trial design is definitive when studying effectiveness of treatment—for instance, when asking, 'Does it work?' in terms of reduction in morbidity or mortality. It can be of limited value when studying unintended effects of treatment, answering questions such as, 'Is it safe?', especially in terms of uncommon side effects. Side effects are difficult to study in clinical trials if they are rare and occur a long time after exposure to treatment.

The paradigm of the clinical trial is intended to produce:

- comparability of populations through randomisation;
- comparability of effects through randomisation and the use of placebo; and
- comparability of information through use of randomisation, placebo and double-blind conditions.

It thereby makes the observed effects of the treatment a valid estimate of the therapeutic effects.

The design of clinical trials can vary. In the parallel group design, subjects are allocated in parallel to two or more experimental conditions such as a treatment vs placebo or a new treatment vs an established practice. This is the classic form of clinical trial. Another design is the cross-over trial, in which subjects are allocated randomly to receive each of the experimental conditions in a different sequence. This design is most appropriate when there is large between-patient variation before treatment, and the intervention has a short latent period and short duration of action. It does have some special problems, however, due to the potential for a carry-over effect from one experimental condition to the other.

Two other forms of the clinical trial are the factorial design and the sequential design. The factorial design improves the efficiency of research that estimates the effects of two or more interventions simultaneously. A study in which two interventions are assessed is known as a two-by-two factorial design. Three interventions requires a two-by-two-by-two factorial design. In the sequential trial, pairs of subjects are allocated to the different experimental conditions and a running tally is kept on the directions of 'pair preferences'. Using statistical methods, it is possible to determine when there is sufficient evidence to conclude that one of the experimental conditions is superior.

More on non-experimental research designs

Experimental designs such as the clinical trial are widely regarded as the gold standard of health research due to their high internal validity, but it is not always possible or desirable to perform an experiment. This may be because the intervention is established practice, or shows so much promise that experimentation is unethical. The government or funding authority may be unwilling to wait for experimental evidence due to political pressure to provide a new treatment. The cost of an experiment may be prohibitive. Sometimes treatment outcomes and, even to a greater extent, the adverse effects of treatment are too rare or too long term to be detected in an affordable experiment. While holding strong internal validity, experimental results may have problems with external validity because the conditions under which they are undertaken tend to be more ideal than average.

We wish to assess the broader effects of the intervention within the health system, when it is adopted on a whole-of-population basis.

Under these circumstances, non-experimental research methods, such as cohort or case-control studies, may be used to estimate the effects of interventions and other exposures in populations whose exposure status has been determined by the complex interplays of real life. Cohort studies and case-control studies are epidemiological research, and are described in detail in Andrew Grulich's chapter 6, 'How is our health?'. In a cohort study, naturally occurring groups of exposed and non-exposed subjects are identified from a source population and are followed over time to observe the occurrence of the outcome. Apart from the absence of experimental allocation, randomisation and a placebo and blinding of subjects, a cohort study is similar in design to a clinical trial and the methods of analysis are essentially the same. In the case-control study, the subjects are selected according to the presence of the outcome of interest and not according to exposure. Persons with a given outcome (cases) and persons at risk of the outcome (controls) are selected from either a dynamic population, with changing membership, or a cohort population followed-up after an intervention or baseline measurement. Case-control studies can be less expensive to conduct than cohort studies, typically require fewer subjects to provide adequate precision, can often be completed within a shorter time frame and are often the only practical study design to use in the case of a rare outcome. However, because information on exposure is often collected retrospectively, they can be subject to information bias.

Commencing with Maclure's case-crossover study in 1991,[4] a new type of case-control design has been developed, known as the case distribution study. This design has the distinguishing feature of not using separate control subjects to estimate the distribution of the population at risk according to exposure status. Each case acts as its own control, drawing on variation in exposure experienced over a period of time.

Methodological issues in quantitative research
Type I error, Type II error, and Type III error

A Type I error represents the 'false positive' of health research. Either as a result of bias, confounding or over-enthusiastic and repeated statistical analysis, researchers may find a statistically significant association between variables, permitting rejection of the null hypothesis. However, a Type I error is committed when the 'truth' is that there is no association.

A Type II error can be considered the 'false negative' of health research. While the truth may be that there *is* an association between study and outcome variables, the researcher may not detect this association, leading to a Type II error. Type II errors are frequently due to inadequate statistical power to detect the actual difference.

A Type III error is where, unbeknown to the researcher, the correct inference is made but for entirely the wrong reasons.

Probability of proof

Researchers identify a 'null hypothesis' which they then seek to refute or reject by demonstrating that any subsequent association between study and outcome variables was extremely unlikely to have been due to chance alone.

Sampling

In health research, it invariably occurs that not everyone with the condition of interest can be sampled and approached to participate in research. Therefore, a sampling strategy is an explicit and preplanned procedure to obtain a subsample of the 'reference population' as the larger group to which you seek to apply your research findings. A probability sample uses some kind of random process to assure that each unit of the population has an equal chance of selection. Stratified random sampling and cluster sampling are variations of simple random sampling, whereby you might use random number software to generate numbers for selection of individuals from within a sampling frame.

Consecutive sampling is often used as a pragmatic substitute for health services research. Researchers can compare the characteristics of their recruited sample against the characteristics of the known reference population to check representativeness.

Statistical power

To avoid a Type II error particularly, it is crucial that researchers calculate sample sizes to ensure that the effect size they seek in experimental research or the associations they hypothesise in descriptive research are likely to be detected. Sample sizes for descriptive studies generally are based on the precision with which researchers seek to quantify proportions or rates. As even a descriptive study will generate analytic questions about the relationships between variables studied, educated 'guesstimates' of the plausible distribution of variables among subgroups of the sample will inform sample size calculations. When planning an experimental study, it also is necessary to estimate the size of the difference to be expected between intervention and control groups after administration to the former of the intervention (see worked examples).

However, there is a school of thought in the science of epidemiology that regards a sample size calculation as a technical exercise that may not necessarily take into account the *value* of the information obtained from a study of any particular size.[5] The most important consideration in planning sample size is the trade-off between the cost of the study and its precision. The larger the sample size, the greater the precision of the results (i.e., narrower confidence intervals), but also the greater the cost of gathering the data. Given that most research has some fixed costs and some costs that vary with the number of subjects, there is a minimum practical sample size below which costs remain essentially the same. There is also a maximum practical sample size, above which increasing costs yield very little improvement in precision. The ideal sample size lies between these extremes and should be determined by how much precision is worth purchasing with available research funds. Inevitably however, some research is conducted with limited numbers. For example, if you wish to survey medical oncologists (cancer specialists) about their practices, you will likely need to survey them all, and you cannot increase the sample size. Increasingly complex designs behove involvement of a biostatistician in planning your research. The partnership of a statistician and health researchers in the interpretation of existing data, and in the planning of further research, is illustrated in chapter 8, 'So, how is the treatment going?'.

The worked examples 4.1, 4.2, and 4.3 highlight the importance of power, significance levels and probable sample differences when a 'sample' size is decided on.

Example 4.1

Imagine you are designing a descriptive survey of clinicians about an important health issue and you seek to demonstrate significant differences in attitudes based on respondents' gender. If previous research, conducted in another country for example, has shown that overall 40% of clinicians agree with a specific attitudinal statement, then you will need 107 male respondents and 107 female respondents to show a difference of 20% between the genders at the 5% significance level (alpha) with 80% power. If female clinicians make up about a third of the workforce you seek to survey, then a random sample will yield males to females in a ratio of 3 to 1. Not everyone will reply to your survey. Accepting that the response rate might be 67%, then 430 clinicians will need to be randomly selected in order to obtain a sufficient number of female respondents to compare gender differences in attitudes.

Example 4.2

Imagine you are designing an experiment to evaluate the effect of an intervention on a specific clinical behaviour from its anticipated baseline of 10%. The table below sets out the various sample sizes required, depending on the size of the difference you hope to achieve (80% power, 5% alpha). If the anticipated baseline is 15%, then larger sample sizes are generally needed to demonstrate differences between groups after the intervention.

	20% difference	25% difference	30% difference
Baseline of 10%	72	51	38
Baseline of 15%	98	66	47

Example 4.3

Imagine you are trying to change the behaviour of clinicians working in hospitals. Your intervention involves organisational change and, therefore, you will randomise hospitals rather than individual clinicians to either intervention or control groups. As each hospital represents a 'cluster' where you will target your intervention, you have designed a 'cluster randomisation trial'. It is obvious that clinicians who work in any one of these hospitals will be more alike than those in other hospitals. If you measure outcomes at the level of the individual clinician, you cannot assume that data from those within clusters are independent. Your sample size calculations must incorporate various estimations of 'intracluster correlation coefficients' (ICC). A statistician must be consulted when calculating sample sizes for these sorts of trials. As a rule of thumb, the greater the ICC, the larger the study will need to be.

Qualitative designs

Where scientific enquiry seeks primarily not to assert attribution but rather to elucidate meaning, qualitative methods are most appropriate.[6] Quantitative methods are too 'blunt' for this sort of question. Indeed,

> Qualitative research takes an interpretive, naturalistic approach to its subject matter; qualitative researchers study things in their natural settings, attempting to make sense of, or interpret, phenomena in terms of the meanings that people bring to them. Qualitative research begins by accepting that there is a range of different ways of making sense of the world and is concerned with discovering the meanings seen by those who are being researched and with understanding their view of the world rather than that of the researchers.[7]

Qualitative research is covered extensively in Jan Ritchie's chapter 9, 'Not everything can be reduced to numbers'. You should refer to that chapter for an explanation of qualitative paradigms and methods. The issues are as broad and complex as for quantitative research. Information gathering can be facilitated by case-study, observation, historical or document analysis, ethnography, consensus methods, interviews or focus groups, to name a few.[8] Analysis involves a disciplined analytical approach to the content, and context, of what has been said, observed, or written.

Qualitative research has its own set of methodological criteria that must be met to assure validity and reliability (or their equivalents). Note that Jan Ritchie terms this rigour in her chapter on qualitative research.

Non-probability sampling appeals particularly to qualitative researchers for whom the range of views needs to be ascertained rather than their distribution among the reference population. Thus, purposive sampling is acceptable to ensure specific views are elucidated. Sample sizes are governed not by statistical power but by decisions relating to thematic exhaustion, redundancy or repetition of observations. Non-probability sampling is inappropriate if researchers seek to generalise quantitative conclusions to a reference population.

Qualitative versus quantitative?

Currently, an unnecessary and unhelpful divide between quantitative and qualitative methods discourages interaction and dialogue between the camps.[9] The contrasts are more apparent than real. Indeed, as subsequent chapters of this book will reveal, the diversity of methods ensures that the complexity of health problems can be tackled with valid and reliable methods. The strength of health research stems from this rich range of methods:

> because of its applied nature, much [health] research is driven, not by the theoretical stance of the researchers, but by the specific practical problem which is turned into a research question ... the choice of method and how it is used can perfectly well be matched to what is being studied rather than to the disciplinary or methodological leanings of the researcher.[10]

Neither camp has an inherent methodological superiority in absolute terms. If you are an experienced quantitative researcher, you will need to collaborate with a qualitative researcher when you seek to understand and explain contextual phenomena. If you are a qualitative researcher seeking to estimate the prevalence of particular views or phenomena, you will need to collaborate with a quantitative researcher. Examples of how both approaches can be used within a study are provided by Jan Ritchie, in chapter 9, from a predominantly qualitative perspective, and by Deborah Saltman and Natalie O'Dea in chapter 10, 'Quality and quantity', in which quantitative methods are emphasised.

Resources

Health research places demands on resources of many types, including physical, human, information and financial resources. Researchers needs physical space and access to equipment such as tape recorders, computers, telephones, and cars as necessary. Subjects as well as members of the research team all are human beings, deserving sound human resources management, communication skills, and, occasionally, conflict management strategies. Researchers need access to library, health databases, electronic publication databases and dedicated research archives such as the National Information Service in Australia. Obvious costs typically included in research grants comprise salaries, printing, postage and telephone bills, but remember to estimate labour on-costs, software licences, meetings and miscellaneous infrastructure.

An insider's view on resource issues in the conduct of research is offered by Alix Magney, Elizabeth O'Brien and Vanessa Traynor in chapter 11, 'Assistants and mentors'. In that chapter, the researchers give some tips on how to negotiate use of resources, and how to make the most of resources that are available for each project. They also address the human resource issue of being managed with respect, and having the opportunity to develop their skills. They speak from their experiences as research assistants.

Planning achievable research

Only research that is focused, driven by a refined and specific research question, is feasible to conduct. This might prove frustrating for some. If it helps, store your 'big ideas' in another place, revisiting them after your first research project is complete. Experienced and successful health researchers patiently compose a research agenda, carving off achievable research questions and answering them study by study, knowing that the larger insight will emerge in due course.

Planning health research is an iterative process. Be prepared to consult, receive constructive criticisms and modify your specific research question and methods. At the end of your planning deliberations, you should have a protocol or plan which others can read and readily understand. Suggested elements of this plan are:

- *Background to the study:* This summarises your groundwork, how you decided the research was timely and relevant; key findings from previous research, and shortcomings or gaps in the extant knowledge base. In this section of the plan, explain how the variables will be measured and justify measurements, tools, and intervals to be deployed. Summarise psychometric properties and sources of published instruments.
- *Aims:* This can be the research question itself and, additionally, subsidiary aims or specific objectives for the research.
- *Method:* This should describe clearly and justify the sampling procedure; methods of obtain consent; data collection procedures; strategies to demonstrate reliability and data integrity.

- *Task allocation*: If a large team is involved, describe and allocate tasks in advance of commencing the study as a means of clarifying expectations and responsibilities.
- *Resources*: This can be a budget outline, as well as an explanation of the human resource contributions to be made by researchers themselves or other consumables required to make the research happen.
- *Statistical analysis*: If your data set is likely to be large and complex, you need to be explicit about data management issues such as data entry, cleaning and processing prior to analysis. With regard to analysis, some 'dummy tables' may help to identify the way to approach analyses. A technical 'recipe', explaining the statistical tests to be undertaken, is recommended. Sample size calculations can be specified here.
- *Anticipated benefits*: Here, you can specify the public utility of your research: who will gain from its insights?; who ought to know about the study?; how will it improve upon current knowledge?
- *Publication options/dissemination strategies*: By anticipating possible journals and other publications outlets, you can better prepare manuscript writing and develop a dissemination plan. Anticipate how you will apply the research findings yourself and/or encourage others to do so.
- *Ethics*: All research should be subjected to scrutiny by an appropriately constituted ethics committee. Documentation of final approval should be readily accessible to researchers, participants and users of research. The process of submitting proposals to ethics committees is explained in chapter 12.

In your planning, remember that: vague research questions are the bane of health research; overinterpretation of preliminary research or findings from less rigorous designs potentially undermines the evolutionary pursuit of knowledge; research questions must drive the choice of research method, not vice versa; good research typically requires funding, patience and recognition of the backdrop of research which preceded it; multidisciplinary input enhances protocol development, relevance and likelihood of effective dissemination;[11] good research also represents a springboard for future research which confirms, refutes, enhances or transforms previous understanding; causality is best determined using experimental designs; and users of research may not fully appreciate methodological limitations of any individual study. This chapter has demonstrated the importance of planning. Planning is, in essence, anticipation of the process of inquiry, so that proper analysis and interpretation can be conducted. The next few chapters present the basic issues in measurement and statistical analysis of data. Statistics need not be too overwhelming, as you will see in Deborah Black's introductory chapter, chapter 5, 'Numbers and more'.

5
Numbers and more

DEBORAH BLACK

This chapter provides an outline of common techniques used in statistical analyses of quantitative data. The strengths and limitations of the use of quantitative data to measure health issues within and between groups of people are discussed. The first section defines 'statistics' and ways of classifying data. The second section emphasises the importance of descriptive statistics in health research. Inferential statistics are introduced and their use is explained by illustration of various inferential statistical techniques including t-tests, ANOVAs, χ^2 and regression. The last section summarises the types of hypotheses which may be tested using different measures and the application of statistical tests to measurements which are collected. This chapter is presented in a narrative style with worked examples for ease of reading, rather than in a more mathematical style.

What is 'statistics'?

Statistics is the science of collecting, organising and interpreting data—that is, transforming data into information. The data elements, or variables, are defined and discussed. The key steps in applying statistics are collecting, organising and interpreting data.

Collecting data

Data collection is described as a *census* if all items in a population are enumerated. However, this is usually not possible in health research because of time and/or resource constraints. A *sample* refers to data collection from a subset of items from the population. The ideal sampling method is when each item in the population has an equal chance of selection in the sample. This is known as simple random sampling. This type of sampling may not always be appropriate when population subgroups of interest are underrepresented in the population. Discussion of specific sampling techniques and sample size determination is included in Jeanette Ward and D'Arcy Holman's chapter 4, 'Who needs to plan?'. Further detailed discussions of sampling are found in Levy and Lemeshow,[1] and information on sample size determination is presented in Lwanga and Lemeshow.[2]

Organising data

Data can be organised and subsequently described in words, in tables or in graphs. This process is described as *descriptive statistics*. Examples of the use of descriptive statistics in health research are presented in the next section.

Interpreting data

Interpreting data refers to drawing inferences to the target population based on the organisation of the data, that is, inferential statistics. Inferential statistics is the analysis of a subset of items from a population and hence making inferences about the population based on the sample. Because samples do not enumerate the total population, there remains a chance of error in the population estimate. Results of analyses must report the size of the error in the estimate or the level of confidence in the estimate. Both the confidence level and the error size will depend on the sample size and the dispersion of the sample data. Large sample sizes with little dispersion will result in better confidence levels about the estimate and smaller error levels. Inferential statistical techniques are discussed later in this chapter.

What is a variable?

Variables are characteristics associated with each item or case in a population. These characteristics are simply recorded as variables in the data. They are called *variables* because they vary, or can be different for different people. The ages of people attending a community health centre on a given day may be recorded. The variable is age.

Age is a *quantitative variable*, meaning it can be measured or counted. Quantitative variables can be classified as continuous or discrete. Age is a continuous variable—it has an uninterrupted range of measures. Although generally measured in years, age can be measured in months, days, hours, minutes and seconds. Other examples of continuous variables include weight and height. A discrete variable is one that can be counted. Discrete variables take only integer ('whole-number') values. Two examples of discrete variables are the number of visits to a general practitioner in a year and the number of patients on a waiting list.

Qualitative variables do not have numerical values. Examples include gender and blood group. Qualitative variables can be ordinal, nominal and dichotomous. These are essentially numbers or codes assigned to concepts to aid in summary and comparison.

Ordinal variables have a number of categories that are ordered. For example, a patient satisfaction survey may have the categories 'most dissatisfied', 'dissatisfied', 'don't know', 'satisfied', and 'very satisfied'. These variables imply a ranking or order which is logical and in which categories are consecutive.

Nominal variables have no natural order, such as causes of death may be cancer, cardiothoracic disease, motor vehicle accident and so on.

Dichotomous variables have only two categories such as male/female, disease present/disease absent, dead/alive and yes/no. Figure 5.1 illustrates the different ways in which variables can be classified.

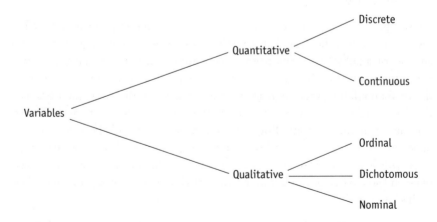

Figure 5.1 Types of variables

Exercise 5.1 Categorising variables

Variable	Quantitative/qualitative	Continuous/discrete or ordinal/ nominal/dichotomous
Gender	Qualitative	Dichotomous
Pain measured on a scale from 1 to 5		
Systolic blood pressure		
Blood group		
Whether you are a smoker or not		
Eye colour		
Number of cigarettes smoked per day		

Try exercise 5.1 to practise your understanding of these key differences in the classification of variables. You could do this exercise alone, or in a small group.

It is not unusual for continuous variables, such as age, to be put into categories. It might be asked why data are placed in categories. The next section, on descriptive statistics, explains why data are presented in different ways rather than as raw figures.

Descriptive statistics

Another term for descriptive statistics is *exploratory data analyses*. Exploratory data analyses should begin with examination of each variable individually, and then look at relationships between variables. It is best to start with graphical presentation.

Let us take an example of 100 people who died on a given day in a specified geographical area. Table 5.1 presents the raw data.

Analyses should begin by looking at each variable individually. A simple pie chart demonstrates that over half of those who died were male (see figure 5.2). Further analyses reveal that around 75% of deaths occur after age 65 (figure 5.3). The most frequent cause of death is diseases of the circulatory system. Figure 5.4 presents the distribution of deaths by cause of death.

Table 5.1 Raw data on people who died

ID no.	Sex	Age	Cause of death
1	Male	81	Diseases of circulatory system
2	Male	22	External causes
3	Female	93	Diseases of the respiratory system
.	.	.	.
.	.	.	.
.	.	.	.
97	Male	65	Neoplasms
98	Female	79	Neoplasms
99	Female	83	Diseases of the circulatory system
100	Male	59	Diseases of the respiratory system

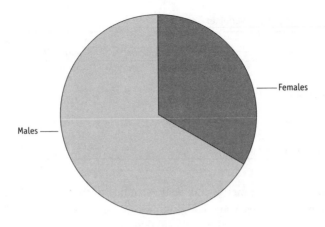

Figure 5.2 Pie chart on sex of those who died

A health researcher might then ask whether the distributions of deaths by age and cause of death were the same for males and females. The information can again be presented graphically (figure 5.5). The graph giving the distribution of deaths by sex and age (figure 5.6) shows that males are more likely to die at a younger age than females. Around 30% of males are dead before the age of 65 compared to only 15% of females.

Figure 5.6 presents a comparison between the proportions of females dying in each category of cause of death and the proportions of males dying from the corresponding category of cause of death. The main cause for both males and females was diseases of the circulatory system, with almost half of the females dying from this cause compared to almost 4 in 10 of the males. The graph also shows that

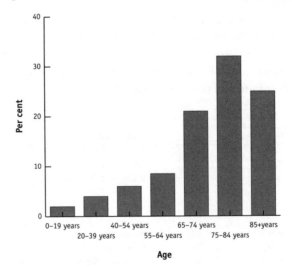

Figure 5.3 Distribution of deaths by age

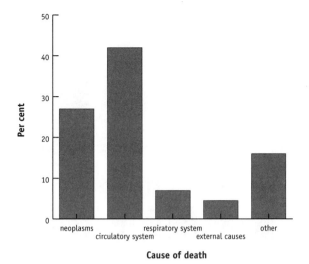

Figure 5.4 Distribution of deaths by cause of death

around 8% of males die from external causes such as suicide and motor vehicle accidents while the proportion of females dying of this cause is less than 1%.

It is not appropriate to compare the age of death and cause of death graphically because of the large number of categories in each variable. It is better to present a single *measure of centrality* for age for each category of cause of death. Measures of centrality can take three forms: mean, median and mode. The mean takes the average of the scores by adding up each of the scores and dividing by the number of scores. The score in the middle is the median. The mode is the score

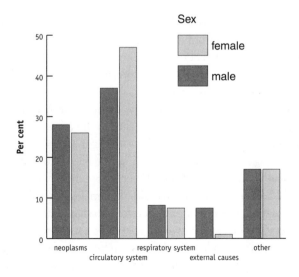

Figure 5.5 Distribution of cause of death by sex

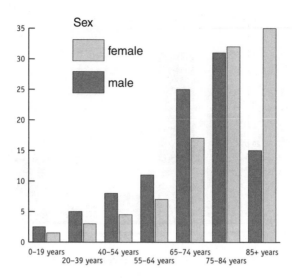

Figure 5.6   Distribution of deaths by age and sex

that occurs most frequently. Using the same data for deaths of 100 people who died on a given day, 5 died of external causes. Their ages were 21, 22, 22, 24 and 26. The mean is

$$\frac{21+22+22+24+26}{5} = 23$$

The mode is 22 and the median is also 22. Calculated using the same method, the mean for the 42 people who died of diseases of the circulatory system is 71. If the mean of age of those who died from external causes is compared with the mean age of those who died from diseases of the circulatory system, a large difference is observed. Similar calculations and comparisons can be made for the other causes of death. Descriptive statistics, therefore, uses both graphical and summary data to provide a picture of raw data.

Without the population sizes in each age group for males and females in the specified geographic area, the rates of mortality in the age/sex cohorts cannot be calculated. If, for instance, the geographic area is a location where the major employer is a mining company, then males might make up 70% of the population. Although the death data show that only 47% of those dying were female, the mortality rate would be much higher for females than males if females constitute only 30% of the population. It is important, therefore, to standardise mortality rates for both age and sex. Comparisons between geographic areas can be made using standardised mortality rates. Similar calculations can be made for fertility rates.

Although in medical research there is great emphasis on case-controlled trials, many important discoveries have been made by exploring raw data. One example of the use of descriptive statistics that was to have major implications for health research was the observation by the Center for Disease Control (CDC) in the USA in 1981 that 5 young homosexual men were being treated for or had died from pneumocystic pneumonia.[3] A later article in 1981 reported that a further 10 homosexual men diagnosed with this disease.[4] The same article reported the unusual occurrence of Kaposi's sarcoma, a disease normally confined to older men, in 26 young homosexual men in New York City (20 cases) and in California (6 cases). This was the first recognition of the AIDS epidemic through observation of routinely collected data.

Two important publishers of descriptive statistical information for health researchers in Australia are the Australian Bureau of Statistics and the Australian Institute of Health and Welfare. The Australian Bureau of Statistics' *Catalogue of Publications and Products* provides a list of publications for both routine and ad hoc surveys by the ABS.[5] Routine data collections include the Census of Population and Housing and the National Health Survey. Another important source of descriptive statistics for health researchers is *Australia's Heath 1998.*[6]

Descriptive statistics provide health researchers with a picture of the mortality and morbidity of their target population. However, in most cases of health research, more specific questions cannot be answered by pre-existing databases. If, for example, patterns of relatively higher morbidity or mortality are observed in the target population after standardisation for age and sex, the health researcher might ask why this has occurred. The researcher would then formulate hypotheses about the target population's lifestyle behaviours and demographic characteristics (other than age and sex) that are associated with their morbidity and mortality. To test the hypotheses, it is almost always impossible to survey all individuals (i.e., take a census), and so a sample is selected to represent the population. On the basis of the sample results, inferences are drawn about the target population. This method of anlaysis is *inferential statistics*.

Inferential statistics

Inferential statistics uses samples to draw conclusions about populations. As samples do not enumerate all items in the population, there is a chance of error in the population estimates. This error is determined, in part, by the spread or *dispersion* in the sample data. One measure of dispersion is the range, which is the difference between the highest and lowest scores in the sample. Another measure of dispersion is the sample variance. This is calculated by taking the sum of the square of difference from the mean of each sample value and dividing by the sample size less one. The standard deviation is the square root of the variance.

In the table 5.2 samples of men with cardiovascular disease, Sample 1 has a range of 25 while Sample 2 has a range of 8. The mean for both Sample 1 and

Table 5.2   Ages of two samples of people

Sample 1 Ages	Sample 2 Ages
50	59
53	60
57	62
61	62
65	62
66	63
66	64
67	65
70	66
75	67

Sample 2 is 63 years while their respective measures of dispersion, the sample standard deviations, are 7.7 and 2.5 years. For both samples, you would infer that the population mean was 63. However, as both samples are of equal size ($n = 10$), you would be far less confident about the accuracy of your estimate in Sample 1 because of the greater dispersion in that sample. Greater dispersion leads to a greater chance of error in the estimate. The sample size, n, and the standard deviation determine the accuracy of the population estimate.

Try exercise 5.2 to check that you understand how to calculate a mean.

Exercise 5.2

Add two additional people to the samples shown in table 5.2. Add a person aged 72 years old to Sample 1, and a person aged 56 to Sample 2. Recalculate the mean age (in years) of each of the samples, using the process described in this chapter.

If you want to go further with this exercise, you could consider how the standard deviations might change, given the additional data.

The normal curve

To determine the size of the error in population estimates, it is necessary to determine how the data are distributed. The curve defining the distribution is called the *probability density curve*. The curve plots the data values on the horizontal axis and the probability of the data values occurring on the vertical axis. The area under the curve is 1. A simple example of 50 undergraduate nursing students' systolic blood pressures is given in table 5.3.

Plotting blood pressures along the horizontal axis with their relative frequency on the vertical axis pattern produces some peaks and troughs but also shows a tendency towards a peak in the middle, the mode, and lower frequencies as systolic blood pressures move away from the mode at 110mmHg (figure 5.6). If the

Table 5.3 Systolic blood pressures of 50 nursing students

Systolic BP (mmHg)	Frequency	Proportion
86	1	.02
91	1	.02
97	2	.04
102	2	.04
103	3	.06
105	3	.06
106	4	.08
108	5	.10
110	8	.16
112	5	.10
119	5	.10
125	4	.08
130	3	.06
132	2	.04
135	1	.02
136	1	.02

number of readings taken increases to thousands, the curve becomes smooth without the peaks and troughs and is described as the *normal curve*. The normal curve (shown in figure 5.7) has perfect symmetry about the mean 110mmHg. The symmetry implies that 50% of the observations are below the mean and 50% are above the mean. The mean is also the median and the mode. A more detailed explanation of the normal curve is presented in *Statistics without Tears: A Primer for Non-mathematicians*.[7]

The mean and the standard deviation determine the shape of the normal curve. One standard deviation either side of the mean accounts for 68% of the

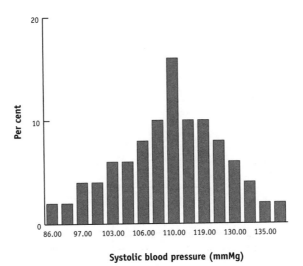

Figure 5.7 Students' blood pressure distribution

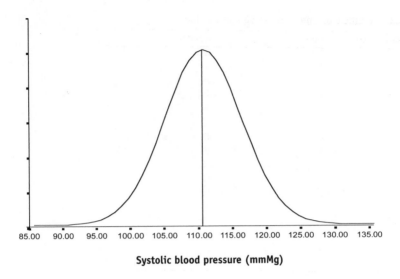

85.00   90.00   95.00   100.00   105.00   110.00   115.00   120.00   125.00   130.00   135.00

Systolic blood pressure (mmMg)

Figure 5.8   Systolic blood pressure

area under the curve. Two standard deviations either side of the mean covers around 95% of the area under the curve. Three standard deviations either side of the mean accounts for most of the area under the curve (99.7%).

The t-distribution has the same symmetrical shape as the normal distribution but varies in its spread according to the sample size. Smaller sample sizes have a t-distribution with greater spread. For 'large' samples (30 or more) the t-distribution is approximately equal to the normal distribution.

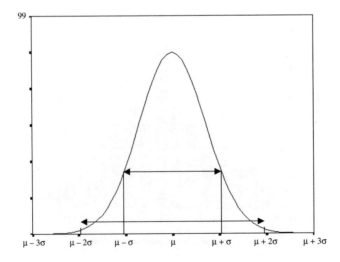

μ – 3σ   μ – 2σ   μ – σ   μ   μ + σ   μ + 2σ   μ + 3σ

Figure 5.9   Normal curve

Central Limit Theorem

The Central Limit Theorem states that if large random samples are taken, then the sample mean will be distributed normally with a mean equal to the population mean and standard deviation equal to the population standard deviation divided by the square root of the sample size, n. The Central Limit Theorem may seem trivial, but it forms the basis of what is described as parametric statistics. Using the Central Limit Theorem, it is possible to calculate upper and lower limits for population estimates (confidence intervals for population estimates), test whether there is a difference between measures from two or more population (t-tests and ANOVAs), and identify relationships between two or more variables (correlation and regression).

Confidence intervals

Returning to the sample of 50 undergraduate nurses' systolic blood pressures, the mean systolic blood pressure of the sample is 112.5 mm/Hg with a sample standard deviation of 11.25 mm/Hg. Using the Central Limit Theorem, it can be inferred that a 95% confidence interval for the mean systolic blood pressure for the total population of undergraduate nurses is between 109.4 to 115.6 mm/Hg.

Similarly the Central Limit Theorem is used to estimate confidence intervals for the population mean age from the two samples of men with cardiovascular disease (table 5.2). For sample 1, the 95% confidence interval for the population mean age of men with cardiovascular disease has a lower limit of 57.5 years and an upper limit of 68.5 years. The 95% confidence interval for the population mean age of men with cardiovascular disease for sample 2 is 61.2 years to 64.8 years. The second sample with much less spread produces a much narrower confidence interval and therefore the population mean is estimated with greater confidence.

Testing hypotheses about population means

Hypothesis testing is an important area of health research. A past population study may have shown that the average age when boys start smoking is 15 years. A health researcher might form a hypothesis that boys are now starting to smoke at a younger age. To test the hypothesis the researcher takes a random sample of young male smokers and calculates the average age at which they commenced smoking. This average is compared to the known population average. In this example, the researcher is dealing with a single population. A health researcher might know that 10% of girls aged 14 to 17 years across Australia smoke. The researcher may wish to test whether the proportion of girls smoking in this age group in a population located in a defined geographic area is greater than the proportion in the Australian population. Again the researcher is testing an hypothesis about a single population.

However, it is more common in health research to test whether there is a difference between measures taken from two populations. If a sample from one population receives an intervention, it is described as the intervention group. If a sample from another population does not receive the intervention, it is described as the control group.

For example, a researcher might wish to test whether an exercise program for men with hypertension will reduce systolic blood pressure. The intervention group takes half an aspirin and attends an exercise program twice a week for six weeks. The control group receives only the same dosage of aspirin for six weeks. Commonsense implies that the men in the control group should have similar ages to those in the intervention group and have similar pre-intervention systolic blood pressures to those in the intervention group. The health researcher's hypothesis is that the intervention group will have a lower mean systolic blood pressure following the intervention compared to the mean systolic blood pressure of the control group. The difference between the groups that is to be tested is defined as the alternative hypothesis (H_1). The null (meaning no difference) hypothesis (H_0) states that there is no difference between the mean post-intervention systolic blood pressures of the control and intervention group.

The alternative hypothesis is tested by taking a sample of men with hypertension in a defined age group, then assigning them randomly to either the intervention or the control group. It should be ensured that the two samples are reasonably well-matched for age and pre-intervention systolic blood pressures.

Of course, because samples are taken, there is always a chance that an error might occur in inferences drawn. If the hypothesis is tested and it is concluded that there is no difference in the population mean systolic blood pressures for the intervention and the control groups and this is true of the population, then there is no error. However, an error occurs if it is concluded that the population mean systolic blood pressures of the intervention group is less than the mean population systolic blood pressure of the control group when there is, in fact, no difference between the means. This type of error—when the null hypothesis is rejected when it is true—is called a Type I error. If it is concluded that the mean population systolic blood pressure for the intervention group is less than the mean population systolic pressure of the control group and this is true, there is no error. An error occurs if it is concluded there is no difference between the population means when in fact the mean for the intervention is less than the mean for the control. This error is called a Type II error. Table 5.4 presents the possible outcomes.

Table 5.4   Outcomes of testing the null hypothesis

	Accept H_0	Reject H_0
The null hypothesis (H_0) is true	OK	Type I error
The null hypothesis (H_0) is false	Type II error	OK

Table 5.5   Post-intervention systolic blood pressures

Intervention systolic blood pressure	Control systolic blood pressure
143.00	169.00
144.00	170.00
145.00	172.00
150.00	176.00
153.00	177.00
154.00	177.00
155.00	177.00
155.00	177.00
156.00	181.00
159.00	182.00
159.00	182.00
160.00	182.00
162.00	183.00
165.00	183.00
165.00	183.00
165.00	184.00
166.00	185.00
166.00	186.00
166.00	188.00
167.00	188.00
167.00	188.00
167.00	188.00
167.00	189.00
168.00	191.00
168.00	191.00
170.00	191.00
170.00	191.00
171.00	192.00
172.00	195.00
173.00	201.00

The chance or probability of a Type I error is controlled for in hypothesis testing and is described as the level of significance or α. The level of significance is often set at 0.05 in health research. In other words, the chance of rejecting the null hypothesis when it is in fact true is 5%. The chance or probability of making a Type II error is called β. The power of a test is $1 - \beta$ and is used in estimating sample sizes. Power has no conventional level in health research but is usually set at 80% or more.

Continuing the example of the intervention program for men with hypertension, suppose a sample is collected of 60 men with hypertension aged 50 to 64 years. Thirty men are assigned to the intervention (exercise and aspirin) and 30 men to the control (aspirin only). Table 5.5 set out the post-intervention systolic blood pressures follows.

Following the intervention of half an aspirin and the prescribed exercise program for 6 weeks, the mean systolic blood pressure of the intervention group was

161.6 Hg/mm with a standard deviation of 8.5 Hg/mm. The mean and standard deviation for the control group who took only aspirin were 183.0 Hg/mm and 7.5 Hg/mm respectively. A t-test is used to test if there is a statistically significant difference in the mean systolic blood pressures. In this example, there is a difference at the 5% level of significance. The chance of rejecting the null hypothesis when it is in fact true is less than 0.001. This is known as the p-value. A smaller p-value indicates less chance of rejecting the null hypothesis when it is in fact true or, in other words, a greater significance, in statistical terms, of the difference. The convention in reporting results is to note, after stating whether a difference occurs, the calculated t-value, the degrees of freedom and the p-value: $(t = 10.84, df = 58, p < .001)$.

This intervention could have been tested another way. Only one group of men could take the aspirin for 6 weeks. At the end of the 6 weeks, their systolic blood pressures would be measured. For the following 6 weeks, the men take both the aspirin and undertake the prescribed exercise program. Their post-intervention systolic blood pressures are then taken. The men, therefore, form their own controls. The mean difference between pre- and post-intervention systolic blood pressures is tested using a pairwise t-test.

Often in health research, more than two groups are tested for differences in their means. Assume that in the study of hypertensive men, another 30 men were randomly assigned to a placebo aspirin. There are now 3 groups: the placebo group (Group 1), the aspirin only group (Group 2) and the aspirin and exercise group (Group 3).

The differences between the means could be tested using a t-test to test the difference in means between Group 1 and 2, then between Group 1 and 3 and, finally, between Group 2 and 3. Four groups would require 6 t-tests. There is, however, a statistical test which tests whether there is a difference between 3 or more means: the ANOVA (analysis of variance). The ANOVA uses a test of significance called the F-test. The F-statistic tests the alternative hypothesis that not all means are equal. If it is concluded that not all means are equal, a further test is required to determine which groups have significantly different means.

This section on comparing means has discussed only quantitative, not qualitative data. Similar comparisons between populations can be made with proportions. Returning to the population of men with hypertension as an example, a smoking cessation intervention is to be tested on the smokers in the study. The intervention was a nicotine patch. The control group received a placebo patch. Whether the men are smokers or not is a qualitative variable so the statistic in this study is the proportion of men who are non-smokers at the end of 6 months. The alternative hypothesis is that the proportion of non-smokers in the intervention is greater than the proportion of non-smokers in the control group. This can be tested using a t-test of significance.

The discussion of statistical inference has been limited to estimates of a single variable up to this point. The next section outlines some statistical techniques that are applied when examining the relationship between two variables.

Table 5.6 Ages and systolic blood pressures

Age in years (x)	Systolic blood pressure (y)
50	151
61	152
62	162
45	147
35	134
55	151
66	170
49	150
51	148
39	139

The relationship between two variables

The statistical procedure used in the analysis of relationships between two variables depends on whether the data are quantitative or qualitative. If the data are quantitative, a technique that may be used is simple linear regression. With qualitative data, the chi-square test of a contingency table is used.

Simple linear regression assumes the relationship between two variables follows a straight line. One variable is defined as y, the dependent variable, and is plotted on the vertical axis. The other variable is defined as x, the independent variable, and is plotted on the horizontal axis. As an example, take systolic blood pressure in a sample of 10 adult men as the dependent variable y and their age as the independent variable x. Table 5.6 lists the ages and systolic blood pressures.

A scatterplot can be used to examine the relationship between the variables. The scatterplot shows that as age increases the systolic blood pressure tends to increase (figure 5.10). This is described as a positive relationship. A

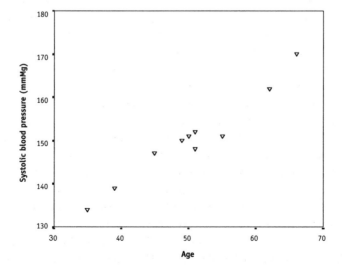

Figure 5.10 Scatterplot of age and systolic blood pressure

negative relationship is said to occur if increases in the independent variable result in a pattern of decreases in the dependent variable. Those readers who have studied any economics will recall the negative relationship between supply and demand curves.

Simple linear regression fits a line described as the 'line of best fit'. The line of best fit is the equation of a line on the scatterplot that minimises the square of the distance between each plotted point and the line. This is called the method of least squares. As this example uses a sample, there may be errors in the estimated equation of the line:

$$\hat{y} = ax + b$$

where $\hat{y}$ called y-hat, is the estimated dependent variable. For the age (x) and systolic blood pressure (y) example the equation is:

$$\hat{y} = 97.2 + 1.1x$$

This represents a positive relationship between age and systolic blood pressure. The strength of the relationship is measured by the correlation, which in this case is .90.

To demonstrate a negative correlation, a comparison between hours of exercise per week (the independent variable x) and systolic blood pressure (the dependent variable y) is made (table 5.7). The scatterplot of hours of exercise per week against systolic blood pressure shows a clear negative relationship between the two variables (figure 5.11). In this case the correlation is negative and equal to $-.97$.

In these two examples, there was a strong positive or negative correlation. In some cases, a scatterplot reveals very little correlation between the dependent and independent variable. As an example, take the years of formal school education as the independent variable and systolic blood pressure as the dependent variable. The data are presented in table 5.8 and figure 5.12. The pattern observed in the data is of no particular positive or negative trend, and in fact the correlation is a very small negative value of $-.35$.

In regression analysis it is not possible to say that the independent variable 'causes' the variation in the dependent variable. If regression analysis was used to determine the relationship between the systolic blood pressure of a man and the age of his partner, a strong positive correlation may be revealed. This does not mean that a younger partner 'causes' systolic blood pressure in the man to be lower. It is more likely to be that the age of their partner is a good predictor of the age of the man. This correlation is described as *spurious correlation*. An excellent predictor of the dependent variable systolic blood pressure is the independent variable diastolic blood pressure. However, this is not helpful in trying to determine risk factors for systolic blood pressure. This type of correlation is described as

Table 5.7   Hours of exercise and systolic blood pressure

Hours of exercise/week (x)	Systolic blood pressure (y)
0.0	180
1.0	168
2.5	155
0.0	190
3.0	145
7.0	110
10.0	100
4.0	135
5.5	130
2.0	161

autocorrelation. It is rare in health research that one independent variable, say age, will explain all of the variation in the dependent variable, say systolic blood pressure. A number of explanatory or independent variables may explain systolic blood pressure. When there is more than one independent variable, regression analysis is described as multivariate regression. A review of multivariate regression is beyond the scope of this book. If more detail on multiple regression is required, there are a number of appropriate references for health researchers including *Statistical Methods in Medical Research.*[8]

Another important application of regression analysis is *trend analysis.* In trend analysis the independent variable is time. Trend analysis has important applications in health services research. Figure 5.13 shows the estimated number of people aged 85 years or more in the Australian population in the census years from 1976 to 1996.[9] The positive trend of increasing numbers of people aged 85

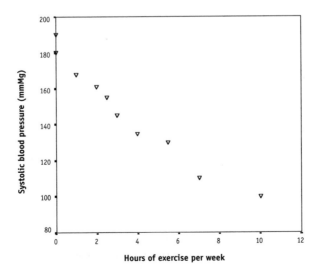

Figure 5.11   Scatterplot of hours of exercise and systolic blood pressure

Table 5.8 Years of education and systolic blood pressure

Years of formal school education (x)	Systolic blood pressure (y)
12	180
5	168
10	155
5	190
13	145
8	110
12	100
7	135
10	130
8	161

years or more with time is apparent. It is possible, therefore, to predict the number of people aged 85 years or more from the regression equation.

The discussion of regression has been limited to simple linear regression where there is a single independent variable and where both the dependent and independent variables are quantitative data. When trying to determine the relationship between two variables that are qualitative, one technique that can be used is the chi-square of contingency tables.

The two variables in this case are categorical and may be nominal, dichotomous or ordinal categories. A chi-square contingency table places each of the categories of one of the variables in the rows, and each of the categories of the other variable in the columns. Table 5.9 sets out an example. The men from a sample of 100 men aged 65 years or more were classified as a current smoker, past smoker or had never smoked. The other variable was whether or not cardiovascular disease was present.

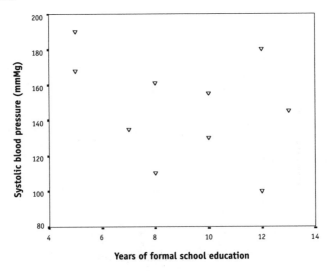

Figure 5.12 Scatterplot of years of education and systolic blood pressure

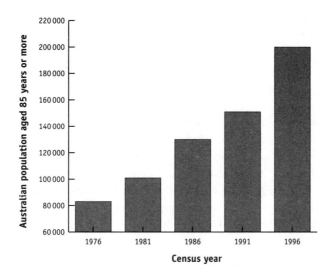

Figure 5.13 Australian population by selected census years

Of the 30 current smokers, 15 or 50% had cardiovascular disease. Of the 15 past smokers, one-third had cardiovascular disease. Less than 1 in 10 of the men who had never smoked had cardiovascular disease. If smoking status did not have a relationship with the presence of cardiovascular disease in men aged 65 years or more, it would be expected that approximately the same proportion of men would have cardiovascular disease in each smoking status category. The difference in what is observed in each of the cells and what would be expected in each cell

Table 5.9 Cross-tabulation of smoking status and CVD

	CVD present	CVD absent
Current smoker	15	15
Past smoker	5	10
Never smoked	5	50

Table 5.10 Range of statistical tests for univariate data

	Hypothesis about a single population	Hypothesis about 2 populations	Comparing more than 2 populations	Relationships between 2 variables
Quantitative	Test hypothesis about population mean	Test hypothesis about a difference in 2 population means	Analysis of variance	Simple linear regression
Qualitative	Test hypothesis about population proportion	(i) Test hypothesis about a difference in 2 proportions (ii) chi-square (χ^2) test of contingency table	chi-square (χ^2) test of contingency table	chi-square (χ^2) test of contingency table

Table 5.11   Range of statistical tests for multivariate data

Explanatory/independent	Quantitative	Dependent	
		Dichotomous	Qualitative with > 2 categories
Quantitative	Multiple regression	Discriminant analysis	Discriminant analysis
Qualitative	Analysis of variance	Logistic regression	Polytomous logistic regression

given no association between smoking status and presence or absence of cardio-vascular disease is squared and divided by the expected value. The aggregate of this score from each cell is used to determine the critical chi-square value. The larger the difference in the observed and expected values, the greater the chi-square value, indicating a more statistically significant result. The determination of the critical chi-square value and its interpretation is discussed in more detail in chapter 7, which deals with categorical data.

Summary of choices

This chapter has presented an overview of what statistics means in the context of health research. It has provided examples of appropriate use of existing databases to present descriptive statistics and has also provided an introduction to inferential statistics. The previous section describes statistical techniques to use when the relationship between two variables is examined. Table 5.10 (adapted from Keller and Warrack[10]) sets out the techniques to be applied to quantitative and qualitative data.

In most cases of health research, more than one explanatory or independent variable will be used to determine variability in a dependent variable. In these cases multivariate analyses techniques should be applied. A simple guide to the appropriate multivariate statistical technique to use for different types of dependent variables and different types of independent or explanatory variables is presented in table 5.11. Discussion of complex statistical manipulations is also included in chapter 8, 'So how is the treatment going?'.

6

How is our health?

ANDREW GRULICH

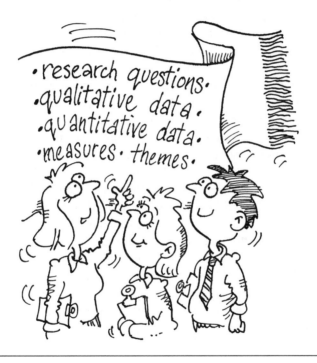

This chapter could also be called 'examining quantitative disease–exposure associations'. It provides an epidemiological perspective on assessing health. Epidemiology concentrates on the health of populations. Statistics which suit large numbers are relied on, and the primary focus is on observational measures which have been applied to large groups of people. The measures may be the same as those which you read about in chapters 4 and 5, and frequently two groups are compared on those measures. This chapter continues the theme of posing sensible and relevant questions, and using appropriate research methods in each health inquiry.

Formulating and answering quantitative questions

In this chapter we address a question that is frequently asked in health research: 'Is exposure x associated with disease y?'

An exposure, such as mobile phone use, or radiation dose, obesity, or smoking, is rarely associated with a disease outcome, such as brain cancer, leukaemia, stroke or emphysema, in every individual. If there were a one-to-one relationship of exposure to outcome, then the association would very quickly become obvious and there would be no need for research. Rather, we usually want to know: 'Does exposure x increase the probability of disease y?'

For example, there is considerable debate over whether hormone replacement therapy increases breast cancer risk. A recent review of all studies that have looked at this question found that the use of hormone replacement therapy might increase breast cancer risk by 2 or 3%.[1] This is a very small effect, but hormone replacement therapy is widely used, and breast cancer is a common disease, so it is still an effect that may be of some public health importance. Other risk–exposure relationships can be very strong indeed. For example, chronic infection with hepatitis B virus raises the risk of liver cancer by about 50 times (i.e., 5000%).[2] Even in this case, however, the majority of people with the exposure (chronic hepatitis B infection) do not develop the disease in question (liver cancer). Some examples of exposure–disease relationships are given in table 6.1.

When an exposure does not lead to disease in every individual, one must assess the strength of the relationship in probabilistic terms. In other words, the question becomes: 'By how much does exposure x increase the risk of disease y?'

To answer this question, one must have a background of unexposed individuals, meaning that the disease-exposure relationship must be studied in a population. In this chapter, we will look at examples of research questions that lend themselves to quantitative, population-based research, to demonstrate the process of hypothesis formulation and study design that comes out of the original curiosity to perform a research study.

An HIV and cancer inquiry

Human immunodeficiency virus (HIV) is the virus that causes acquired immune deficiency syndrome (AIDS). AIDS is characterised by immune deficiency and

Table 6.1   Examples of exposure–disease relationships in health research

Exposure	Disease	Magnitude of association
Hormone replacement therapy	Breast cancer	Increases risk by 2–3%
Smoking	Heart disease	Increases risk by 100–300%
	Lung cancer	Increases risk by 500–1000%
Hepatitis B infection	Liver cancer	Increases risk by 5000%

opportunistic infections which are related to a breakdown in normal immune defences. In the absence of treatment, AIDS usually results in death.

There has been a suggestion that different forms of cancer appear in groups of people with HIV and AIDS. This has roused the curiosity and concern of many health carers and researchers. It is a compelling research area for them to focus on. Their initial study question may be: 'Is HIV/AIDS associated with an increased risk of cancer?'

To begin the inquiry, an understanding of the conditions and their context is needed. This becomes the 'background' to the research question.

Background

The occurrence of clusters of one type of pigmented skin cancer, Kaposi's sarcoma (KS), among male homosexuals in New York and California was a harbinger of the AIDS epidemic.[3] This gave an indication that at least some types of cancer were associated with this new form of immune deficiency. Since then, it has been estimated that at least one in three people with AIDS will develop cancer during their illness. With tens of millions of people living with AIDS around the world, this is obviously a major public health problem, and the definition of what types of cancer occur in people with AIDS is important for their clinical care.

In addition, the occurrence of cancer in people with AIDS is of interest in teasing out the causes of cancer. Prior to AIDS, there had been suggestions that immune deficiency was associated with cancer. When organ transplantation was first made possible by the development of pharmacological means of immune suppression, it was quickly noticed that a couple of forms of cancer, mainly non-Hodgkin's lymphoma (NHL) and KS, occurred at greatly increased rates in these individuals. In addition, it was known that NHL occurred at greatly increased rates in children with certain congenital immune deficiencies.[4] Initially, this was taken as providing evidence that 'immune surveillance' protected against cancer. This hypothesis states that the immune system is responsible for the detection of early cancer and the elimination of the potential malignant clone through an immune response.[5] However, as data on transplant-associated malignancies grew, it became apparent that only a minority of cancer types, mainly those believed to have an infectious cause, were increased in people with immune deficiency. As people with AIDS also have immune deficiency, they are another population researchers may find useful to study in the search for causes of cancer.

Making the research question an answerable hypothesis

A research question will often start out as very general, such as 'Are people with AIDS at increased risk of cancer?' Before a study is designed, it is crucial that the initial question is broken down into a series of *answerable hypotheses*. This will direct the research effort at questions that one is able to answer. It may be that the research question will change a little during the study, as new results from other work comes to light, but it is crucial to have answerable hypotheses before the study design begins. A first step in this process is to define precisely the 'exposures' and 'outcomes' of interest.

Defining the exposure: AIDS, HIV or immune deficiency?
In epidemiological research, it is essential to define what the exposure is. In summary, HIV (the human immunodeficiency virus) is the virus that causes AIDS. AIDS (acquired immune deficiency syndrome) is a clinical syndrome that comprises HIV infection, plus one of a variety of opportunistic infections and cancers that are indicative of severe immune deficiency.[6]

Prior to the introduction of combination anti-retroviral therapies in the mid 1990s, AIDS developed on average ten years after HIV infection. For the first few years after HIV infection, immune deficiency is rather mild.

This information helps the epidemiologist to decide what group should be focused on. Taking the usual course of the condition into consideration, if one wishes to study the effects of severe immune deficiency, then it would be inappropriate to include people with early HIV infection as part of the exposed population. In such a situation, one would like to use a marker of severe immune deficiency. This might be diagnosis of AIDS, or a more precise marker of immune function in people with AIDS such as CD4 positive lymphocyte count. Alternatively, if the research question concerned a direct effect of HIV rather than immune deficiency, then the answerable question would not be dependent on immune deficiency. In this case, as previous evidence points to an important role of immune deficiency we will note AIDS as the exposure of interest.

Defining the outcome: how is cancer defined?
Epidemiologists must also define the outcome that they will focus on. Cancer is a leading cause of death in industrialised countries. Although commonly thought of as 'a disease', there are in fact many types of cancer with many different causes.[7]

These differences affect the way an epidemiologist defines the outcome variables. If a study is investigating a possible aetiological relationship between an exposure and an outcome, then it makes good sense to define diseases in *aetiologically homogeneous categories*. For example, it would not make sense to group together cancers of the lung and colon as outcomes, because we know that they have very different aetiologies. Lung cancer is predominantly related to smoking, and colon cancer is predominantly related to diet, at least in industrialised countries. It might make sense, however, to group cancers of the colon and rectum, as they are known to have similar aetiologies. The outcome groupings have to make good clinical sense.

Thus, in the current study it would make sense to separate cancer types individually, using a predetermined classification scheme. For many diseases, the best accepted classification scheme is the *International Classification of Disease*, published by the World Health Organization and reviewed approximately every twenty years.[8]

After considering this background information, an initial hypothesis, which can be phrased as an answerable question, is: 'People with AIDS are at increased risk of individual cancer types, as defined by the international classification of disease'.

This hypothesis is then pursued, beginning with a literature review. Notice that the literature review can be focused, given that the initial hypothesis has been properly defined.

The literature review

After the germ of an idea has been implanted for a research project, the first stop should be the library and the Internet. It is usually the case that you will not be the first person to think of this research question! You can further refine a research question, and thus your choice of research methodology, by first finding out what others have done in the area.

In this research area, a literature review in the early 1980s would tell us that Kaposi's sarcoma (KS) and non-Hodgkin's lymphoma (NHL) occurred at increased rates in transplant recipients receiving immune suppressive therapies. NHL, but not KS, occurred at increased rates in children with congenital immune deficiency. In addition, reviews of the first several case series of people with AIDS would tell us that there were many cases of KS,[9] which was previously an extremely rare cancer in Western countries.

What routinely collected data are available to look at this question?

Having formulated a research question, there may be routinely collected sources of data that are available that might allow your research question to be examined without conducting any specific data collection. Epidemiologists frequently use data that has already been collected. They conduct analyses of that information. That is just as valid as collecting the information and analysing it. Both forms of data collection have issues of validity and reliability which must be considered. You may like to review these concepts in chapter 4, 'Who needs to plan?'

In the case of HIV, AIDS and cancer, there are already large population data-bases of incidence, and of some other clinical and demographic measures for each person who has been diagnosed with the conditions. In some circumstances, a disease may be perceived as a public health or health services issue by the government, and is classified as a 'notifiable' condition under legislation.

HIV/AIDS registration

AIDS, like many infectious diseases, is a notifiable disease in many parts of the world. The notification of AIDS, and in fewer countries, of HIV infection, is used to help plan health services and prevention campaigns, and to assess the impact of HIV/AIDS on the population. In Australia, data are collated and published every year.[10]

Cancer registration

Throughout much of the world, the registration of new cases of cancer with a centralised registry is mandated by legislation.[11] In Australia, each state and territory has its own cancer registry, and forwards data to the National Cancer Statistics Clearing House. Data are collected on area of residence, age, sex, and country of birth of the person with cancer, as well as the location and cell type of cancer. This allows rates of cancer to be calculated for the population, and these rates can be standardised for age to allow the comparison of rates of cancer between populations with different age structures.

The availability of these data makes a significant difference to the type of study that an epidemiologist can conduct. Examples of specific study types are described below. However, it is sometimes possible to deduce some information about a disease–exposure relationship from routinely collected data. For example, HIV was initially an infection that affected mainly homosexual men, so data on cancer rates in unmarried men were used as a surrogate for data on cancer incidence in HIV-infected homosexual men.[12] This approach relied on the assumption that a large proportion of young never married men were HIV-infected homosexuals. This assumption was only reasonably accurate in the centres of the AIDS epidemic in the US. For example, in San Francisco it was estimated that about one-third of never married men aged 25 to 54 years were homosexual or bisexual, and that nearly half of these were HIV infected in 1984.[13] These studies found that incidence of NHL was up to 10 times higher in never married men compared to married men, and the incidence of KS was 1000 times higher in this group.

Ecological studies: comparing rates of exposures and diseases

In an *ecological study*, population levels of an exposure are compared to population rates of a disease. So, in this example, the rate of AIDS is the population level of an exposure, and this is compared to cancer rates, which is the population rate of a disease. Examining the rates of AIDS and of cancer over the years since the beginning of the AIDS epidemic might shed some light on possible relationships.

In figure 6.1, we see that the incidence of NHL was increasing rapidly in New South Wales over the period of the HIV epidemic.[14] However, rates of NHL were also increasing in women, in whom HIV is uncommon in Australia, so there must be other reasons for this increase, even if HIV is part of the reason.

Plotting the incidence and mortality in this way will lead to further questions. For instance, the researcher may wonder about geographic location and incidence.

If both AIDS and cancer are registered in the same geographic areas, time trends in the two can be compared by area. For example, in New South Wales, it is

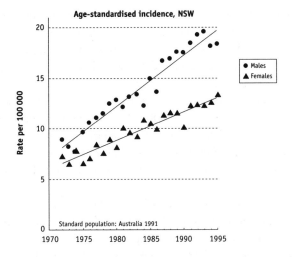

Figure 6.1 Incidence and mortality of non-Hodgkin's lymphoma, 1972–95
Source: M.S. Coates and B.K. Armstrong, *Cancer in New South Wales: Incidence and Mortality 1995*, Sydney, NSW Cancer Council Sydney, 1998.

known that rates of HIV and AIDS are much higher in eastern Sydney. In figure 6.2, one can see that rates of NHL increased markedly in men in eastern Sydney compared to men elsewhere in the state in the late 1980s, suggesting an association between HIV and NHL rates.

Ecological studies are comparatively weak studies to answer a hypothesis, as they report on associations of average measures of exposures and disease in populations, rather than connecting exposure and disease in individuals. For example, there was no way of knowing in the eastern Sydney data whether it was the men with HIV who were developing NHL, or whether it was another exposure.

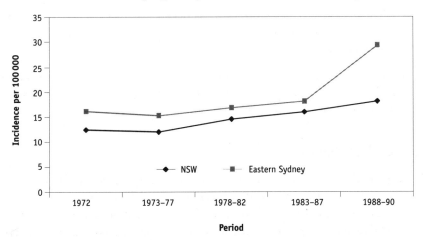

Figure 6.2 Age-standardised incidence per 100 000 of non-Hodgkin's lymphoma in males in eastern Sydney, and in New South Wales, 1972–90
Source: M. McCredie, M. Coates, S. Chu, and R. Taylor, *Trends in Cancer Incidence by Region, New South Wales 1972–1990*, Sydney, New South Wales Cancer Council, 1992.

It is unusual that an ecological study can answer a hypothesis, but in this case, because the relationships were so strong, even a comparatively weak study design such as an ecological study was successful in confirming the hypothesis. Indeed, KS was part of the original case definition of AIDS, and NHL was added a few years later.

Although an association was confirmed, it was well known that not everyone with HIV infection developed KS or HIV. In the registration of AIDS, data are collected on the risk behaviour that has led to HIV infection, and on whether or not people develop KS or NHL at AIDS diagnosis. This was an obvious source of data to look at associations between individual risk behaviours and risk of KS and NHL.

A review of these data for people with AIDS registered in the US found that 15% of people with AIDS developed KS as their first AIDS defining illness, but that this ranged from 1% in haemophiliacs to 21% in homosexual or bisexual men. The prevalence of KS at AIDS was much lower in women, but was four times more common among women reported to have sex with bisexual men than in women whose partners were injecting drug users.[15]

These data were interpreted as suggesting that KS might be due to a sexually transmitted infection. In contrast, data on people with AIDS with NHL revealed little difference in risk among risk groups.[16] The relative constancy of risk across transmission groups for NHL suggested that it was unlikely to be related to a sexually transmitted or blood borne agent.

Thus, without collecting any original data, researchers were able to confirm an association between KS and NHL and AIDS, and suggest that KS may be related to a sexually transmissible agent. These details led to two new answerable hypotheses:

- Is AIDS associated with an increased risk of cancers other than NHL and KS?
- Is a sexually transmissible agent associated with an increased risk of KS in people with AIDS?

To answer these questions, it will now be necessary to collect new data in analytic epidemiologic studies. The methods for these epidemiological studies are described in the following sections.

Case-control studies

As introduced in chapter 4, 'Who needs to plan?', case-control studies compare the past exposures of a person with a disease (a case) with a person who does not have the disease in question (a control). Ideally, a case-control study includes all of, or a random sample of, people with disease in a population, and a random sample of those without the disease.

Case-control studies are popular studies because they are relatively inexpensive and quick to perform compared with other epidemiological study designs. However, despite these attractions, case-control studies are probably the most complex epidemiological study design, and are prone to a variety of biases.

First, it can be difficult to exclude the fact that a disease may have led to an exposure, rather than the other way around. For example, diet may be altered by early disease symptoms, so asking a person about their current diet may not reflect the diet that a person with a disease has been consuming for years prior. While this may be somewhat ameliorated by asking about the relevant period, deficiencies in recall frequently make this a difficult process.

Second, the presence of disease may make a person more likely to recall past exposures. This is called 'recall bias'. The issue of recall was featured in chapter 4. It is a concern in all research in which data are collected, and is not particular to epidemiological research methods.

Third, it is frequently difficult to organise randomly sampled cases and controls. This can lead to unpredictable biases. For example, hospital-based patients are frequently used as sources of cases and controls, and yet it is known that they do not represent the general population. People in hospital are much more likely to drink alcohol to excess, to smoke cigarettes, and to report a variety of activities that are detrimental to health than the general population. Using such a population in a case-control study may lead to serious biases. For example, researchers may wish to examine alcohol consumption as a risk factor for patients hospitalised with a newly described liver disease, and may use emergency department attendees as controls. Such controls would be a biased sample of the general population, because many are likely to be presenting to emergency because of alcohol-related accidents and illnesses. This would lead to a masking of any true association between alcohol and the liver disease in question.

There are different ways of testing hypotheses that cancers other than KS and NHL are associated with AIDS. The case-control study has not been popular in industrialised countries in studying associations between specific cancers and HIV/AIDS. In those countries, higher quality, and more costly, cohort studies have been possible. However, in Africa, where the infrastructure to perform cohort studies is frequently not available, case-control studies of associations between HIV and cancer have been performed.

These studies have generally compared the HIV prevalence among patients with a specific cancer (cases) to the HIV prevalence in patients with all other cancers apart from KS and NHL (the controls). This study design relies on an assumption that people with all other cancers will have a HIV prevalence that is similar to that of the general population. Such studies have identified one more cancer that is strongly associated with HIV, that is, cancer of the conjunctiva of the eye.[17] This relationship has since been confirmed in cohort studies in the US.[18]

The case-control design has been much more extensively used in looking for sexual risk factors for KS in people with AIDS. In these studies, people who develop KS are compared with people who develop manifestations of AIDS other than KS. These people are questioned about their past sexual behaviour and their history of sexually transmitted diseases. These studies have found that people with KS report a history of more sexual partners, and of more sexually transmissible infections, than controls. This has been interpreted as supporting the hypothesis that KS might be due to a sexually transmitted agent.[19]

Indeed, this work stimulated basic scientists to search for such a pathogen, and in 1995 a previously undescribed herpesvirus, now termed human herpesvirus 8, was discovered in KS tissue.[20] Since then, epidemiologists have confirmed that this is the cause of KS.[21] Epidemiologists have also confirmed that the agent is indeed sexually transmitted.[22]

To summarise, epidemiologists can use case-control methods to test ideas of associations, or to confirm associations.

Cohort studies

In a cohort study, a group of people with an exposure are followed through time and compared with a group of people who do not have that exposure. People with the disease of interest at baseline are excluded. The rate of disease development in those who are exposed is compared to those who are not exposed.

Methodologically, cohort studies are a strong research design, as the exclusion of people with disease at baseline makes it likely that the exposure has preceded the disease and not vice versa. The downside of such a design is that studies using it tend to be very expensive, and take a long time to answer a research question.

Further, a disease must be relatively common to be studied using the cohort design. It is impractical to study causes of rare diseases using a cohort design as an enormous population would have to be followed, for a very long time, to give the study enough statistical power to address the study hypothesis.

Like case-control studies, cohort studies are subject to some biases. The most important is loss to follow up. If there is a substantial degree of loss to follow up, then it is difficult to interpret the results of a cohort study. This is because the disease–exposure relationship may be different in those lost to follow up than in the population who have remained under follow up.

Many cohort studies have been performed of cancer in people with HIV infection. However, because of the relative rarity of cancers other than NHL and KS, these cancers have had limited statistical power to detect HIV–cancer relationships. You will remember how important power is from chapter 4 'Who needs to plan?', and you may wish to reread the section in chapter 4 on power and error to understand the significance of numbers of people being studied to the statistical significance of results that can be obtained.

A variety of cancers have been suggested to occur in people with AIDS at increased rates in cohort studies, but there has been little consistency among the studies, and a clear picture of what cancers occur at increased rates has not emerged from these studies.[23]

However, because both AIDS and cancer are registered in some jurisdictions, it is possible to perform a variant of a cohort study called a *linkage study*. In this type of study, data from more than one database are linked. In this case, people who appear on the AIDS register are linked to data from a cancer register, and this allows the calculation of cancer rates in people diagnosed with AIDS. Such a study follows, albeit passively, all individuals who are registered with AIDS. The rate of cancer in the general population forms the comparison rate. It assumes that all individuals remain under observation for the period of the study, so it is only useful with relatively stable populations, in which there is little emigration outside the study area. Three such studies have been performed, and have consistently found that higher rates of one cancer type, Hodgkin's disease, are found in people with AIDS.[24]

Intervention studies

The ultimate proof that an exposure is causally related to disease is that removal of exposure will decrease the risk of disease. This may be studied in cohort studies, where removal of exposure should be followed by a decrease in disease risk. However, alternative explanations are usually possible because the exposure of interest is not the only exposure that changes. More rigorously, the hypotheses can be tested by randomly allocating individuals to an intervention that removes the exposure. You will remember from chapter 4 that this is termed a randomised controlled trial.

As the process of removing exposure is random, other differences between the groups will tend to balance out, and the only difference between the populations will be the intervention. Randomised controlled trials are the highest quality epidemiological study design, but are frequently not possible for practical or ethical reasons.

Clearly, it would be unethical to randomly allocate people to receive HIV infection! Nevertheless, sometimes a 'natural experiment' may occur. In the case of HIV, as one instance, there has been the introduction, since the mid 1990s, of combination anti-retroviral therapies. These therapies have been effective in partially restoring the immune system in most people with HIV infection, and thus they have led to at least a partial removal of the immune deficiency that is believed to lead to cancer.

Data collected since the introduction of these therapies suggest that this has been associated with major reductions in the incidence of AIDS-associated KS and more modest reductions in the incidence of AIDS-associated NHL.[25]

To address the hypothesis that human herpesvirus 8 is truly the cause of KS, a randomised controlled trial would have to randomise removal of the virus from infected people to see if this decreased the risk of KS. Such a trial was recently performed, although the trial was not designed to look at prevention of KS. The study was a randomised controlled trial of the anti-herpes drug ganciclovir in people with AIDS, which was designed to look at the prevention of a disease caused by another member of the herpesvirus family, cytomegalovirus. This drug also has activity against human herpesvirus 8, and the study demonstrated that ganciclovir reduced the incidence of KS by more than 70%.[26] This final piece of evidence suggests that human herpesvirus 8 truly is the cause of KS.

In this chapter, I have used the example of AIDS-associated cancer studies to demonstrate the process of analytical epidemiological research, and the variety of study designs that are possible. The choice of study design depends not only on what study is most appropriate for the disease–exposure relationship in question, but also on what studies have been performed previously. If a well-designed randomised controlled trial addressing your research question has already been performed, then it is likely that a case-control study of the same question will add little information. If there is no previous research in this area, then any reasoned inquiry process will add something to the area. Like other inquiry pursuits and methods demonstrated in this text, a reflective process of working with the context of clinical data as well as the numbers is crucial.

7
Meaningful categories

MARY PHIPPS AND DUSAN HADZI-PAVLOVIC

This chapter explores number comparisons that are based on categorical and ordinal measures. These are both non-parametric approaches to using number comparisons. Examples which use small numbers of people are highlighted here, as ordinal statistics are frequently used with very small group sizes. As in the other statistics chapters, when statistical tools are mentioned, their interpretation is covered as well as their use.

Two authors have contributed the different sections: 'Categorical data analysis' is by Mary Phipps, a statistician, and 'Analysis of ordinal data' is by Dusan Hadzi-Pavlovic, a research psychologist. They offer practical tips, and give examples from their own experience of working with health data. More formulae are included in this chapter, to give you a sense of the number manipulations which occur when you run certain statistical tests, often 'unseen' when computer programs perform the tests for you. You will notice that the formulae or the interpretation of the result can be quite different, depending on the assumptions that you make about the data. This reinforces how important it is to choose your statistical manipulations carefully, depending on the type of data which you draw on.

You may care to revise the concept of frequencies in chapter 5, 'Numbers and more', by Deborah Black before you read this chapter. Knowing what categories can be applied to individuals, and what group those individuals belong to, is essential before applying categorical data analysis.

Categorical data analysis
MARY PHIPPS

In many medical applications, we encounter situations in which n individuals have been classified into k mutually exclusive categories. Counting the individuals in each category produces a set of frequencies, called *categorical data*.

The appropriate statistical analysis of categorical data depends on the way in which the data are obtained. The data may arise from cross-classifying a single random sample of n individuals by two different criteria (blood group and eye colour perhaps). Alternatively, two independent random samples (for example a control group and an independent treatment group) may both be classified into a set of distinct categories. Although a chi-square (χ^2) test is used to analyse the data in each case, the questions answered by the tests differ. Accordingly, the presentation of the statistical analysis of categorical data will be introduced with the discussion of an illustrative example in each of the following sampling situations:

- one random sample classified by one criterion
  - goodness of fit of fully specified model
  - goodness of fit of incompletely specified model
- one random sample cross-classified
  - independence test
- observational studies, prospective and retrospective
  - odds ratio and relative risk
- independent random samples
  - test of homogeneity of proportions
- matched pairs

Variations or generalisations of these situations may be found in advanced textbooks on the analysis of categorical data, but will not be discussed here. For further reading see Agresti,[1] and Andersen.[2] To begin with, some examples of categorical data are provided to help illustrate different sampling situations. Understanding the type of data you have is essential in deciding on your statistical tests, and then, in the interpretation of the results of those tests.

Categorical data examples

Example 7.1 A single sample, split into two categories of a single criterion

From a sample of 54 at risk patients who have undergone tests for testicular cancer, results show that 32 are 'cases' and the remainder are 'non-cases'.

Example 7.1 is the simplest type of categorical data, resulting when a single random sample (here of size $n = 54$) is obtained and is split into k mutually exclusive categories (here there are two categories, 'case' and 'non-case', so $k = 2$). The categorical data are the two frequencies 32 and 22. Observing these frequencies may prompt you to ask whether these frequencies would normally be found in an 'at risk' population for which the ratio of 'cases' to 'non-cases' is, say, 2:1. This question will be answered using χ^2 methods later in this chapter.

Example 7.2 A single sample, cross-classified by two criteria

The records for 70 kidney patients at a hospital include information on the observed level of Henoch's HSP condition ('severe', 'mild', 'HSP –ve'). The observed frequencies are displayed in table 7.1.

Table 7.1   Kidney patients cross-classified by sex and level of HSP

HSP level	Severe	Mild	HSP -ve
Sex			
Male	12	20	10
Female	10	15	3

In example 7.2, a single random sample of $n = 70$ has been cross-classified by two criteria, sex and level of HSP, into $k = 6$ categories, and the categorical data are displayed in a 2×3 table known as a 2×3 *contingency table*. The following question may be asked: is there strong evidence from the data of independence of sex and HSP level in the population of kidney patients sampled? This question will also be answered later in this chapter using χ^2 methods.

When there are two criteria of classification as in example 7.2, but one of these has r and the other has c mutually exclusive categories (or levels), the n individuals in the random sample can be cross-classified into $k(= r \times c)$ categories. The frequencies become the entries in the resulting $r \times c$ contingency table, and the table is used to test for independence of the row and column criteria in the population which was sampled. At the next level of generalisation, a single sample may be cross-classified by more than two criteria, with interest in the independence of criteria in pairs, triples, and so on.

It is important to be aware that the type of contingency table shown in table 7.1, in which a single sample is cross-classified by two criteria, is often confused with categorical data obtained from two independent samples for which the *same* criterion is of interest for each sample. Consider example 7.3.

Example 7.3 Two independent samples, each classified by a single criterion

In a variation of example 7.2, suppose a random sample of 42 male kidney patients and an *independent* random sample of 28 female kidney patients are diagnosed as severe, mild or non- HSP, and suppose that the results are as in table 7.1.

Two populations (male kidney patients and female kidney patients) have been independently sampled here. It is not appropriate now to test for independence of sex and HSP level in the combined population of kidney patients, since it is not this population which has been sampled. Instead, we might ask whether the two populations (male and female kidney patients) have the same breakdown by HSP levels.

Examples 7.2 and 7.3 illustrate the importance of understanding the nature of the data. If we are presented with data in the form of table 7.1, we need to establish whether the data arose from a *single* cross-classified sample or from *two* independent samples. Once this is done, we can ask the appropriate question and carry out the correct analysis.

Example 7.4 Matched pairs, classified by a single criterion

A study by Canaris and Jurd on alcohol-related brain damage (ARBD) contains information on 32 patients who were classified by the admitting doctor either as ARBD (+) or as non-ARBD (−).[3] Later, they were reclassified by a neuropsychological assessment (NP test) on discharge from hospital. Tables 7.2a, 7.2b and 7.2c present the data in different ways.

The paired structure of the data is evident in table 7.2a, but if the data are condensed, as in table 7.2b, we might be tempted to analyse the results as if they resulted from two independent samples. This would be incorrect because the researchers did not use two independent samples of 32. Instead, they

Table 7.2a ARBD (+/–) as diagnosed by doctor (MD) and by NP test (NP)

Patient	MD	NP	Patient	MD	NP	Patient	MD	NP	Patient	MD	NP
1	+	–	9	–	+	17	–	+	25	+	+
2	–	–	10	–	–	18	–	+	26	–	–
3	–	+	11	+	+	19	–	–	27	+	+
4	–	+	12	+	+	20	–	+	28	–	–
5	+	+	13	–	–	21	–	+	29	–	–
6	–	–	14	+	–	22	+	+	30	–	+
7	–	–	15	–	–	23	–	+	31	–	+
8	–	+	16	–	–	24	–	–	32	–	–

Table 7.2b Diagnosis vs method of diagnosis

Diagnosis by	ARBD	Non-ARBD	Total
Doctor	8	24	32
NP test	17	15	32

Table 7.2c Doctor's diagnosis vs NP test diagnosis

Diagnosis by doctor Diagnosis by NP test	ARBD	Non-ARBD	Total
ARBD	6	11	17
Non-ARBD	2	13	15
Total	8	24	32

recorded results for 32 patients, each of whom was diagnosed twice. Clearly the samples are not independent. Each patient has been self-matched.

In contrast, if the data appear as in table 7.2c, there might be a temptation to analyse the data for independence of row and column classifications. Again, this would be the wrong analysis as the sample was not cross-classified by two different criteria, but rather was measured by two different methods for the presence or absence of a single criterion, alcohol-related brain damage (ARBD). The appropriate question is whether or not there is a real difference in diagnosis by the doctor and by the NP test. The analysis uses the correlation structure in the matched pairs, focusing on the 'discordant pairs', which in this case are the 13 (= 11 + 2) patients for whom the diagnoses differ. This example illustrates the importance of establishing the nature of the categorical data before setting up and testing a hypothesis about the population (or populations) sampled. A test of independence of rows and columns would be meaningless here.

One random sample—classified by one criterion

You will remember that example 7.1 was based on a single random sample split into two categories, 'case' and 'non-case'. Suppose we decide to question the suggested hypothesis of a 2:1 ratio of cases to non-cases in the 'at risk' population sampled.

This is an example of a fully specified model in which we expect on average two-thirds of a random sample to be 'cases' and the remaining third to be 'non-cases'. We write this hypothesis as:

$$H_0 = P(\text{case}) = \frac{2}{3}$$

The probability model is:

Case	Non-case
$\frac{2}{3}$	$\frac{1}{3}$

For a sample of size $n = 54$, this means that the expected number of 'cases' is 36 (i.e. $\frac{2}{3} \times 54 = 36$) when H_0 is true. The question asked might then be whether the observed frequency of 32 is consistent with this hypothesis. The appropriate analysis is a *goodness of fit* test with a fully specified model and with $k = 2$ categories. The following description of this test will use example 7.1 as an illustration.

Goodness of fit test—fully specified model

Notation: The notation we shall use for the expected frequency in category i is E_i, with O_i for the corresponding observed frequency. For the data of example 7.1, we first compare these values visually.

i:	Cases	Non-cases	Total
O_i	32	22	54
E_i	36	18	54

Test statistic: The test statistic we use is X^2, with the formula:

$$X^2 = \sum_{i=1}^{k} \frac{(O_i - E_i)^2}{E_i}$$

and for this example the calculated value of X^2 is:

$$X^2 = \frac{(32-36)^2}{36} + \frac{(22-18)^2}{18} = 0.444 + 0.889 = 1.333$$

Notice that X^2 would have been zero if the observed frequencies had been exactly equal to the expected frequencies (i.e. if $O_i = E_i$ for each i). Conversely, X^2 would have been larger than 1.333 if there had been a greater discrepancy between the observed and expected frequencies. In fact, the larger the value of X^2, the stronger the evidence from the sample against the hypothesised ratio of 2:1.

Use of χ^2 tables: How do we decide when X^2 is large enough to indicate that the hypothesised ratio is dubious for the population sampled? We use the fact that, even when the model is correct, different samples will yield different calculated values of X^2, some more likely than others. For a fully specified model with k categories, these values of X^2 are known to follow an approximate χ^2_v probability distribution when H_0 is true, with $v = k-1$. The upper tail of this probability distribution is tabulated in the Appendix; table 7.3 presents an extract.[4]

Table 7.3 Extract from the χ^2 table

p	0.99	0.95	0.90	0.10	0.05	0.025	0.01
v							
1	0.000	0.004	0.016	2.706	3.841	5.024	6.635
2	0.020	0.103	0.211	4.605	5.991	7.378	9.210
3	0.115	0.352	0.584	6.251	7.815	9.348	11.345
4	0.297	0.711	1.064	7.779	9.488	11.143	13.277

The entries are the values x such that $P(\chi^2_v \geq x) = p$. For example, to find the value of $P(\chi^2_4 \geq 8.1)$, we enter the table in row $v = 4$, and locate values near 8.1. From the table we can see that $0.05 < P(\chi^2_4 \geq 8.1) < 0.10$.

Example 7.1 continued (A goodness of fit test with fully specified model)

Since $k = 2$ use $v = k - 1 = 1$. Assuming H_0 is true, we now use the fact that X^2 has the χ^2_1 distribution. To calculate how unusual it would be to obtain a value of χ^2_1 as large or larger than 1.333 (the calculated X^2), we enter the table in the row labelled $v = 1$ and notice that $P(\chi^2_1 \geq 2.706) = 0.10$. Therefore, $P(\chi^2_1 \geq 1.333) > 0.10$. What does this probability tell us? We assumed that H_0 was true in the sampled population so more than 10% of samples arising from such a population would result in frequencies just as extreme as those we actually observed. As this is not very unusual, our data can be considered quite consistent with the hypothesis H_0: $P(\text{case}) = \frac{2}{3}$

---

p-value

The tail probability from the χ^2_v table, $P(\chi^2_v \geq X^2)$, is called the *p-value* of the test. From the tables, the p-value exceeds 0.10 in example 7.1. If a statistical computer package is used, the exact value (here, 0.25) would be given. It is up to you to base your findings on this p-value, so the interpretation of the p-value is crucial.

Clearly, the smaller the p-value, the stronger the evidence against H_0. The p-value is a measurement between 0 and 1 and it measures how unusual it would be to obtain data at least as extreme as yours if H_0 were indeed true, i.e.,

the smaller the p-value, the stronger the evidence against H_0.

As a general rule, a p-value of 0.05 or lower is usually taken as strong evidence against H_0, but of course does not prove H_0 to be false. A p-value greater than 0.05 means that the data are quite consistent with H_0 in the sense that 5% or more of samples in the long run would produce such extreme frequencies when H_0 is actually true.

Example 7.1 continued
In this example we found a p-value exceeding 0.1. This is not small enough to constitute evidence against the model that the ratio of cases to non-cases is 2:1.

Warning Any category with $E_i < 5$ should be combined with an adjacent category before using the χ^2 test. The reduced number of categories is then treated as k. Also, for small samples ($n < 20$), the χ^2 test is not appropriate.

The procedure which you should follow in applying a 'goodness of fit' test is summarised here. As you can see, the process is a reasoned series of steps, with close attention being given to the type of sampling method used.

Procedure for a 'goodness of fit' test—Fully specified model
Step 1: State your hypothesis H_0 about the probability model for the categories.

Step 2: Calculate all E_i under H_0 and set the E_i out against the O_i. If necessary, combine categories so that $E_i \geq 5$. The final number of categories is written as k.

Step 3: Calculate $X^2 = \sum_{i=1}^{k} \frac{(O_i - E_i)^2}{E_i}$

Step 4: Use χ^2_v tables with $v = k - 1$ to find the *p-value* $= P(\chi^2_v \geq X^2)$.
Step 5: Interpret the p-value and state your findings.

The following is a worked example of a goodness of fit test for a fully specified model, step by step.

Assume that in a genetics experiment involving two factors A and B, 114 progeny were classified into four categories:

$$
\begin{array}{ccccc}
\text{AB} & \text{Ab} & \text{aB} & \text{ab} & \text{Total} \\
75 & 15 & 14 & 10 & 114
\end{array}
$$

Imagine that you were to examine the hypothesis that the categories are in the ratio 9:3:3:1 in the population which produced the categorical data. The steps you would need to follow are those outlined in the boxed procedure which you have already read. Note that steps 2, 3, and 4 could be calculated by a computer program for you, but steps 1 and 5 need your active instruction and interpretation.

As an exercise, you could try to do this example yourself, before looking at the working provided.

Step 1: H_0: Probability distribution of the categories is:

$$
\begin{array}{cccc}
\text{AB} & \text{Ab} & \text{aB} & \text{ab} \\
\frac{9}{16} & \frac{3}{16} & \frac{3}{16} & \frac{1}{16}
\end{array}
$$

Step 2: Since $\frac{1}{16} \times 114 = 7.125$, the observed and expected frequencies are

$$
\begin{array}{ccccc}
 & \text{AB} & \text{Ab} & \text{aB} & \text{ab} \\
O_i: & 75 & 15 & 14 & 10 \\
E_i: & 64.125 & 21.375 & 21.375 & 7.125
\end{array}
$$

Step 3:
$$
X^2 = \sum_{i=1}^{4} \frac{(O_i - E_i)^2}{E_i}
$$
$$
= \frac{(75-64.125)^2}{64.125} + \frac{(15-21.375)^2}{21.375} + \frac{(14-21.375)^2}{21.375} + \frac{(10-7.125)^2}{7.125} = 7.45
$$

Step 4: Since $k = 4$ categories, we use $v = 4 - 1 = 3$, and find the p-value from the χ^2_3 table. The p-value $= P(\chi^2_3 \geq 7.45)$. Entering the table in row $v = 3$, we see that the p-value is between 0.05 and 0.10.

Step 5: The p-value is not very small. We conclude that the data are consistent with the theory that the categories are in the ratio 9:3:3:1 for the population sampled.

If a computer package is used, steps 2 to 4 are performed for you, and a p-value is provided. The interpretation depends on the nature of the data. Here, the data is from a single sample with a specified model. Steps 1 and 5 are not done for you on the computer.

Goodness of fit test—Incompletely specified model

Sometimes we may wish to test the form of the model, but we need to use the data to estimate b unknown and unrelated parameters before the model can be completely specified. In this case, we say our model is incompletely specified. *Maximum likelihood methods* are used to estimate the parameters first. This is beyond the scope of this book but for illustration, a worked example is given, in which the appropriate estimate is suggested. The steps for the test are the same as for the fully specified model, but now we use $k - b - 1$ for v instead of $k - 1$.

Procedure for 'goodness of fit' test—Incompletely specified model

Step 1: State your hypothesis H_0 about the probability model for the categories, estimating the b unknown parameters from the data.

Step 2: Calculate all E_i under H_0. If necessary, combine categories so that $E_i \geq 5$. The final number of categories is written as k.

Step 3: Calculate $X^2 = \sum_{i=1}^{k} \frac{(O_i - E_i)^2}{E_i}$

Step 4: Use χ^2_v tables with $v = k - b - 1$ to find the *p-value* $= P(\chi^2_v \geq X^2)$.

Step 5: Interpret the p-value and state your findings.

These steps are applied in the following example of a goodness of fit test for an incompletely specified model. Plato et al. reported the following data on haptoglobin type (Hp1-1, Hp1-2, Hp2-2) in a random sample of 190 villagers in Cyprus.[5]

Table 7.4 Haptoglobin genotype

Hp1-1	Hp1-2	Hp2-2	Total
10	68	112	190

Quite often, assertions are tested using available data. For instance, you may assume for this example that the Hardy-Weinberg Law states that if gene frequencies are in equilibrium, these genotypes occur in the long run in the ratio $(1 - \theta)^2 : 2\theta(1 - \theta) : \theta^2$. Then, you could feel that you wanted to test the adequacy of this model for the population of Cyprus villagers. You could do that, as described step by step below.

We first need an appropriate estimate of θ, the unknown parameter required to specify the model fully. Intuitively it seems that

$$\frac{112}{190} + \frac{68}{2 \times 190} = 0.768421$$

would make a reasonable estimate, and this is the maximum likelihood estimate.

Step 1: H_0 : Model is $(1 - \theta)^2 : 2\theta(1 - \theta) : \theta^2$ with θ unspecified.

Step 2: Using 0.768421 to estimate θ, substitute in the model to give:
$$0.05363 : 0.35590 : 0.59047$$

Multiplying by 190 gives the expected frequencies, and the $O_i(E_i)$ are:

$$10\ (10.19)\quad 68\ (67.62)\quad 112\ (112.19)$$

Step 3: $X^2 = \frac{(10-10.19)^2}{10.19} + \frac{(68-67.62)^2}{67.62} + \frac{(112-112.19)^2}{112.19}$

$$= 0.004 + 0.002 + 0.000 = 0.006$$

Step 4: Since $k = 3$ and $b = 1$, we have $v = k - b - 1$, and the p-value is $P(\chi^2_1 \geq 0.006)$. Thus, from the table, the p-value is between 0.90 and 0.95.

Step 5: The p-value is so large that we conclude the model is a very good fit. One common error is to conclude that 'there is a 90 to 95% chance that H_0 is true'. This is not the correct interpretation of a p-value. Instead, a p-value in the range 0.90 to 0.95 means that the frequencies we observed were typical under the assumption that gene frequencies are in equilibrium (H_0).

One random sample—cross-classifed by two criteria

When a random sample is drawn and then cross-classified into r levels of one criterion and c levels of another, the data can be summarised as a contingency table with $k = r \times c$ mutually exclusive categories. We may wish to test for independence of the two criteria. This is illustrated using categorical data example 7.2.

Example 7.2 (continued)

Recall that a sample of 70 patients was cross-classified by sex and HSP level. There were 6 categories in the 2×3 contingency table (table 7.5). The data are reproduced here for convenience.

The row and column totals are not fixed in advance, but are the result of classifying the sample of 70 once it has been selected. This is a common feature of categorical data used to test for independence of row and column classifications. That is, a single sample is cross-classified.

Table 7.5 Contingency table

HSP level	Severe	Mild	Non-HSP	Total
Sex				
Male	12	20	10	42
Female	10	15	3	28
Total	22	35	13	70

Test of independence

If sex and HSP level were truly independent, we would expect the frequency of the 'male, severe' category for samples of 70 to be

$$70 \times \frac{22}{70} \times \frac{42}{70} = \frac{22 \times 42}{70} = 13.20$$

More generally, if R_i is the total for row i and C_j is the total for column j, the expected frequency E_{ij}, corresponding to the observed frequency O_{ij} in the row i and column j position is:

$$E_{ij} = \frac{R_i \times C_j}{n}$$

Thus in example 7.2, $E_{11} = \frac{42 \times 22}{70} = 13.20$, $E_{12} = \frac{42 \times 35}{70} = 21.00$, and so on. Continuing in this way, we can complete a table of expected frequencies. They are displayed below in brackets beside the corresponding observed frequencies for this example as $O_{ij}(E_{ij})$:

$$12(13.2) \quad 20(21.0) \quad 10(7.8)$$
$$10(8.8) \quad 15(14.0) \quad 3(5.2)$$

Recall that the expected frequencies have been calculated under the model of independence. This model is not fully specified. It requires $\frac{42}{70}$ as an estimate of the proportion of male kidney patients in the population sampled. The proportion of female kidney patients does not need to be estimated independently, since it is obviously $1 - \frac{42}{70}$. Similarly, $\frac{22}{70}$ and $\frac{35}{70}$ are estimates of the proportion of severe and mild HSP cases respectively. The proportion of 'HSP $-$ve' is then obviously estimated by $1 - (\frac{22}{70} + \frac{35}{70})$. Thus the number of parameters estimated *independently* for the model is $b = 3$ and since $k = 6$ we can therefore use the X^2 test statistic and the χ^2_ν table with $\nu = k - b - 1 = 6 - 3 - 1 = 2$. This example is continued after a few notes of general importance.

Tips:

- An easier way to find ν (when χ^2_ν is appropriate) is to calculate $\nu = (r-1)(c-1)$. In this example, $(r-1)(c-1) = (2-1)(3-1) = 2$ and so $\nu = 2$.
- *Computer packages* If a statistical computer package is used to perform the χ^2 test, you should choose the Pearson chi-square option. You may also be given the option of a Yates's corrected p-value. We do not recommend this more conservative approach.
- *Small expected frequencies* The χ^2 test for independence is not appropriate unless all cells have $E_{ij} > 1$ and no more than 20% of them have $E_{ij} < 5$. This is Cochran's rule.[6]
- *Small sample procedure* For the case of a 2 × 2 contingency table with small sample size, the χ^2 approximation is not appropriate, and a different approach is needed. Rosner for example gives details of the numerical calculations needed for small 2 × 2 tables.[7] Refer to Rosner if you are using a hand calculator, otherwise a statistical computer package is suggested. If your package gives

a choice of Fisher's Exact Test and the mid-p, we recommend the mid-p be used, as it has been well documented that Fisher's Exact Test is overly conservative, giving larger p-values than warranted by the data.

Procedure for test of independence of two criteria

Step 1: State your hypothesis H_0 of independence of row and column criteria.

Step 2: Calculate all $E_{ij} = \dfrac{R_i \times C_j}{n}$ under H_0. Check that all $E_{ij} > 1$ and that no more than 20% of the $E_{ij} < 5$.

Step 3: Calculate $X^2 = \sum \dfrac{(O_{ij} - E_{ij})^2}{E_{ij}}$

Step 4: Use χ^2_v tables with $v = (r - 1)(c - 1)$ to find the *p-value* = $P(\chi^2_v \geq X^2)$.

Step 5: Interpret the p-value and state your findings.

Example 7.2 continued (Test for independence)

Step 1: H_0: Sex and HSP level are independent.

Step 2: The E_{ij} have already been calculated and Cochran's rule is satisfied.

Step 3: $X^2 = \sum \dfrac{(O_{ij} - E_{ij})^2}{E_{ij}}$

$$= \frac{(12-13.2)^2}{13.2} + \frac{(20-21)^2}{21} + \frac{(10-7.8)^2}{7.8} + \frac{(10-8.8)^2}{8.8} + \frac{(15-14)^2}{14} + \frac{(3-5.2)^2}{5.2}$$

$$= 0.109 + 0.048 + 0.621 + 0.164 + 0.071 + 0.931 = 1.944$$

Step 4: Since $r = 2$ and $c = 3$, we have $v = (r-1)(c-1) = (2-1)(3-1) = 2$ and we find the p-value from the χ^2_2 table to be $P(\chi^2_2 \geq 1.944) > 0.10$.

Step 5: Since the p-value is large, it appears that the data are consistent with the hypothesis of independence, and we conclude that the severity of HSP is not related to the sex of the kidney patients in the population sampled.

Another worked example follows, illustrating a test for independence of factors. In a large study into the prevalence of byssinosis among workers exposed to cotton dust, Higgins and Koch classified 5419 workers in the cotton textile industry by several factors.[8] A cross-classification by length of employment and byssinosis reduces to table 7.6, a 2 × 2 contingency table. The question is prompted: Are these factors independent? The steps outlined above can be followed.

Table 7.6 Incidence of bysinossis and employment (in years)

Employment	less than 10	at least 10	Total
Byssinosis			
Yes	63	102	165
No	2666	2588	5254
Total	2729	2680	5419

- **Step 1**: H_0: Incidence of byssinosis is independent of the length of employment in the cotton textile industry (i.e. length of exposure to cotton dust).
- **Steps 2, 3 and 4,** if done using computer software or calculated by hand, result in a p-value of $P(\chi_1^2 \geq 9.87) < 0.01$.
- **Step 5:** The p-value is very small, indicating very strong evidence of a relationship between length of employment and incidence of byssinosis among workers in the cotton textile industry.

Observational studies

The last worked example is an illustration of an observational study. Here, the criteria of classification can be considered as risk factor (cotton dust exposure +/–) and response (byssinosis +/–), with the risk/response status being *observed* for each subject.

Other types of observational studies are *prospective* or *retrospective* studies. In a prospective study, the risk status (+/–) of subjects is identified and independent samples from each of these groups are followed forward in time with the purpose of examining the effect of the risk factor on the response. If however, a positive response is quite rare, it may well happen that the study might result in all negative responses. In such cases it is usual to identify subjects instead by response status (+/–) and to follow independent samples from each group back in time (retrospective study) classifying the subjects by initial risk status. This ensures that rare responses are represented in the categorical data.

A chi-square test of independence of risk and response was discussed for cross-classified data as in the byssinosis example; before discussing the appropriate chi-square analysis for independent samples (such as those arising from a prospective or retrospective study) we will look at two measures of the association between the risk and the response, the *relative risk* and the *odds ratio*. Suppose the risk factors (+ /–) are given in the rows of a 2 × 2 table (see table 7.7) and the responses or disease status (+/–) are given in the columns.

Table 7.7 Typical risk factor and disease status table

		Disease status		
		+	–	Total
Risk factor	+	a	b	a+b
	–	c	d	c+d
	Total	a+c	b+d	a+b+c+d

Odds ratio and relative risk

The *relative risk* is the ratio of the chance of contracting the disease among those with the risk factor to the corresponding chance among those without the risk factor. It can be estimated directly from a *prospective study*.

Calculation of relative risk from a prospective study

An estimate of the chance of disease among those with the risk factor is based on the observed number $(a + b)$ with the risk factor and so is $\dfrac{a}{a+b}$. The corresponding chance among the observed number $(c + d)$ without the risk factor is $\dfrac{c}{c+d}$. The ratio of these is

$$\frac{a}{a+b} \div \frac{c}{c+d} = \frac{a(c+d)}{c(a+b)}.$$

We write this as our estimate $(\hat{R}R)$ of the relative risk:

$$\hat{R}R = \frac{a(c+d)}{c(a+b)}$$

To interpret this, a relative risk of 3 indicates that an individual with the risk factor is estimated to be 3 times more likely to contract the disease than an individual without the risk factor. An alternative measure of association is the *odds ratio*.

Calculation of odds ratio from a prospective study

We can estimate from a typical table the odds of having the disease to not having the disease among individuals with the risk factor as $\dfrac{a}{b}$. The corresponding odds among individuals without the risk factor is $\dfrac{c}{d}$. The ratio of these odds is

$$\frac{a}{b} \div \frac{c}{d} = \frac{ad}{cb}$$

We write this as our estimate $(\hat{O}R)$ of the odds ratio:

$$\hat{O}R = \frac{ad}{cb}$$

Tip: Notice that for rare diseases, when both a and c are small relative to b and d respectively, $c + d \cong d$ and $a + b \cong b$, so that $\dfrac{a(c+d)}{c(a+b)} \cong \dfrac{ad}{cb}$. Hence the relative risk and the odds ratio are approximately equal *in the case of rare diseases*.

Calculation of odds ratio from a retrospective study

In a retrospective study, we should condition on the disease status rather than on the risk factor. This means that we can estimate from a typical table the odds of having had the risk factor to not having had it among individuals with the disease as $\frac{a}{c}$. The corresponding odds among individuals without the disease is $\frac{b}{d}$. The ratio of these odds is

$$\frac{a}{c} \div \frac{b}{d} = \frac{ad}{cb}$$

which is identical to the calculation of $\hat{OR}$ from a prospective study. This equivalence means that, even in a retrospective study, we can use the odds ratio as an approximation to the relative risk *in the case of rare diseases*.

The byssinosis example can be reworked as an example of the estimate of odds ratio and approximate relative risk. The data from that example in table 7.6 is rearranged in table 7.8 to correspond with the typical table. The risk factor ('+' = at least ten years exposure) appears in the first row and the response or disease status ('+' = byssinosis present) appears in the first column. It is then easy to identify a, b, c and d.

Table 7.8   Byssinosis: Disease status and risk factor

		Disease status	
		+	−
Risk factor	+	102	2588
	−	63	2666

The disease byssinosis is rare (notice that 102 is small compared with 2588, and 63 is small compared with 2666). Thus we can use the odds ratio to estimate the relative risk by calculating

$$\hat{OR} = \frac{102 \times 2666}{2588 \times 63} = 1.67.$$

This indicates that the risk of byssinosis is almost twice as great for workers exposed to cotton dust for a long time as it is for those exposed for a shorter period of time.

Independent random samples

An illustrative example is presented as a worked explanation of testing for homogeneity of proportions from independent random samples. In the mid 1970s, Byar et al. conducted a clinical trial on patients with superficial bladder tumours.[9]

Patients were randomly assigned to one of three treatments, 48 to a placebo, 32 to pyridoxene and 38 to thiotepa. The numbers of patients who remained tumour free (–) for each treatment throughout the trial (see table 7.9) are summarised in Andrews and Herzberg.[10]

Table 7.9 Tumour status: Absent (–) or present (+) after treatment

Tumour status	–	+	Total
Treatment			
Placebo	19	29	48
Pyrixdoxene	17	15	32
Thiotepa	20	18	38
Total	56	62	118

The question is prompted: Is there a common success rate (proportion of negative results) for the three treatments? The appropriate test is known as a test for homogeneity of proportions over the three treatments.

Test for homogeneity of proportions

The common success rate under this hypothesis is estimated by the observed success rate, $\frac{56}{118} = 0.475$ (the overall proportion who are tumour free) and the expected frequency E_{11} is therefore $E_{11} = \frac{56}{118} \times 48 = 22.781$. Notice that E_{11} can also be expressed as $E_{ij} = \frac{R_1 \times C_1}{n}$, and that the other expected frequencies are obtained similarly. The general result for E_{ij} is:

$$E_{ij} = \frac{R_i \times C_j}{n}$$

Thus, the same method for calculating E_{ij} is used (although the reasoning differs) for both this situation (independent samples) and the situation of the previous section (single sample cross-classified). Apart from the statement of the hypothesis and the conclusion, the arithmetic for the two tests is identical.

Procedure for test of homogeneity

Step 1: State your hypothesis H_0 of homogeneity of proportions over the populations.

Step 2: Calculate all $E_{ij} = \frac{R_i \times C_j}{n}$ under H_0. Check that all $E_{ij} > 1$ and that no more than 20% of the $E_{ij} < 5$.

Step 3: Calculate $X^2 = \sum \dfrac{(O_{ij} - E_{ij})^2}{E_{ij}}$.

Step 4: Use χ^2_ν tables with $\nu = (r-1)(c-1)$ to find the *p-value* $= P(\chi^2_\nu \geq X^2)$.

Step 5: Interpret the p-value and state your findings.

These steps, when applied to the bladder tumour example, form a test of homogeneity, as follows.

Step 1: H_0: The three treatments have a common success probability in the populations sampled.

Step 2: Assuming H_0, $E_{ij} = \dfrac{R_i \times C_j}{n}$. The O_{ij} (E_{ij}) are written:

$$19\,(22.78) \quad 29\,(25.22)$$
$$17\,(15.19) \quad 15\,(16.81)$$
$$20\,(18.03) \quad 18\,(19.97)$$

Step 3:

$$X^2 = \frac{(19-22.78)^2}{22.78} + \frac{(29-25.22)^2}{25.22} + \frac{(17-15.19)^2}{15.19} + \frac{(15-16.81)^2}{16.81} + \frac{(20-18.03)^2}{18.03} + \frac{(18-19.97)^2}{19.97}$$
$$= 0.627 + 0.567 + 0.216 + 0.195 + 0.215 + 0.194 = 2.014$$

Step 4: Since $r = 3$ and $c = 2$, we have $\nu = (r-1)(c-1) = 2 \times 1 = 2$, and we find the p-value from the χ^2_2 table to be $P(\chi^2_2 \geq 2.014) > 0.10$.

Step 5: Since the p-value is large, the data are consistent with the hypothesis of a common success probability for the three treatments in the population sampled.

A further worked example of a test for homogeneity follows. A study was undertaken in Tasmania on the possible difference between the sexes in complying with the national target for sodium intake for the year 2000.[11] Independent samples of 87 men and 107 women (systematically sampled from the Australian Commonwealth Electoral Roll) were surveyed and the results are in table 7.10.

Table 7.10　Compliance with Australian sodium intake for year 2000

Compliance Sex	Yes	No	Total
Male	5	82	87
Female	39	68	107
Total	44	150	194

Step 1: H_0: The proportions complying with the target are the same for men and women in the Australian Commonwealth Electoral Roll.

Step 2, 3, and 4 *as calculated by a statistics computer program, result in*: a p-value of $P(\chi^2_1 \geq 25.79) < 0.01$.

Step 5: The p-value is small and so we conclude there is very strong evidence of a difference in compliance for men and women.

Tips:

- *Small samples* Rosner gives details of the numerical calculations needed for 2×2 small tables.[12] Refer to Rosner if you are using a hand calculator, otherwise a statistical computer package is suggested. If your package gives a choice of Fisher's Exact Test and the mid-p, we recommend the mid-p be used, as it has been well documented that Fisher's Exact Test is overly conservative, giving larger p-values than warranted by the data.
- *Observational studies* Often several independent samples are followed over time (prospective studies) or back through time (retrospective studies). They can be analysed by the method of this section.

Matched pairs

The use of the same individual 'before' and 'after' a treatment may help to control for extraneous sources of variability when interest is in the possible effect of the treatment. Similarly, carefully matched pairs of individuals may be classified by a single criterion as in the next example of matched pairs analysis.

In a study to investigate the possibility that tonsils may be a type of protective barrier against Hodgkin's disease, Johnson and Johnson selected 85 Hodgkin's patients who had a sibling (within 5 years) of the same sex who was free of Hodgkin's disease.[13] Each member of the pair was classified according to whether or not a tonsillectomy had been performed earlier in life (see table 7.11).

Table 7.11 Tonsil status of 85 paired patients

Sibling Hodgkin's patient	No tonsillectomy	Tonsillectomy	Total
No tonsillectomy	37	7	44
Tonsillectomy	15	26	41
Total	52	33	85

The key interest is in the observed proportion of tonsillectomies in the Hodgkin's group $(\frac{41}{85} = 0.482)$ compared with the proportion in the non-Hodgkin's (sibling) group $(\frac{33}{85} = 0.388)$. A test of homogeneity for independent samples is inappropriate since we do not have two independent samples. Instead, we have a sample of matched pairs. The matching indicates the presence of a correlation structure in the data. If the structure is ignored and independence wrongly assumed, the analysis is meaningless. There are 63 *concordant pairs*: 37 pairs in which both members of the pair have not had a tonsillectomy and 26 pairs in which both have a history of tonsillectomy. The *discordant pairs* are the remaining 22 (= 7 + 15) pairs.

McNemar's test for equal proportions (of which 0.482 and 0.388 are our observed proportions) is a χ^2_1 test based on the discordant pairs.[14]

In general, for a paired table with $b + c$ discordant pairs,

$$
\begin{array}{ccc}
 & + & - \\
+ & a & b \\
- & c & d \\
\end{array}
$$

the test statistic is:

$$X^2 = \frac{(b-c)^2}{(b+c)}$$

which has an approximate χ^2_1 probability distribution, with p-value = $P(\chi^2_1 \geq X^2)$ under the hypothesis of equal proportions. For the above example,

$$X^2 = \frac{(7-15)^2}{(7+15)} = 2.91$$

and the p-value is approximately $P(\chi^2_1 \geq 2.91)$. From the tables, 0.05 < p-value < 0.10. (A computer package gives the exact value as 0.09.) So, there is some evidence, but it is not convincing evidence, that the proportions of tonsillectomies differ for individuals matched in this way. We conclude that the sample is consistent with no protection barrier due to tonsils.

It is useful to note here that some authors and computer packages use a 'correction for continuity', which has the effect of making the test overly conservative, giving larger p-values than warranted by the data.

To further illustrate the use of McNemar's test, we can return to the categorical data example 7.4, which you will remember was on alcohol-related brain

Table 7.12 ARBD (+/–) as diagnosed by doctor (MD) and by test (NP)

Patient	MD	NP	Patient	MD	NP	Patient	MD	NP	Patient	MD	NP
1	+	–	9	–	+	17	–	+	25	+	+
2	–	–	10	–	–	18	–	+	26	–	–
3	–	+	11	+	+	19	–	–	27	+	+
4	–	+	12	+	+	20	–	+	28	–	–
5	+	+	13	–	–	21	–	+	29	–	–
6	–	–	14	+	–	22	+	+	30	–	+
7	–	–	15	–	–	23	–	+	31	–	+
8	–	+	16	–	–	24	–	–	32	–	–

damage. For convenience, we reproduce in Table 7.12 the matched data of Canaris and Jurd on the diagnosis of ARBD (alcohol-related brain damage) in the same patient, by the admitting doctor (MD) and by a neuropsychological assessment (NP) on discharge (see table 7.12).[15]

Table 7.13   MD and NP diagnosis

	+	–
+	6	11
–	2	13

Each patient has been self-matched and the diagnosis of ARBD (+/–) is summarised in table 7.13 with MD diagnosis in columns vs. NP diagnosis in rows.

Recognising the paired nature of the data, we perform McNemar's test for H_0: Equal proportions of positive diagnoses by both methods in the population sampled.

From the data,

$$X^2 = \frac{(11-2)^2}{(11+2)} = 6.23$$

The p-value is approximately $P(\chi^2_1 \geq 6.23)$ and from the tables, we find that $0.01 <$ p-value < 0.025. The p-value is very small indicating strong evidence that the diagnoses by the two methods differ more than would be expected by chance alone if the two methods give the same diagnosis in the long run.

Tip: The χ^2 test is an approximation only to the exact (conditional) binomial test and the approximation is quite rough if the number of discordant pairs is small ($<$ 20) as in this example. Rosner gives details of the numerical calculations needed for the binomial test with small 2×2 tables.[16] Refer to that text if you are using a hand calculator, otherwise a statistical computer package is suggested, selecting the McNemar option if it is available. Note, however, that this test is conservative, particularly for small samples, because it is a conditional test.

In conclusion, we stress again the importance of identifying the nature of the categorical data. A 2×2 table of data for example might have arisen: from a cross-classification of a single sample by two criteria with two categories each, or; from two independent samples, each condensed into two categories of a single criterion, or; from matched pairs. The hypothesis (i.e., the question asked) and hence the conclusion drawn, depends on the sampling method. Just because the data are in the 2×2 form does not mean that a test of independence is appropriate. We also stress the importance of understanding the meaning of a p-value: the smaller it is, the stronger the evidence against the H_0.

Analysis of ordinal data
DUSAN HADZI-PAVLOVIC

Just as in the previous section, this section emphasises the nature of the data before choice of statistical test. The relationship between categories is a key focus.

Ordinal data examples

In some research settings, when we measure or assess people on a certain property, we feel able to say that one person has more of the property than some other person (or less of it, or the same amount of it), but we feel unable to say how much more (or less) of it the person has. The data arising from such measurements are usually referred to as *ordinal* data. The word 'ordinal' is used because the most we can do is order or rank people. Some ordinal data look very much like the categorical data discussed earlier in this chapter, and they can be analysed using those methods. It is possible, however, to also analyse them in a way that uses the fact that the categories (or levels) of the variables are ordinal. Other ordinal data look like the continuous data discussed in Deborah Black's chapter 5 'Numbers and more', but the methods for continuous data are typically thought to be inappropriate for ordinal data.

Ordinal data can come about in a number of ways, but it is simplest to say that they come about either because we deliberately set out to collect ordinal data, or because some other type of data has had to be transformed into ordinal data. Consider examples 7.5–7.8.

Examples 7.5–7.8 differ not only in how the data were generated, but in the information that they provide. Examples 7.5 and 7.6 tell us about the breadth of severity, but remove a lot of the differences between people. There will be patients, assigned to the same category, whom we know are not the same in their illness, perhaps even non-trivially so. They are in the same category either because our measuring device (ruler, mind, etc.) cannot distinguish between them, or because we do not want to distinguish between. The next examples (7.7 and 7.8)

Example 7.5

Physicians assess a group of patients and assign each to one of the following categories of illness severity: **1**: *mild*, **2**: *moderate*, **3**: *severe*, **4**: *very severe*. The data are ordinal because (i) for any two individuals we can determine whether the illness of one is more severe, less severe, or as severe as the illness of the other; and (ii) the distance between the categories would usually be regarded as unequal.

Example 7.6

These data could have arisen in another way. Originally the physicians had worked with a 10-point scale and each patient was given a score from 1 to 10. It was decided that the scale was difficult to use consistently and that the values should be grouped into four categories (**1**: 1–2, **2**: 3–5, **3**: 6–8, **4**: 9–10). While the data look similar, they have been produced not by an explicit assignment, but by a transformation.

Example 7.7

A physician is provided with case notes and asked to rank the patients on severity. The patient with the most severe illness is assigned a '1', the next most severe a '2' and so on. If two or more patients cannot be distinguished, they are given the same rank. Again, the data are ordinal; patients are ordered and we know that patients with different ranks differ, but nothing about the degree of inter-rank differences. It is important to note that while patients have been assigned numbers (ranks) we do not attach any meaning to the numbers beyond the order they provide.

Example 7.8

These data too could have arisen differently. A test was used (perhaps a laboratory test, or a task for patients to perform) which purports to measure the severity of the illness, with scores on this test taking on values in the range 0–100: 23.0, 40.5, 88.1 and so on. The intention had been to analyse the data using a statistical test which assumed a normal distribution for the dependent variable, but the data were found to be so far from this requirement that it was decided to analyse them after turning the scores into ranks, the patient(s) with the lowest score receiving a rank of 1 and so on. Instead of being produced by an explicit ranking, the ranks have resulted from the transformation of interval data.

show data which tell us nothing about how ill the patients are, only about their relative standing, though in doing so they might introduce differences that are unimportant since there will be patients who are a number of ranks apart, but whom we know are only trivially different.

Imagine now that the patients described in examples 7.5–7.8 were actually from two arms of a clinical trial comparing standard treatment against a novel treatment, and the physicians, blind to the treatment received, had provided the ratings as part of the end-of-treatment evaluation. If the data from example 7.5 showed a similar proportion of patients from both groups in each of the categories, we would conclude that the two treatments were equally effective (or ineffective). Yet if the categories were broad, and within categories subjects from one group were generally ranked lower than those from the other, then one could feel that some evidence for a difference between treatments was being missed. If the data from example 7.7 showed a marked difference between the two groups (patients receiving one treatment tended to be ranked much higher that those receiving the other treatment), it would nevertheless be possible for all the patients to still be in the *very severe* category, thus suggesting little, if any, actual improvement.

Sources of ordinal data

Data that could be considered as ordinal arise in various situations. Some common situations in which ordinal data arises follow. In various areas of general social research, the following situations are common:

- *Examination results* These are often reported as *fail, pass, credit, distinction* and *high distinction.*While someone with a *pass* is regarded as having performed less well than someone with a *credit* and so on, the difference between a *pass* and a *credit* is not held to be the same as that between a *distinction* and a *high distinction.* When these grades are based on 'continuous' marks (say out of 100), they represent an instance when we have thrown information away, choosing, for example, to ignore the difference between 75 (just a *credit*) and 84 (nearly a *distinction*). Sometimes this is true, but the convenience of five categories is preferred. The risk is that sometimes it represents a belief that the difference between 75 and 84 provides no useful information.
- *Social class* Assignment into social classes (e.g., *low, middle* and *upper*) is a classic example of measurement regarded as ordinal, though one for which, on closer examination, the basis of the ordering is perhaps not as clear as is thought.
- *Level of achievement* Those responsible for an education program might be interested to know the level of knowledge achieved by the participants. They might be rated as to whether they have *minimal knowledge, good knowledge, but minimal practical skills* or *good knowledge and practical skills.* These ratings are frequently used in health education programs.

In health research, the following examples are common:

- *Stage of disease* A patient's condition might be classified as being in the *prodromal, acute,* or *chronic* stage of a disease.

- *Presence of disease* Pathologists grade tumours according to various schemes, neurologists rate brain scans for the degree of atrophy and so on. One's data might consist of biopsies rated as *benign, possible disease, probable disease*, and *definite disease*.

- *Illness severity* Following a treatment patients are classified as much worse, worse, unchanged, better and much better. In such research, even if the categories are defined, it is rarely the case that the categories are taken to mean that a patient is 'better' than someone in the category just below by as much as they are 'worse' than the person in the category just above.

- *Rating scale of frequency of symptom occurrence* A sample of people are asked to rate the frequency of each of a set of symptoms using the following scale: *some of the time or never, a good part of the time* and *most of the time*. The original Likert scale is another example.

- *Continuous-like ordinal measures* Finally, note that the ordering or ranking usually follows implicitly from assigning people to categories or assigning a rank to a score. It is rare for data to represent an ordering created by explicitly comparing individuals since such a task is time consuming. The physician who ranked patients in example 7.7 would not have found it easy to do so for 100 patients. There are methods, however, that involve explicit comparisons. For instance, paired-comparisons can be used in situations when the relative taste or smell of objects like foodstuffs is of interest. You can easily decide whether one taste is preferable to another, and then move on to see if is still preferable to the next paired comparison. The listing of all comparison decisions then yields the ranking of all items.

Assessing ordinal data

In S.S. Stevens's system of scale types, ordinal data is one step up from nominal data (where we cannot order people), but one step below interval data where both people are ordered and the distances between categories are known. Among statisticians there is still considerable discussion about the utility and validity of his system, but even if the implications for statistical inference are not as major as is sometimes said, it does serve to focus our attention on the meaning of our numbers.

Within the health sciences there is often a *laissez-faire* attitude to whether data are interval or ordinal. Ordinal data are analysed as if they were interval, and interval data are sometimes transformed in a manner that destroys the interval properties, for instance via a logarithmic transformation to normalise them. Ordinality is foremost a property of the data, and the data are the result of our measurements, be they rulers, laboratory tests or clinical judgments. Just because a set of categories looks ordinal it does not mean that the people providing the data have an ordinal model in their mind when they use those categories. If we are serious about using ordinal data as such, then the opportunity to examine whether data really are ordinal should be followed up when it arises.

The analysis of rating scale data using *item response models* such as *Rasch scaling* provides an interesting example. Imagine that subjects rate a number of items on a four-point scale of symptom frequency 1–4, where the symptoms are associated with a particular disorder. If the categories are ordinal then we would expect the probability of someone answering '1' to be maximal for individuals with the lowest severity; as severity increases the probability of '1' decreases and that of '2' increases until '2' becomes the most likely response; similarly from '2' through to '3' and '3' to '4'. Some item response software can estimate for each item how the probability of a particular response varies as a function of severity. After fitting such a model we sometimes find that the expected progression is violated: category '3' becomes most likely after '1' and not after '2' for example. Sometimes, this is related to poorly worded items. But sometimes it can be alerting us to the fact that our 'frequency of symptoms' measure is not related to the underlying disorder as we had thought—some symptoms become more likely early on in the disorder, but then become less likely. This lack of ordinality makes it less reasonable, for example, to simply add up items to obtain a severity score since a '3' is sometimes less severe than a '2'.

Analysis of ordered categorical data

The analysis of ordinal data is presented by way of a series of examples. As with categorical analysis, the nature and source of the data is a prime focus before statistics are applied.

The data in table 7.14 were collected in the middle of the nineteenth century on 9039 patients who had amputations performed.[17] They represent a cross-classification of outcome (lived, died) by location of amputation. Since location is defined primarily by the number of beds, it largely makes sense to treat location as ordinal, even though the first category is somewhat inconsistent with that and the last category is likely be an amalgamation of widely different-sized hospitals. Note also that the distances between the categories are not constant. With only two levels of outcome the nominal–ordinal distinction does not need to be made since it does not affect the analysis.

One way of analysing these data would be to carry out a chi-square test for independence (or no association). You will recall that chi-square was covered in considerable detail earlier in this chapter. Such a test would be significant ($\chi^2 = 331.0$ df 5, $p < 0.001$), and would allow us to conclude that the probability of dying varies according to location. Of itself, however, it would not allow us to infer what looks fairly obvious from the table, namely, that there is a steady increase in the death rate as hospital size increases. Such a pattern of increase (or decrease) is often referred to as a *linear trend*. There is a specific statistical test for

Table 7.14 Amputation location and outcome

| Location | Outcome of amputation | | Total | Odds of death | Adjacent odds ratios |
	Lived	Died			
At home	2098	228	2326	0.109	
	90.2%	9.8%	100.0%		
< 26 beds	143	20	163	0.140	1.28
	87.7%	12.3%	100.0%		
26–100 beds	761	134	895	0.176	1.26
	85.0%	15.0%	100.0%		
101–200 beds	1370	310	1680	0.226	1.28
	81.5%	18.5%	100.0%		
201–300 beds	803	228	1031	0.284	1.26
	77.9%	22.1%	100.0%		
> 300 beds	2089	855	2944	0.409	1.44
	71.0%	29.0%	100.0%		
Total	7264	1775	9039	0.244	
	80.4%	19.6%	100.0%		

linear trend called the Cochran-Armitage test. Carrying out this test produces a statistic: $T = -17.89$ (with $p < 0.001$) which allows us to infer that there is a linear trend, though not necessarily only a linear trend.

An alternative to this analysis can be built around one of the basic elements of a contingency table, namely odds and odds ratios. This approach arises from a more advanced method of analysis of contingency tables, log-linear models, which involves natural logarithms of cell frequencies and odds. The linear trend in the percentages of deaths can be seen in the 'odds of death' column, which makes sense since the odds are just a re-expression of the percentages. For any pair of adjacent rows we can calculate an odds ratio for the implied 2×2 table, so that, for example, the odds ratio for the table with 'At home' and '< 26 beds' as its rows equals $0.140/0.109 = 1.28$, and we can calculate another four such odds ratios (see column 'Adjacent odds ratios'). Another feature suggested by the table is that steadily increasing odds of death are paralleled by constant odds ratios, and it turns out that a convenient way of expressing linear trend in a table is as linear trend in the log of the odds. If the logs of the odds (here logs of the odds of death) lie on a straight line, then odds ratios are all equal. The odds themselves or the percentages will tend to be linear but will also have a curvilinear trend. If the odds ratios are all equal to 1 this is equivalent to the hypothesis of no association (5 odds ratios and 5 df is no coincidence). Applying the relevant calculations to table 7.1 we find that the hypothesis of constant odds ratio has $(\chi^2 = 1.91$, df 4 ($p = 0.75$). The non-significant chi-square is what we want to find since it tells us that the model fits the data well. The estimate of the constant odds ratio is 1.30 (95% confidence interval = 1.27–1.35) and it implies, for example, that if the odds for 'At home' are 0.109 then those for '> 300 beds' should be $0.109 \times 1.30 \times 1.30 \times 1.30 \times 1.30 \times 1.30 = 0.405$, which is quite close to the observed value. By utilising the ordinal nature of location, which is ignored by the usual chi-square test, the analysis has provided us with a much more useful inference about the relationship between location and outcome, and in doing so has only used up one more degree of freedom.

The data in table 7.15 were reported by James Cowles Prichard in his *A Treatise on Insanity and Other Disorders Affecting the Mind*,[18] and describe outcome in admissions to an asylum called The Retreat, near York, England, for the years 1812–33. The rows represent patient type defined by the duration of the illness prior to admission, while the columns show outcome. The statistical question to be examined in the analysis of the data is whether there is a relationship between duration of illness at the time of admission and outcome. Whether any conclusions should be limited to The Retreat, or applied more generally, is less a statistical question and more one of drawing conclusions given the principles of (psychiatric) epidemiology and nosology.

These principles would help us to define the data set to be analysed. The use of the data under 'died', as Prichard's source of the data noted, is questionable. We know that some deaths arise from phenomena due to the disorder (for instance, suicide, psychotic exhaustion, or self-neglect) and so could be taken to reflect upon the treatment, whereas some arise from the causes of a disorder (for instance, cerebrovascular disease producing a dementia) and reflect less on treatment of the disorder per se. Since we are contemplating analysing these data as ordinal, we need to examine the data closely and ask: 'Are these rows (columns) ordinal?' Duration is obviously a mixture of severity, intractability, and the social factors influencing admission. We could also ask whether someone who is

Table 7.15   Outcome of admissions to The Retreat

| Illness | Died | Remain | Condition when removed | | Recovered | Total |
			Unimproved	Improved		
< 3 mths	8	1	1	2	51	63
	12.7%	1.6%	1.6%	3.2%	81.0%	
3–12 mths	10	18	6	3	28	65
	15.4%	27.7%	9.2%	4.6%	43.1%	
> 12 mths	15	34	17	4	31	101
	14.9%	33.7%	16.8%	4.0%	30.7%	
Readmission	17	16	13	1	58	105
	16.2%	15.2%	12.4%	1.0%	55.2%	
Total	50	69	37	10	168	334
	15.0%	20.7%	11.1%	3.0%	50.3%	

removed by friends in an 'unimproved' condition is really better than one who remains, or just someone who has friends to remove them? How should we regard readmission: as indication of a disorder of long-standing, or one of short-standing where past experience has prompted a quick admission? The small frequencies in a few of the cells raise the issue of collapsing some of the columns. For the purpose of analysis we will leave 'died' as the worst outcome, collapse columns 2–3 into an 'unimproved' outcome and columns 4–5 into an 'improved' outcome and we will move the 'readmission' row to lie immediately after '< 3 mths'. This is somewhat post hoc for the purpose of the chapter, but a proper ordering is not always obvious, and judgment, uninfluenced by the data themselves, will be needed, including the decision to not presume that the data are ordinal.

The figures show the percentage who are dying as being fairly constant while the proportion who are improving decreases with illness duration, except for 'readmission'.

The process of thinking about a table in terms of odds ratios, and of the 2×2 tables within that table, can be used here as well. There are $(4 - 1 = 3) \times (3 - 1 = 2) = 6$ such odds ratios here, of which the first is $(53 \times 29)/(59 \times 2) = 13.0$ and the last is $(15 \times 24)/(10 \times 51) = 0.706$ (see rows labelled Adjacent OR in the table 7.16). The test for no association, which says that these odds ratios are all equal to 1, is significant ($\chi^2 = 47.21$, df 6, p < 0.001) so there is evidence of an association between duration and outcome.

The log-linear model for linear trend above can be extended to when both the number of rows and columns is greater than two. It is usually called the test for *uniform* or *linear-by-linear association* and says that the odds ratios for the 6 sets of adjacent 2×2 tables are all equal but greater than 1 (less than 1). Bear in mind that the linear-by-linear model is actually a number of different models for which the obtained odds ratio is determined by how the columns and rows are scored when fitting the model. Uniform is the special case where the scores are one unit apart. This would imply that as we go down the columns and across the rows, then the percentages should increase (decrease). The estimated common odds ratio is 1.35 and the test of this hypothesis is significant ($\chi^2 = 37.19$, df 5, p < 0.001) indicating that the model does not fit the data well.

Table 7.16 Illness duration and outcome

Illness duration	Improved	Unimproved	Died
< 3 mths	53	2	8
Adjacent OR		13.0	0.147
Readmission	59	29	17
Adjacent OR		1.58	0.711
3–12 months	31	24	10
Adjacent OR		1.88	0.706
> 12 mths	35	51	15

Table 7.17   Odds ratios from applying the uniform, row and column effects models to table 7.16

	Uniform		Row effects		Column effects	
	Col 1–2	Col 2–3	Col 1–2	Col 2–3	Col 1–2	Col 2–3
Row 1–2	1.35	1.35	2.21	2.21	2.26	0.613
Row 2–3	1.35	1.35	1.15	1.15	2.26	0.613
Row 3–4	1.35	1.35	1.24	1.24	2.26	0.613

With the uniform model asserting constant odds ratios as we go across the columns and down the rows, one way of relaxing this assumption is to have the odds ratios only constant across the rows, or only down the columns. This leads to the *row effects* (R) model where the odds ratio is the same within a row but differs from row to row, and the *column effects* (C) model where it is the same within a column but different from column to column. The R model also fails to fit the data ($\chi^2 = 32.92$, df 3, p < 0.001) and when we compare the adjacent odds ratios fitted by the model (see table 7.17) with the actual data we can see why this is a poor hypothesis. The C model provides a much better fit to the data ($\chi^2 = 7.79$, df 4, p = 0.0997). The odds ratios have been expressed in way which shows the odds favouring a better outcome for a shorter duration so that the column effects model says that the odds of 'improved' for the first row are 2.26 times those in the second, those in the second 2.26 times those in the third and so on. On the other hand the odds of 'unimproved' for the first row are 0.613 times those in the second, those in the second 0.613 times those in the third and so on, which actually means that 'died' becomes more likely than 'unimproved' as duration increases. It is also possible to fit more complex models but that lies outside the scope of this discussion. Finally, it is worth noting that the cell with only 2 cases makes a good fit more difficult since it results in the wayward odds ratio of 13.0 and the largest source of lack of good fit is associated with that cell.

Analysis of ordered data using ranks

The data in panel I of table 7.18 are scores from two independent groups, perhaps people with the same diagnosis who have received different treatments. Assuming that low scores indicate a low level of disorder, both groups have some subjects with a near complete recovery, but group B is distinguished by having a larger number with a moderate to severe disorder. A conventional analysis of the data, using the t-test for independent groups, allows us to infer that group B is more disordered than group A (t = 2.44, df 20, p = 0.024).

However, the t-test assumes that the data within groups are 'normally distributed'. As you will recall from earlier chapters, this assumption actually follows from the more basic assumption that the error component of the linear model has a normal distribution. The t-test also has the important assumptions that the observations are independent and that the variances across groups are equal. In this case, this assumptions of normal distribution does not appear to be true. This observation is supported when we carry out a test for normality (such as Lilliefors's version of the Kolmogorov-Smirnov test, or the Shapiro-Wilks test).

If one wanted to persist with the t-test for such data, a number of avenues are open. First, one could appeal to the robustness of the t-test against minor departures from normality. Robustness means that the test continues to produce the expected number (roughly) of correct decisions. Departure from normality can come in many forms and unless the particular departure in a set of data corresponds to a form for which the t-test has been shown to be robust, the appeal is arguably weak. Second, one could transform the data so that it more closely approximates normality, though this will not always work and it means that we now have to talk about the transformed scores, something which might not be useful, or which would make comparisons with other research difficult. Third, one could use a t-test-like procedure which allows an error distribution other than just the normal (procedures called generalised linear models). The data may still not fall within the available range.

The alternative is to use methods that do not make the sort of assumptions the t-test does, that allow us to make the sort of inferences we want to about the data, and that use as much of the information in the data as possible. Such procedures are called *nonparametric* or *distribution-free* methods, and in the situation we are looking at, they employ ranks, that is, they use the ordinal information in the data, to enable inferences about differences between groups. Nonparametric is the more common term though distribution-free is also used. The appropriateness of these terms has been argued about, in part because some nonparametric tests involve parameters and because often there are some assumptions about the distribution of the data. It is best to think of them as involving fewer or less stringent assumptions.

Because they use ranks, these methods are also suitable for data we have decided to treat as ordinal for reasons other than to do with assumptions. In the data under consideration, we could imagine them to be based upon some laboratory test where such tests can show considerable variability, which one would not want to attribute to a corresponding degree of variability in the underlying condition.

For the data in table 7.18, we can use the Wilcoxon rank sum test or its equivalent, the Mann-Whitney test (WMW). The null hypothesis that is tested is whether the data in the two groups come from populations with identical distributions; no assumptions are made about the shape of the distribution, but it is assumed that the distributions are continuous. Two distributions will fail to be identical either because they have different shapes or because they have different means or medians (sometimes referred to as different *locations*). If the WMW test is significant, we can reject the null hypothesis of identical distributions and, provided we are willing to make the assumption that the shapes are similar, we can infer that the two groups differ in their locations (mean or median). It is important to see that we are going from data that consist of ranks, and that tell us nothing about the value of the means, to making an inference about whether a difference exists between means, though without estimating the size of that difference. In table 7.18, we can see the ranks given to the scores, based on combining the two groups, that are used by the test and how adjustments are made for scores which are ties. The Mann-Whitney form of the test does not need the explicit ranks. Carrying out the WMW test we are able to reject the null hypothesis of identical distributions and, assuming similar shapes, of equal means ($z = 2.50$, $p = 0.013$), the same conclusions as with the t-test.

If we go to panel II of table 7.18, we find that group A has two additional observations, values which are the two largest for that group. If we now carry out the t-test, we find that the reduction in the mean difference and the increase in the variance of group A leave us unable to reject the null hypothesis ($t = 1.76$, df 22, $p = 0.092$). In contrast, the WMW test still results in a rejection of the null hypothesis ($z = 2.07$, $p = 0.039$) since the ranks have not been as altered by the addition of the two observations. In other words, changes in scores (or the addition or deletion of cases) will tend to leave the WMW test unaltered provided the ranks do not shift by much, even if those same changes make substantial differences to the means and standard deviations. The reason for this is that ranks ignore

Table 7.18   Independent group scores

| | Panel I | | | | Panel II | | | |
| | Group A | | Group B | | Group A | | Group B | |
	Score	Rank	Score	Rank	Score	Rank	Score	Rank
1	1	2.5	1	2.5	1	2.5	1	2.5
2	1	2.5	2	6.5	1	2.5	2	6.5
3	1	2.5	2	6.5	1	2.5	2	6.5
4	2	6.5	14	13.5	2	6.5	14	13.5
5	2	6.5	14	13.5	2	6.5	14	13.5
6	10	9.0	15	16.0	10	9.0	15	16.0
7	11	10.0	19	17.0	11	10.0	19	18.0
8	12	11.0	20	18.5	12	11.0	20	20.0
9	14	13.5	20	18.5	14	13.5	20	20.0
10	14	13.5	21	20.0	14	13.5	21	22.0
11	—		22	21.5	18	17.0	22	23.5
12	—		22	21.5	20	20.0	22	23.5
N	10		12		12		12	
Mean	6.8		14.3		8.8		14.3	
SD	5.8		8.2		7.1		8.2	

the information contained in the relative size of the scores (doubling the value of the largest score, for example, leaves the ranks unchanged) and this is as it should be since in using ranks we are only using order. Finally, note that the ranks could have come from a situation where all the subjects had been considered as one group and then explicitly ranked against each other.

The case of two independent groups can be extended to three or more independent groups (nonparametric analysis of variance) through the use of the Kruskal-Wallis test. Another case is that of two dependent groups. Recall that two dependent groups typically involve people measured on two occasions (say, pre- and post-treatment) or groups where each person from one group has been matched (say, for age and sex) with another person who then goes to make up the other group (dependent pairs). The data from a pre–post study is given in table 7.19 and we have expressed the difference (or change from pre to post) in two ways: as the number obtained by subtracting post from pre and as a direction (higher, lower, unchanged). If we felt unable to use the parametric dependent groups t-test because of violation of assumptions, then the difference–size data can be used to test the null hypothesis of no change via the nonparametric Wilcoxon signed rank test. Two of the assumptions for this test are that the distribution of the differences is symmetric and that the differences have meaning (i.e., that they are interval scores) since the test needs to rank the differences. This second assumption is of course a difficulty if we only have ordinal data. We can agree that subject 4 (score of 8) was more severe at the start than subject 1 (7) and also more severe at the end (5 versus 4), but if the data are only ordinal we cannot say strictly that $8 - 5 = 3$ is the same difference as $7 - 4 = 3$. If we remain true to the ordinal nature of the data we have to rely only on the difference–direction data, for which we can use the *sign* test. Carrying out these tests we find that the Wilcoxon rejects the null hypothesis ($z = -2.33$, p = 0.020) whereas the sign test does not (p = 0.180). In this small sample, the 7 '+' outcomes and 2 '–' outcomes are not sufficient for the sign test to reject the null, but if we use the information about the magnitude of the changes we do have enough subjects.

The preceding examples will have highlighted that behind the 'results', there is often considerable activity: decisions are made on how to measure; on how to re-express measurements when things 'do not work out'; and on what to use as

Table 7.19 Pre–post study data

	Subjects									
	1	*2*	*3*	*4*	*5*	*6*	*7*	*8*	*9*	*10*
Pre-treatment score	7	7	8	8	8	9	9	10	10	10
Post-treatment score	4	8	2	5	9	6	3	5	4	10
Difference–size	3	−1	6	3	−1	3	6	5	6	0
Difference–direction	+	−	+	+	−	+	+	+	+	tie

the final variables for analysis. As you become more familiar with statistical methods, you will see that choices also have to be made about which statistical tests to use, or which models, out of many possible ones, to fit and test. Further texts may help you.[19]

Published articles are a compressed product so that such activity is not always apparent, or is glossed over, but it is sensible to assume that some of it has been going on when you critically read an article. With a categorical variable, for example, you should ask how appropriate were the levels used, and how contingent might the results be either on the chosen levels or on the way they have been grouped for analysis. If a paper says, for example, that due to non-normality the data were analysed as ranks, then you should think about what it might mean that the data were non-normal: might it be the result of a poorly drawn sample of subjects, or the product of a faulty laboratory procedure?

Try exercise 7.1, by yourself, or in a group, as you think further about meaningful categories.

Exercise 7.1

Consider a rating scale for decline or improvement where the five ordered anchor points for each item are: much worse, worse, unchanged, better, much better.

Write some alternative anchor points that could be used.

Examine how the suitability of alternative anchor points might vary across different disorders, patient groups, or raters.

Or:

In a study, patients and their relatives rate their satisfaction with a health service on a scale of 1–10 and you wish to compare the two groups. Consider the appropriateness of, and issues in, analysing the data as:

- continuous scores
- ordinal ratings (ranks)
- responses on a categorical variable with 10 levels; *or*
- responses on a categorical variable with 4 levels where you need to decide how to group the original scores running 1–10 into scores running 1–4.

8

So, how is the treatment going?

DEBORAH BLACK AND SUSAN IRVINE

This chapter is aimed at the health care workers who need to understand research so that they can bring the best knowledge to their practice of health care, and is also targeted at beginning researchers. This chapter seeks to unravel and explain some of the complexity and debate that surrounds the seemingly simple question, 'So, how is the treatment going?'. This can also be asked as 'So, does the treatment work?' It will examine why researchers ask questions about treatments, and describes how a health researcher might go about researching the effectiveness of a particular intervention for a specific problem.

This chapter is co-written by a statistician and clinician, to highlight how essential both clinical and analytical reasoning skills are in making sense of research and research results, and in becoming generators of health research. It is a practical demonstration of the task set by Phillip Godwin in chapter 2, 'Using research in practice', of beginning to inquire into a health issue and make sense of available information and prior research. Asthma is the topic used in a demonstration of that process. The chapter also presents an example of how clinicians and a statistician can form a useful partnership to investigate a clinical issue, in this case, a research project on cardiac surgery and outcome. That project involved measures as varied as categorical, ordinal and parametric. Making sense of the data demanded sophisticated critical analysis skills, from both the clinicians and the statistician.

Health and illness are complex ideas that cannot be easily measured or assessed. They have different meanings for different people and the goals of successful treatment can differ among patients, among health care providers and among members of society.

Professionals often develop models to simplify complex concepts and to make it possible to solve problems about one aspect of the concept. These models are value laden. Many models and approaches have been developed in health and health care, such as the 'medical model', or 'the primary health care model'. Various models or approaches can be used to research the effectiveness of interventions. We have proposed a 'health outcomes' approach. This text has previously noted the influence of the outcomes approach in modern health care and health research, particularly in chapter 2, 'Using research in practice', and in Jeanette Ward and D'Arcy Holman's chapter 4, 'Who needs to plan?'. You may like to revise the issues of measurement and comparison, in chapters 4 and 5, before you read this chapter.

Identifying the goal of inquiry

Health researchers beginning a journey of inquiry into treatment effectiveness, whatever their primary goal of that inquiry, will be confronted by an enormous quantity of literature that was published during the 1990s. An analysis of the use of certain keywords in health and medical electronic databases over time is pre-

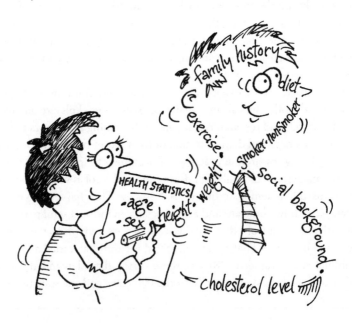

Table 8.1   Increase in 'effectiveness' citations

Keyword	1988	1992	Inc. factor 1988–92	1996	Inc. factor 1992–96
Evidence-based med.	0	2	*	230	115 times
Health outcomes	20	75	3.8 times	215	2.9 times
Quality	2000	3335	1.7 times	4291	1.3 times
Clinical pathways	0	2	*	319	160 times
Managed care	210	511	2.4 times	2938	5.7 times
Clinical guidelines	8	183	22.9 times	1315	7.2 times

sented in table 8.1. The keywords in the table are associated with the increasing emphasis on assessing the effectiveness of interventions. This increase has been matched by an increase in textbooks offering tools and instruments to make the inquiry easier, by prescribing scales and questionnaires to accommodate the various steps in measuring clinical outcomes.[1]

The health researcher may wonder why there is this apparent increase in the need to know whether interventions are effective or not and why. Linder provides one extreme point of view for the increasing emphasis on outcome measurement in the United States as a remedy for an ineffective system, in which professionals may deliver less than adequate services, and 'customers' cannot tell what they are getting.[2]

Another possibility is that today's patients are far more informed about treatments and their outcomes than their counterparts of twenty years ago, and want to be. They can access good information electronically and many want to have a part in the clinical decisions which are made. This has led to recent literature with an increasing focus on whether the patient is free of symptoms and signs, and what impact the treatment has had on his or her quality of life. In other words, the effect of the treatment needs to be assessed in terms of the patient's social, economic and psychological supports, and in terms of the patient's value preferences and personality motivations.[3]

A recent approach committed to asking 'does the treatment work?' is seen in the Cochrane Collaboration.[4] Archie Cochrane emphasised the importance of care rather than cure, a philosophy based on his experiences as a doctor in a German prisoner-of-war camp. Advocating that treatments should be 'evidence based', the Cochrane Database of Systematic Reviews has as its objective, the provision of information for clinical decisions. The Collaboration is made up of international groups of individuals who have a commitment to prepare, maintain and disseminate systematic reviews from the scientific literature of the effects of health care for specific diseases. The reviews are limited to the results of clinical trials, and do not include routinely collected patient data. Hayward acknowledges the problem in evidence-based medicine of attributing the treatment to the outcome.[5] Another problem with this type of systematic review is discussed by Walters and Walters,[6] as members of the Cochrane Airways Group, who cite problems in 80 per cent of published papers where results presented

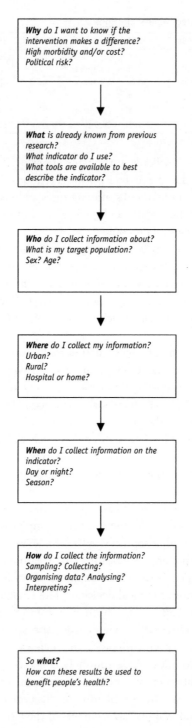

Figure 8.1 Question flow chart

are derivative, giving only changes from the baseline, or only reporting p-values. Essentially, these papers are illustrating the problem of providing links between practice and research. The statistical results which are presented in such peer-review papers are brief, and the data are condensed to what the researchers interpreted as meaningful results.

In summary, the motivation for assessing the effectiveness of treatment includes political, economic and consumer elements. The health professional is only one player in a large team. The process a researcher can follow to answer specific questions about treatment is summarised in figure 8.1.

Before they can start their processes of inquiry, researchers need to address the question: 'Why do I want to know whether this intervention makes a difference?' A decision-maker or manager (evaluator) needs to solve a problem or make a decision now, and wants to know which strategies and interventions used in the past were useful or not in a particular context, and which to use next time. A scientific researcher wants to add to knowledge about human life and other aspects of the natural world. Scientific research and service evaluation have different goals, but confusion often arises in people's minds about the differences between them. This may be because many of the methods used (gathering information, organising information, analysing information, interpreting information) are the same. Scientific researchers have traditionally answered this question by saying that they want to add to knowledge about the natural world and to describe links between things that happen. In this instance, treatment pathways could become better understood and more predictable. Research should be generalisable—that is, it should be able to be applied in contexts other than that in which the actual research was conducted. This differentiates research from evaluation. Research findings can be used to influence health policy and service development, to plan new services or discontinue services, to discontinue ineffective treatments, and to modify treatments for individuals. Yet, there are basic human dilemmas that research cannot solve for us any more than any other process can. Often what is good for one individual may harm another. Benefit to a few individuals may not be any benefit to the population or society as a whole. Any research study has an opportunity cost, in that when resources are directed to answer one question, those hours, professional expertise, building facilities, and financial resources are not available to answer another question. These issues must be acknowledged before any research starts. Researchers should be able to identify the value-based decisions that preceded the formulation of their health research questions. This can give a research team the dedication it may need to stay committed to a difficult and long process, which research studies can often be. The researcher should be able to say, 'As a researcher I can accept that, by choosing to look at this question this way, I am choosing to ignore other aspects of this problem. As a researcher, I accept that, in choosing to ask this question,

I am preventing these resources being used to answer another question that is very important to someone else.'

No research question or research finding is context free. No research question (and therefore research finding) is value free. For example, you may suggest that funding priority in paediatric research should be given to conditions and diseases that impose a heavy burden of suffering, for which mainstream therapies are insufficient, and in which the research has a reasonable likelihood of being help-ful. Thus, the 'why' question will direct the researcher's focus to a choice about which of several interesting questions should be answered first. It will influence the way the health problem and the treatments are defined, and the paradigm that is chosen as the theoretical underpinning of the research approach.

An asthma inquiry

Asthma has been identified as one of six priorities by the Commonwealth, state and territory governments in Australia as National Health Priority Areas. The Aus-tralian Institute of Health and Welfare stated that asthma cost approximately $447 million in the financial year 1993/94 and that there were 730 deaths in 1996. Recognising the difficulties of defining asthma, they state that a 'recent wheeze' (in the last 12 months) was reported by around 25 per cent of school age children in Australia and that there is good evidence that this trend has been increasing. Also, asthma affects one in ten adults and one in seven teenagers.[7] The Australian Institute of Health and Welfare in *Australia's Children—Their Health and Wellbeing* stated that childhood asthma prevalence rates place Australia in the top two or three countries.[8] In a media release from the Australian Health Minis-ter's Conference on 4 August 1999, the Australian Capital Territory's Health Min-ister, Mr Michael Moore stated that asthma was a 'prevalent disease, which affects so many young people, and is now a matter of top priority for all Governments'. Thus, asthma is common and debilitating, with a high burden of suffering and huge community costs. Past research findings have answered some questions. While we cannot predict the exact causes of asthma, we do understand some of its risk factors and its pathological processes. There has been enough success in treat-ments research to justify the likelihood that new treatment regimens are feasible. That is, research questions can be formulated that are neither overwhelmingly dif-ficult or too trivial to justify scientific study. From the health researcher's perspec-tive, asthma raises questions relevant to preventive and curative care, clinical and population health, and physical and psychosocial interventions. In brief, asthma is believed to justify the considerable research attention it receives at present and a researcher can readily explain why this is the case.

The inquirer will wonder: What is already known from previous research? What is the direction of my research? What is my 'hunch' about the links between the health problem and the treatment? Can I state this as a specific hypothesis? The initial goal is to formulate a specific research statement, which clearly states the problem on the one hand, the treatment on the other, and the indicator which has been chosen to demonstrate whether there is a predictable link between the two. This initial stage of inquiry is complete when the researcher can document:

- the definition chosen to describe the specific disease or health problem
- the definition chosen to describe the specific treatment or intervention
- the statement defining the difference the researcher is seeking to document
- and a hunch or feeling about why the treatment may or may not make a difference.

Defining the disease

It is known that asthma is an inflammatory disease affecting the airways (bronchi and bronchioles) leading into the lungs. Asthma occurs when the airways become narrow because the tissue lining them swells and secretes mucus. This is an allergic reaction, that is, the body is overresponding to a supposedly damaging invader. There is one key clinical symptom and sign: a wheezing or whistling in the chest in the last twelve months, which can be reported by the children themselves.[9] Some of the things that matter about asthma in children, the 'variables' in research jargon, are: the impact of the same pathological process (the narrowing of airways) is greater in children than in adults because of their anatomically smaller tubes; and its incidence is increasing, especially in temperate climates. Gels and Banks compare current epidemiological knowledge about asthma to that of cancer a few decades ago: 'these studies revealed striking international differences that gave rise to many new hypotheses, tested in further epidemiological studies that identified previously unknown risk factors for cancer.'[10] These risk factors may not have been in the hypotheses investigated if the initial international comparisons had been confined to few Western countries. More specifically, Rose has noted that whole populations may be exposed to risk factors, for instance, high exposure to house-dust mite allergen, and the patterns may be apparent only when comparisons are made between rather than within populations.[11] Further, 'viral infections are the most common cause of asthma exacerbation in adults and children and contribute substantially to asthma-related absenteeism and admission to hospital.'[12]

Defining treatments

Accepted treatments include pharmacotherapy, alternative or complementary medicine, environmental control, patient education and treatment plans. 'There is increasing interest in the idea that earlier intervention with inhaled corticosteroids as first-line therapy might possibly avoid irreversible airway obstruction and hence favourably alter the natural history of the disease.'[13] A common aim in treatment research is to test whether asthma exacerbation had the same peak expiratory flow characteristics as poor asthma control.[14]

Choosing indicators

The next set of inquiry questions are: What information do I need to collect to demonstrate whether there is a predictable link between the problem I have chosen and the treatment I have chosen? What tools are available to help me choose this outcome? In this chapter, we have chosen the tool of health outcome measures to demonstrate the research process. At first, it seems that the health outcome goal of a health intervention must be so obvious that it hardly needs restating. Surely it must be to improve people's health, which is that state of complete physical, mental and social well-being, and not merely the absence of disease or infirmity. Like many obvious statements, there is enormous complexity for the person who is actually trying to define a research hypothesis or statement that might in the future help solve a problem. Does a good outcome mean that the treatment will lead to people having fewer symptoms and signs of illness, or that people feel satisfied with their health, or that fewer resources are used in achieving an acceptable outcome? In health research, the term 'health outcome' is used to describe a measure to evaluate treatment. Health outcome measurement can range from death and disease to emotional health and patient satisfaction. Fries and Spitz describe health outcomes as multi-dimensional: 'Patient health outcome usually refers to a final health status measurement after the passage of time and the application of treatment. In the future, patient outcome will be increasingly described by a cumulative series of health status measurements'.[15]

The simplest measure that can be used to assess treatment is whether the patient is dead or alive. An often used measure of how cancer treatment is going is five-year survival rates, that is, what proportion of treated patients are still alive five years after treatment commenced? Although this may appear to be a straightforward measurement, caution should be taken in making comparisons between mortality rates without standardisation for risk factors such as age and sex as discussed in chapter 5, 'Numbers and more'. Another simple measure of how a treatment is going is whether an individual who presents with signs and symptoms is free of them following treatment. Again, this measure must be viewed in context, that is, ensuring that the social, emotional and physical side effects of the treatment are not worse than the symptoms. The comprehensive approach to measuring how the treatment has been going in terms of quality of life has been the subject of considerable debate in health and medical journals.[16] At one extreme, Leplege and Hunt state that making inferences about outcomes from 'a variety of indicators [of quality of life] may tell us something about life but nothing about quality'.[17] The authors further argue that the objective of measuring outcome 'is to select the health policy and medical intervention that maximises benefits at the collective (or individual) level'. This is a utilitarian approach. However, they state, an existential approach reflects the views of lay people, in that the preferences or values of one person may be different from others. In summary, the authors state that quality of life should be replaced by subjective health status, which gives little insight to their quality of life.

A number of writers support this notion that quality of life, although important, cannot be measured.[18] Gulliford states that 'unequivocal measurement of health outcomes can only be made in clinical trials'.[19] At the other extreme, Gill and Feinstein argue that measurement of quality of life has developed into 'a small cottage industry' which has been aiming at the wrong target with too much emphasis on what the 'experts' perceive as measures of quality of life and not enough input from lay people. The authors point out that there is a 'multiplicity of new and complex instruments that often lack face validity' and that patients' quality of life can only be measured through patients' opinions, which add to or replace instruments developed by experts. They question 'whether the academic psychometric principles, although perhaps elegant statistically, are satisfactory for the clinical goal of indicating what clinicians and patients perceive as quality of life'.[20] Others also support the measurement of quality of life based on patients' perceptions.[21]

With regard to asthma treatments and outcomes

Research on asthma and treatment outcomes has used a combination of indicators, in asking the primary questions: does it work?, what are the adverse effects?, and how much does it cost? A further question has been: if mainstream mediations have unacceptable costs or side effects for diseases that are largely self-limited, is it worth offering an untested but inexpensive, non-toxic placebo instead? Answering these questions requires sophisticated, critical, and creative cost–benefit analyses.

Outcomes measured include costs, adverse events, and patient preferences. Tools to measure health outcomes, such as the SF36, include clinical, functional, social and economic measures. These are summarised below.

> *Clinical measures* have included: avoidance of adverse effects/side effects; improvement in pulmonary function; improvement in symptom scores; improvement in patient compliance/adherence; reduction in bronchial hyperreactiveness; reduction in disease markers; reduction in frequency of exacerbation; reduction in frequency of respiratory infections; reduction in incidence of chronic irreversible disease; reduction in medication usage; and reduction in mortality.

Functional measures focus on: improvement in activity levels.

Social measures have included: improvement in patient/family knowledge and skills; limitation of inconvenience or bother; limitation of negative psychosocial impacts; optimisation of quality of life; and patient satisfaction with care.

Economic measures focus on: cost and cost limitation.

Outcomes which are measured can include more than the traditional measures of morbidity, mortality, cost of care, and patient satisfaction. They can also focus on the impact of care on family cohesiveness, cultural identity, spiritual beliefs, resilience, coping and self-efficacy. Additional outcome measures may need to be developed to address the quality of life and the concept of health rather than just the absence of disease.

Another model, quality assurance, uses health outcomes as a component of a clinical and managerial framework that commits staff to producing a systematic continuous process of evaluating agreed levels of care and service provision. The objectives of a quality assurance program, as stated by a WHO working group, are:

> to assure that each patient receives such a mix of diagnostic and therapeutic health services as is most likely to produce the optimum achievable health care outcome for that patient, consistent with the state of the art of medical science, and with biological factors such as the patient's age, illness, concomitant secondary diagnoses, compliance with the treatment regimen, and other related factors; with the minimal expenditure of resources necessary to accomplish this result; at the lowest achievable risk of additional injury or disability as a consequence of the treatment; and with maximal patient satisfaction with the process of care, his/her interaction with the health care system, and the results obtained.[22]

This group further stated that under the umbrella term 'quality assurance' there are four particular components which need to be considered. Those components are: patient satisfaction with services provided; professional performance (technical quality); resource use (efficiency); and risk management (the risk of illness or injury associated). The elements of this approach are noted throughout this text, and are discussed in chapter 10, 'Quality and quantity'. The discussion in this chapter will be limited to a health outcomes approach.

Who is the focus?

The first question for a researcher examining how a treatment is going is whether they are concerned with an individual or population. What might be the best treatment for an individual may not be the best treatment for a population. A change in health status for an individual will be measured differently from a change in health status for the group.

A change in baseline of health status or measure for an individual is the clinical interview and the change is measured with clinical evaluation. For a group, the baseline health status measure is based on a survey instrument and the change is based on a health idea.[23] Focusing on measuring how a treatment is going in a group, one of the most important issues in assessing whether a treatment is successful is defining the target population treatment regimens, and recognising that outcomes will vary according to the characteristics of the patient.

Returning to asthma, asthma severity, asthma management and outcome measures such as re-presenting at hospital with a severe asthma, and hospital admissions with asthma will vary with the age of individual. The management of asthma with children will involve parents, not just the patient. If the population is defined as children 14 and under, those under 12 months must be excluded from the target group, if wheezing in babies is defined as the result of 'anatomically small airways rather than true asthma'.[24]

Based on the 1996–97 AIHW Hospital morbidity database, asthma prevalence in 1 to 4 year olds is lower than older age groups, but hospital admission rates are higher in this group than the older group. Asthma hospital admissions for boys was higher than hospital admissions for girls because of the higher prevalence in boys.[25] A study by Goodman and colleagues showed that although the rate of asthma medication in children had increased, the target population, children with severe asthma, had not met use of inhaled anti-inflammatory drugs national guidelines.[26]

It is, therefore, important to ensure that the effect is measured in the target population and not viewed at an aggregate level. In summary, clearly age and sex are important determinants of what the treatment will be, and how it will be assessed.

When do I collect information?

One of the major difficulties facing researchers is that they rarely have the resources (time and money) to assess the effect of an intervention on a sufficiently large group of patients. Therefore, measures will be disease specific, and the assessment of impact is dependent on the stage of disease when the impact is assessed.

For instance, if your measure is whether patients have returned to activities of daily living (ADL), when this question should be asked will vary depending on the intervention they have undergone. For minor surgery, you might expect a patient to return to ADL within two weeks, whereas for more major surgery, this might not be appropriate to measure for twelve months. Time-relevant points with regard to disease and problem include: how quickly do symptoms change?; when will an effect be expected?; does the disease process fluctuate or is it steady?; does the disease progress or not?; is the intervention continuous or intermittent?; do environmental factors such as time of day or season impact on the intervention?. In some cases, results that may be good in the short term, but are dependent, for long-term success, on continued financial or professional support. This again demonstrates that research questions are always context related and the context always must be specified. A time-relevant inquiry on asthma was pursued taking into account these queries, and the reasoning process is presented here.

Air passages narrow in response to many 'triggers' including exercise, pollens, house-dust mites, cold weather and throat and chest infections. Therefore, if your measure of how the treatment is going is hospital admissions of children, you will find seasonal variation in your data. The type of sport or exercise undertaken by children varies with the time of year. Pollens and dust mite pressure varies with season. Similarly, cold weather is a trigger for throat and chest infections. Hospital admission patterns will also vary with the time of day that presentation at the emergency department occurs. Children are more likely to be admitted if they present between 8 am and 6 pm than at other times.[27] Also, peak expiratory flow waves in normal subjects vary throughout the day, which is known as diurnal variation.[28] A recommendation is therefore that asthma guidelines be varied to take more daily observations and to alter the calculation because diurnal variability will be 'grossly underestimated'. In another example, Gels and Banks state that if international guidelines were altered to include earlier intervention with inhaled corticosteroids, this would have an effect on the long-term outcome of childhood asthma.[29] In summary, triggers for asthma vary with time of day and season. Similarly these triggers will vary with location as discussed in the next section.

Where do I collect information?

Where a population lives will impact on climate and other environmental factors, accessibility and health policy. Geographic location is almost always a component in the calculation of indices of socioeconomic status. It is well documented that socioeconomic status is a prime determinant of health status.[30] Gels and Banks state that the worldwide variations in rates, and partly the variations seen within some countries, suggest that environmental factors (in their broadest sense) may be critical to the development of these disorders in childhood.[31]

If we confine our analysis to just one continent, Australia, variations in climate because of latitude, geography and distance from the coast are still significant. Variations exist because of differences in health policies between states. Between rural and urban communities, differences exist in accessibility to health services, ambient air pollution and income. Therefore for the health researcher, it is crucial that the location of their study population be accurately defined.

Asthma provides a good vehicle to demonstrate how differences in triggers and access to services depending on location will impact on both treatment and outcome. In a study by Jalaludin and colleagues of admission rates as an indicator of the prevalence of severe asthma in western Sydney, they caution about inferring to other populations based on their results with the statement, 'our study was conducted in a metropolitan tertiary paediatric hospital. The reliability of hospital admission rates as indicators of the prevalence of severe asthma in other hospital settings, in different population groups and over time remains to be established'.[32]

The triggers for asthma, including cold weather, humidity, pressure of pollens and dust mites, and ambient air quality, will all alter with where the health researcher studies interventions. Geography such as locations in valleys, will impact on respiratory morbidity.[33] A child presenting at an emergency department with severe asthma is far more likely to be admitted if the family live more than fifteen minutes travel time from the hospital. Therefore, hospital admission rates as an outcome measure must be viewed in the light of where the child lives.

How is the information collected?

Having determined factors (who, what, where and when) to take into account when assessing the success of the treatment, how does the health researcher begin the study? There are a number of approaches to research, however the gold standard is the double-blind randomised control where there is one group receiving an intervention (what) and another the control. The participant is not aware if they are receiving the intervention or the control. In double blind experiments the two groups are matched for age and sex (who), they are exposed to the same environmental factors and have access to the same services (where) and are studied at the same time of day and season (when). The participants have an equal chance of being assigned to the control group or the intervention group (random).

How big a difference you wish to measure, the required accuracy of the estimate and the variation in the measure across the population will determine the appropriate sample size for your study. For instance, if you wish to detect a difference in peak flow for children with severe asthma, the smaller the difference that you consider as signficant between the measures for the two groups, the larger the sample required.

It is not always possible to conduct double-blind randomised trials to assess how a treatment is going because of ethical issues, time and cost constraints. The analysis of routinely collected data that have been controlled for confounding variables can provide appropriate answers to research questions about how a treatment is going. In a study in Western Sydney of paediatric admission rates, researchers used routinely collected medical records with an accompanying survey of attending doctors and a survey of parents to conclude that admission rates can be used a proxy measures for the prevalence of severe asthma.[34]

Other study types include meta-analysis where a systematic review of a number of studies to assess how a treatment is going. One such study by Plotnick and Ducharme estimated the therapeutic and adverse effects of the addition of inhaled anticholinergics to β_2 agonists in acute asthma in children and adolescents. The studies included in the meta-analyses were restricted to randomised controlled clinical trials conducted in an emergency department setting.[35]

Various methods can be used to collect data and many studies include several collection methods to validate the data. Data collection methods in assessing how a treatment is going range from: observing, including participant/observation/ethnography; asking, including techniques of face-to-face, telephone, and mail survey and focus groups; and experimenting, ranging from quasi experiment through to action research techniques. These techniques are covered in other chapters. Suffice to say here that the researcher is free to gather information from variety of studies, in various methodological frameworks, and to make use of the information gained from such diverse studies. Sometimes, multiple methodologies are used within one study.

For instance, Gels and Banks conducted a study into the effect of drugs on the long-term outcome of childhood asthma and collected data from a number of sources including: a retrospective review performed on charts of patients, a spirometry, and a completed questionnaire.[36] As another example, the International Study of Asthma and Allergies in Childhood Steering Committee collected data through: children completing self-reported questionnaires, and children viewing five sequences of clinical asthma in different situations and being asked which person best illustrated their breathing.[37] They believed that by showing rather than describing the signs and symptoms of asthma to children, the video questionnaire would provide more accurate recognition of clinical asthma, which would be useful to compare information between populations with different cultures and languages.

How should the data be organised?

Descriptive statistical and qualitative analysis tools are available to help the researcher to organise the data collected. Organising the data into meaningful tables or graphs will depend on the research question which in this chapter is, very broadly, 'How is the treatment going?' Chapter 5, 'Numbers and more', provides a number of different ways of presenting descriptive data in tabular and graphical form to show differences between groups. Organising the data into meaningful 'pictures' not only provides the researcher with an indication of whether the intervention has made a difference, but also identifies other variables that appear to be making a difference to the defined outcome of the treatment. These other variables are termed possible explanatory variables.

Having identified the explanatory variables, the statistical analyses to be conducted will attempt to see whether there is a statistically significant change in the outcome measure when the treatment changes while controlling for other explanatory variables. The statistical technique used will depend on whether the data are categorical or continuous. Chapters 5 and 7 provide some indication of the procedure to use. The study by Jalaludin and associates in Western Sydney[38] used logistic regression, a multivariate technique to determine what variables influence a dichotomous variable. In this case, the dichotomous variable was whether or not a child with asthma was admitted to hospital. The researchers aimed to determine whether the asthma severity was a predictor of admission, while controlling for other confounders.

After deciding on the study design, collecting the data, organising and analysing the data, the researcher must then interpret the results for other health professionals to apply to their clinical setting. In other words, to explain how the treatment is going. They need to explain not only if the intervention did make a statistically significant difference, but also if it could be used in other settings.

How should the significance be explained?

Health research is assumed to be of value to society. Findings are assumed to be able to be applied to develop new services, to manufacture new drugs, to provide new educational materials and health promotion approaches, and to decrease the prevalence of diseases. Therefore, the researcher not only must complete the research process by providing an interpretation of the findings and documenting and distributing this for other researchers to critically analyse, but also ask the vexatious question 'so what?'. 'Having completed my study, can I as a researcher feel confident that these findings can be applied to improve the health status of individuals or populations?' Society can rightly ask whether the researcher has a responsibility to ensure that the research findings are applied to society's benefit.

Health researchers must ensure that interventions that have been successful in a controlled experiment can be applied in a real-life setting. David Berwick, an acknowledged expert on health outcomes, states that while 'journal reviewers demand evidence of proper control and statistical analyses', they ignore the role of what he describes as 'real-time science'[39]—that is, the routine collection of data and the analysis of these in terms of patient outcomes. However, it must be recognised that a surrogate must always be chosen as a measurement of patient outcome in real life.

It should be noted that treatments can be given to individuals or to populations and that the treatments and the difference to be measured will vary accordingly. As an example, the work of Trye and colleagues into hypertension asked: 'are we better to try to move the whole population down a few mm Hg in hypertension or to move some individuals down more units?'[40] Clearly, moving a whole population down an insignificant amount will have less impact than a larger shift in a number of individuals.

Researchers should be aware of the many steps between a research study, and changed health outcomes. If the treatment does work and does make a difference, how long is it sustained? Is it affordable in every context or is it only affordable in some? How will research findings be applied in a particular context? Is this treatment no longer needed because the health problem has diminished because of effective interventions? In summary, the health researcher needs to make a judgment that the intervention can be applied and that the difference measured makes a difference to the patient in different situations.

The seemingly simple question, the title of this chapter, 'How is the treatment going?' cannot be answered so simply. The most important question for any health researcher is why should they conduct a study to see whether a treatment is effective. There are many drivers for such research, but three major ones are: high levels of morbidity in a particular disease, high cost to the community and government initiatives. A review of research on the chosen health issue will assist in deciding *what* you will measure to determine whether the intervention makes a difference. Researchers need to ensure that they specify who the results will apply to, when they can be applied and where they are to be applied. Having determined the target population, researchers need to be able to collect, organise, analyse and interpret their findings. Research about how a treatment is going needs to be generalisable to other groups besides the study group. If not, so what?

This section has demonstrated the partnership of a statistician and a health researcher. The statistician's skills were in synthesising available research results, and interpreting them, and communicating them in relatively simple terms. The health researcher's main role was in considering the relevance of that research for the context under consideration.

A cardiac inquiry

This section demonstrates the sharing of expertise between the health researcher and the statistician in the generation of new research data. The inquiry process involved an exchange of knowledge: the statistician explained the use of appropriate statistical techniques, and the health researcher provided the statistician with an insight into the clinical meaning of the variables. The complexity of the cardiac inquiry was driven by the clinical question. Most clinical outcomes involve several explanatory factors. The statistician's role in this inquiry was to determine those factors that explained most of the variability in the patients' health outcomes after their cardiac surgery. This meant that complex statistical models were used. The acceptable statistical options were only meaningfully generated by the statistician once she understood the clinical process of what was being studied. The statistician should clearly explain to the health researcher how to use the modelling techniques, and how to interpret the validity of the results.

In short, the statistician needs to understand the research question, and its significance for clinical work. The statistician provides the researcher with available and appropriate techniques for the question. Variables can then be chosen which meet both the researcher's and statistician's requirements. The results will then be meaningfully generated.

One of the authors of this chapter, a statistician, Deborah Black, was asked to assist in the analyses of some complex data relating to neurological health outcomes following coronary artery bypass graft (CABG) surgery patients at a large teaching hospital in Sydney. The database, with 3979 records for all patients who had undergone CABG surgery at the study hospital between 1984 and 1992, has been maintained by the perfusionist, an anaesthetic consultant.

The success following CABG surgery is measured in terms of reduced mortality, relief from symptoms and activity limitations, work status, levels of re-hospitalisation and medication use.[41] However, such traditional measures of outcome do not include a measure of psychological outcome. This is a major deficiency in defining outcomes, because studies show 54 per cent of patients following CABG suffered from depression,[42] and 61 per cent of patients suffered neurological complications.[43]

At the study hospital, the perfusionist has concentrated on the symptomatic neurological outcome following CABG, and has produced observable improvements in outcome over time by relating outcome to the perfusion process. The continuous quality improvement (CQI) program implemented by the perfusionist was to plot 3-dimensional graphs at intervals when sufficient data have been collected. The variables analysed in each graph were: various blood gas measurements including pH, PO_2, PCO_2, haemoglobin (on the x-axis); time on bypass measured at time 0, 10 minutes on bypass and then every 20 minutes until 150 minutes (on the y-axis); and average NSUM, a score for neurological damage (on the z-axis). As an example, figure 8.2 presents partial oxygen (PO_2) by time on bypass by mean NSUM.

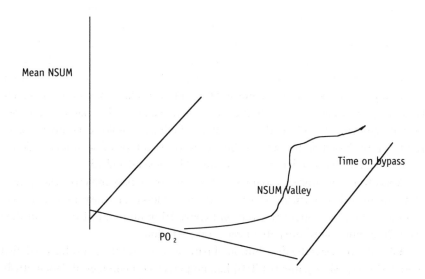

Figure 8.2 Partial oxygen by time on bypass by mean neurological deficit

Peaks occur in the three dimensional graphs where the average NSUM is high. It would therefore be expected that the patients would wish to minimise neurological damage and would prefer to be in the valleys where NSUM is lowest, as illustrated on the graph of figure 8.2. At six monthly intervals, the perfusionist produced such graphs based on the total number of patients at that time for each of the blood gas measurements. Subsequently, he attempted to maintain the blood gas variables in the valleys for all patients. The perfusionist consulted the author for support in data analyses to support the CQI process of maintaining blood gases in the valleys defined by the 3-dimensional graphs.

This database includes details from the hospital's clinical information system, blood gas measurements recorded during bypass, cross clamp time, time on bypass and a measure of patient-assessed physical and neurological outcomes. To measure neurological outcomes that could be attributed to the perfusion process, all patients were interviewed as inpatients pre-surgery and an attempt was made to interview all patients 12 months post-surgery.

The pre-surgery interviews were unstructured and administered in a sympathetic manner by the perfusionist. These interviews ascertained demographic and lifestyle characteristics of the patients, any co-morbidities and details of what their expectations of activities of daily living would be one year post-surgery.

The one year post-surgery follow-up interview was semi-structured and was administered by telephone by an interviewer who was blind to the clinical, demographic and perfusion process characteristics of the interviewee. At least three telephone calls were made at different times in an attempt to follow up all patients.

To elicit details on neurological damage due to the procedure, patients were questioned in relation to their expectations recorded pre-surgery. They were asked whether they had noted any changes in memory, moods, ability to concentrate, levels of depression, irritability and social life. Up to three responses on types of neurological deficits in pre-coded categories were recorded. For each response, they were asked to assess the impact of that deficit on a scale when: 0 = absence or denial of symptoms even if prompted; 1 = a just noticeable or occasional symptom; 2 = a daily noticeable, consistent, but still tolerable, complaint; 3 = severe enough to be of daily annoyance and interfering with functional living; 4 = markedly interfering with enjoyment of life; and 5 = disabling. The final neurological outcome score (NSUM) was based on the sum of the scores for each type of neurological deficit mentioned. NSUM then has possible values of between 0 and 15.

Apart from the process variables such as time on bypass and cross clamp time that are recorded normally during perfusion, blood gas measurements were recorded when the patient was put on bypass, 10 minutes into bypass, and then every 20 minutes until the patient came off perfusion.

Table 8.2 presents the distribution of patient scores for the neurological deficit score (NSUM). Most patients (70%) had no perceived neurological deficit attributable to the surgery with only one patient scoring the maximum of 15 points.

Table 8.2 Distribution of NSUM scores for all patients

NSUM	Frequency	Proportion (%)
0	2768	69.6
1	241	6.1
2	375	9.4
3	112	2.8
4	201	5.1
6	117	2.9
7	35	0.9
8	27	0.2
9	20	0.5
10	6	0.2
11	5	0.1
12	2	0.1
13	0	0.0
14	0	0.0
15	1	0.0
Total	3979	100

The distribution of the neurological deficit scores shows that most patients have either no deficit or minor deficit. Such a skewed distribution is common for health outcomes that measure deficit. The skewed distribution precludes the use of parametric multivariate statistical analyses, such as taking means of the NSUM.

Univariate analyses were conducted to identify variables associated with the presence of some neurological deficit. The data were subsequently analysed using ordered polytomous logistic regression. This is a regression technique which is appropriate when the dependent variable is an ordered qualitative variable. The regression used 5 ordered categories of deficit: none (NSUM = 0), mild (NSUM = 1 to 2), moderate (NSUM = 3 to 4), substantial (NSUM = 5 to 6) and severe (NSUM>6). The table below presents the factors that explained the variable in the neurological deficit categories.

These results show that if patients have angina one year post-surgery, they are approximately 1.9 times more likely to be in a higher NSUM category—that is, the patient has a greater deficit. If they are not in the valley for partial oxygen, then they are 1.6 times more likely to be in a higher category of NSUM. The interaction between age and year of surgery is included because it was included in the model but the odds of being in higher category are only just above one. Patients

Table 8.3 Factors explaining variability using Polytomous Logistic Regression

Factors explaining variability	Odds ratio	95% CI for odds ratio
Presence of angina one year post-surgery	1.86	(1.40–2.48)
Not in the partial oxygen (PO$_2$) valley	1.61	(1.20–2.17)
Interaction between age and year of surgery	1.002	(1.001–1.003)
Year of surgery	0.87	(0.83–0.91)
Time on bypass	1.13	(1.04–2.64)

were less likely to be in a higher NSUM category as year of surgery increased or 1.2 times more likely to be in a higher category if one year earlier. For a 30-minute increase in bypass time, patients were 1.1 times more likely to be in a higher NSUM category.

The unravelling of the story of how the cardiac surgery was going was complex. A reasoned approach was essential, concentrating on meaningful clinical issues, and appropriate statistical manipulation for the types of measures to hand in that clinical context.

9

Not everything can be reduced to numbers

JAN RITCHIE

The research methods outlined so far in this book have well served the health care sector, its technical personnel, and its patients or clients, in providing an approach that helps describe, explain and predict health care issues to the benefit of humankind. As the previous authors have pointed out, particularly in the last few chapters, the way of knowing contributed by quantitative research is defined by certain rules and practices, and has a particular reliance on inference through manipulation of numbers. However, not everything in health or health care can be reduced to numbers. This chapter will discuss what we might describe as another way of knowing. This different approach uses what are called qualitative methods in order to attempt systematically to describe and explain phenomena.

The domain of qualitative research

The term 'qualitative research' encompasses a wide collection of research practices which have certain characteristics, the most definitive of which, as already implied, is production of findings that do not depend on statistical procedures or quantification.[1] Primarily, these approaches appreciate the value-laden nature of inquiry, and seek meaning and understanding ahead of quantifiable measures. They deal with the socially constructed nature of reality, the close relationship between the researcher and the researched, and the frequent necessity to make investigations without stripping the phenomenon under study of its context. Whereas conventional scientific research ultimately seeks causal relationships between variables, in most instances qualitative research ultimately seeks deeper and richer understanding. Qualitative research results are written in narrative with an orientation to language and discourse.

Although the social sciences have long used qualitative methods and regarded them as integral to their knowledge development, medicine and the health sciences have built their research foundation on the positivist, reductionist tradition, referred to generally as scientific method. However, these health disciplines not only deal with physiological and pathological entities that mimic the hard sciences in their predictability, they also deal with people. Human beings are not predetermined in their behaviour, but rather are self-determined. The instinctive response of lower order animals has, in humans, been replaced in most instances with a range of rational, cognitively resolved responses. Yet, one person's rational decision may bear no resemblance to another's. Despite the most carefully constructed study design, the ability causally to predict human behaviour remains, and will always remain, an inexact science.

The acknowledgment by health disciplines that they are founded on the social sciences, in addition to medical science, frees researchers within them to investigate not only the effectiveness of a treatment or intervention physiologically, but also whether the people exposed to this intervention understand what it means, value it and choose to comply with it. It allows investigators to explore people's experiences with different diseases, conditions and treatments. It gives meaning to individual's decisions about, for instance, their food habits when they prioritise social affiliations over healthfulness of their food choices. It permits an exploration of the politics of decision-making in health care that often appear not to follow a logical, rational, scientifically determined pathway.

This acknowledgment does more. In broadening the foundations upon which health research studies are conceived and designed, the opportunity arises to consider the various sets of assumptions underlying decisions about what might constitute the best way to answer the research question posed. Although scientific method has a hierarchy of levels of investigation where prediction is the ultimate goal, the assumption underpinning qualitative research is that this approach *will* describe, and *may* under some circumstances explain a phenomenon, but it is expected that it *will not* predict a cause and effect relationship. Despite the strength of this statement, later sections in this chapter will discuss the fact that useful, important and influential implications may be derived from the descriptions and explanations.

The contribution of inductive reasoning to research

A research study of the conventional biomedical type comes with an explicit theory already positioned, and the research design evolves to test hypotheses concerning relevant relationships within the theory. This is a deductive line of reasoning where the rule or theory is stated and the examples or applications unfold in a way that fits the rule. However, in order to build the theory in the first place, empirical observations are undertaken, providing data which in turn can be examined and categorised, leading to theory development. This, in contrast, is an inductive line of reasoning where similar patterns arising from a series of examples and applications lead together to posit a theory explaining these patterns. As LeCompte and Preissle succinctly state: 'In a sense, deductive researchers hope to find data to match a theory; inductive researchers hope to find a theory that explains their data'.[2]

It is obvious therefore that both lines of reasoning contribute to the wide picture of research understanding, and both are integral to broad knowledge development. Qualitative research can add considerably to the inductive part of the picture which, until recently, had been somewhat neglected in the health sciences.

The methodological revolution

It is important to grasp the difference between the meanings around the qualitative paradigm as a concept, and qualitative method as a set of research techniques.[3] The term 'paradigm' has gained currency in recent decades, particularly through the work of Thomas Kuhn.[4] In his remarkably influential writings, Kuhn suggests that each scientific community has its own way of viewing what constitutes a scientific problem, and consequently determines the appropriate manner in which it should be addressed. He uses the term 'paradigm' to denote a collective view of what constitutes the nature of the world. He suggests that the set of values arising from this world view guides the investigator in the type of research questions that are asked and in the subsequent methods that allow these questions to best be answered.

There are different approaches to qualitative research, which reflect different underlying philosophical orientations. The main orientations include: phenomenology, ethnography, grounded theory process, feminism, and critical social theory approach. Denzin and Lincoln's text summarises the basis of each of these philosophies and their implications for qualitative process.[5]

Within the health arena, there is a distinct polarisation between the dominant, positivist paradigm, regarded by the scientific method investigators as the only legitimate way through which knowledge can be created, and the alternative, interpretative, qualitative paradigm of the social sciences, which acknowledges the inherent value-laden nature of inquiry. Research undertaken from the former perspective recognises only observed, objective phenomenona and positive facts, whereas research embraced within the latter world view seeks to acknowledge the ability of human beings to interpret their world, and to give meaning to their subjective experiences.

Naturally, the methods used to collect and analyse data within the qualitative paradigm tend to be primarily qualitative. However, it is becoming increasingly common for health-related research studies to use a mix of methods. The purpose here is to add social meanings and subjective values to the basic positivist picture. Guba and Lincoln place mixed methods within what they call the postpositivist paradigm, since they suggest that the perspective that this kind of research takes is from the basic world view of positivism, and yet the methods used to bring this subjectivity and social value into the inquiry are qualitative.[6]

Rigour in qualitative research

The greatest problem conventional quantitative researchers have in appraising the different methodology of qualitative researchers is the inability of the latter to meet the same kinds of standards of rigour and soundness as they expect in their own research. This unrealistic expectation at present forms the widest barrier in the development of strong partnerships for multimethod approaches in the health sciences. Hence, in developing discussion in this chapter on application of qualitative research, we will start with considering issues of standard setting and rigour.

It needs to be made clear that all genuine, knowledge-seeking, ethical researchers attempt overtly to demonstrate the trustworthiness of their work. What is required from the beginning is a recognition that qualitative research methods are chosen primarily because they provide the best way of answering the research question posed. They are not a second-class form of investigation that barely meets the standards of conventional research but an alternative form of investigation that has its own set of criteria against which it should be judged.

Since the criteria for what counts as valuable are so different between the two methodologies, using criteria such as 'reliability' and 'validity' in qualitative circles seems ill advised. This is because objective reality is not sought in qualitative research, nor as a rule is generalisability possible, or even anticipated. The terms therefore are relatively meaningless in this different forum as the research goals are not comparable. Thus, in many of the aspects of rigour discussed in this section, it will be noted that different terms have been developed to describe attainment of appropriate criteria.

Selection and sampling

The first aspect of rigour that needs to be considered is that of systematic selection and sampling. Phenomena to be investigated in any form of research may be studied in a way that allows findings to be generalised more widely, or may be considered purely for their own sake. The former (frequently termed 'probability sampling') is more common as a strategy of quantitative research when a smaller sample is chosen to be representative of a whole population. Exploring something for its own sake is the more common approach in qualitative research and, in the words of Miles and Huberman, 'is not unlike detective work'.[7] Here the research seeks to unravel fine details of specific, purposefully chosen foci of interest. Statistical methods of determining sample size are irrelevant when the purpose is deep understanding of a particular, nominated phenomenon. What is chosen to be studied is done so, purposefully, in the expectation that this one item, or this selection of items, will provide the greatest chance of revealing interesting information to answer the posed research question. Just as a detective follows interesting leads as each reveals itself in the course of an investigation, so in each particular instance, the qualitative researcher places attention on where most can be learned. Consequently, it must be emphasised that there is a decided logic in qualitative sampling, which is different, but no less sound, rational and systematic, from that logic used with quantitative designs.[8] Key aspects of this logic relate to decisions about purposeful selection, the size of the sample, flexibility and data saturation.

Purposeful selection refers to the more general process of exerting options around the circumstances of the study, such as when, where and with whom it will take place. Usually, the more refined the research question, the more specific the selection process will be, thus comfortably minimising the options. When selection is straightforward, the researcher need only delineate the relevant population or phenomenon, justifying this choice for whatever reason, such as theoretical considerations, accessibility or ethical aspects to name a few. Rationale for selection is important to be described in instances where there may be investigation of only one, or a few cases. What is interesting in selection in these instances is that, because there is no requirement to generalise findings, there is often an inclination away from the typical and towards the unique, particular and fascinating, since here is where we may learn most.[9]

Sampling is a more specialised form of selection, referring to the systematic extraction of a subset of a larger population.[10] Again it is essential to justify the reasons for choice, but since in qualitative research our samples are usually of the non-probability type, the logic of sampling follows other leads. In choosing our data sets, we primarily choose a sample which we anticipate will allow us to explore what we purposefully want to explore. This is usually termed 'purposeful' or 'purposive' sampling.[11] A similar approach is theoretical sampling, where the logic is based on the researcher's theoretical reasons for undertaking the study.[12] Occasionally, we just sample less discriminately as in convenience or opportunistic sampling. Despite the negative way this approach is often described in the literature,[13] it may be the most appropriate way to answer the research question, given the situation at the time. The inductive nature of most qualitative research means that, in exploring phenomenon new to us, we may have to take advantage of those people or situations that appear before us. This manner of building a picture of a previously non-researched item is highly regarded in the biological sciences, for example in developing understanding of a newly discovered animal species. Again, as long as an adequate rationale is given, it can be as easily justified as other means. Another useful way of seeking hard-to-reach research participants can be through snowball sampling, where the first individuals taking part refer us on to others who possess the particular characteristics relevant to the study. A chain of respondents can evolve in this way.

An important aspect of sampling in much qualitative research is seeking to find and analyse diverse or opposing perceptions or experiences in a study, especially if it is expected that these perceptions may go against the mainstream findings. Choosing negative or discrepant cases as part of our sample allows the potential for richer data through the need to explore contradictions.[14]

For reasons made clear above, the size of the sample is less a consideration than the actual make-up of the sample itself. Again, it depends on the research question. Much qualitative research explores a single case. A larger sample may be made up of a very few individuals but in-depth interviews with these few may produce very rich and revealing results. In a sense, the size of the sample can be viewed as inversely proportional to the depth and detail of the findings.

When seeking clarity about an unclear phenomenon, it is often valuable to continue collecting data until no new information is revealed. This state of closure of new information is known as 'data saturation'. Many factors influence the decision whether to continue until the data saturates: accessibility, time, and cost, to name a few, but the principal influence arises from what the data is revealing. A key characteristic of qualitative sampling therefore is flexibility with the way the study design ends up being dependent on what is found as the study progresses. Whereas conventional quantitative research endeavours at all costs to meet the predetermined sample size as planned, in qualitative research of an inductive nature, the expected sample can appropriately grow or diminish or change with little predictability as the study unfolds.

Trustworthiness

In order to indicate the extent to which the research is sound, credible and trustworthy, some acceptable processes have developed in qualitative research practice. Triangulation is an important one of these, referring to the use of multiple methods within the one study, for the purpose of reaching a deeper understanding of the phenomenon being researched.[15] The term 'triangulation' has been borrowed from land surveying where it refers to a way of confirming the location of a particular point through taking multiple sights from different perspectives. Denzin and Lincoln remind us that its use in qualitative research does not denote a form of validation but instead, an alternative to validation. Denzin's earlier work describes four types of triangulation.[16] Data triangulation refers to the use of various forms of data sources to gain different perspectives, such as might eventuate in interviews with patients, carers and providers about a disease experience. Investigator triangulation refers to the use of several researchers especially in the analysis and interpretation phases of a study. Theory triangulation refers to the use of multiple theoretical perspectives to interpret a single set of data. Finally, methodological triangulation refers to the combined use of various methods, such as observation, interviewing and document perusal, to study a single problem.

Lincoln and Guba suggest some further methods of establishing the trustworthiness of the research.[17] Among others, these include prolonged engagement and persistent observation, providing an audit trail, and member-checking.

Where possible, most qualitative researchers see the value of undertaking prolonged and persistent engagement with the participants and/or in the setting. Sufficient involvement must occur for the researcher to be satisfied that data being collected are relevant and important to allow the research question to be answered. This advice is particularly related to the building of trust and respect between researcher and researched, a relationship which is essential in the self-exposure so often a mark of qualitative research, and which of necessity takes time. It also is a recognition of the importance of context which can best be experienced with prolonged immersion in the field.

A clearly signposted audit trail is another way to demonstrate trustworthy research. The process of the research should be documented in a way that is trackable. This is much more important in this type of study where the flexibility referred to above allows for the possibility of new and unexpected directions to be taken. The sequence of steps taken and the reason for these steps must be available to any reviewer.

Member-checking is a term coined by Guba and Lincoln to refer to verification with participants as to whether what they said has been interpreted with the meaning they ascribed.[18] The check can occur at any time throughout the research process and can be formal or informal, and with individuals or with groups. As well as providing opportunity for participants to check for errors or to offer additional information, it can also contribute to the analysis phase and to systematic organisation of data.

Peer involvement is another useful mechanism for establishing soundness. The investigator triangulation discussed above would entail the greatest involvement of peer researchers and would allow more than one perspective in each phase of the research. However, it is a common acceptable practice to involve a peer at various different steps of the research process, especially in the analysis phase. It is very reassuring to have another person code and categorise one's own collection of narrative data as confirmation that there is a degree of shared interpretation. However, Morse reminds us that there are many instances where there is a risk that the creative nature of qualitative research analysis will be dampened, and the findings reduced in richness if only those codes that are shared are used.[19]

A final method of establishing soundness is through a variety of ways that qualitative researchers use to document their personal reflections on the research process. The nature of this kind of research is such that not only are the subjective perceptions of the participants valued, so too are those of the researcher. These perceptions are usually clearly exposed in the analysis and interpretation phase as described above, but a continuing documentation of self-reflection can enhance understanding by someone external to the study. Memos included in field notes or dedicated research diaries and journals can achieve this purpose constructively. Grbich acknowledges the value of this form of documentation, but takes the process further, describing it as 'reflexivity'.[20] She emphasises the potential contribution of enhanced self-awareness to the building of joint constructions of meaning and to reducing the power differential that so often exists between the researcher and the researched.

Range of methods of collecting qualitative data

Although there exists a wide range of qualitative data collection methods that have derived from the different research schools or methodologies,[21] within the health arena there are four collection methods that are commonly employed. These are:

- individual, in-depth interviewing,
- focus group discussion,
- document interpretation, and
- participant observation.

This section will relatively briefly outline each of these methods, with the expectation that the reader can explore the finer details of implementing these procedures in any of the many texts covering qualitative research in general. Application of these methods and procedures will be illustrated below in the section dealing with strategies of inquiry.

Just as the more general approach to the research is chosen though a consideration of which approach best allows the research question to be answered, so the specific technique of data collection will be chosen with this consideration in mind. Although some studies will gather data very decidedly through one of these techniques alone, it is very common for a qualitative study in the health arena to gather data by nominating a primary technique, but incorporating aspects of other techniques as well. This combining of techniques can occur as a planned form of triangulation where needed, but is also very valuable as a way of illuminating the study context or adding more detailed description as the study unfolds.

In-depth individual interviewing

This section will outline the characteristics of well-designed and managed, unstructured and semi-structured, interactive interviewing. In addition, the limitations and risks of this form of data collection and analysis will be discussed. Discussion of surveys and structured interviews can be found in other parts of this book, and chapter 10 will help clarify where these different methods stand in relation to each other.

In-depth, individual interviews are chosen as the most appropriate method of gathering data when the purpose of the research is to expose beliefs, perceptions, attitudes and opinions that are otherwise hidden in people's minds. This form of interviewing excels when its purpose is to tap personal experiences in order to understand the meaning individuals give to events and relationships in their lives. It needs to be made very clear that the interviewee's subjective view is the paramount aspect sought here. Open-ended questions used in quantitative studies in order to gain a report of factual situations can appropriately be described as collecting secondary data, because the criticism of limitation of recall can be levelled. In these instances, the criticism is that personal reports *to* the researcher take the place of direct, primary observation *by* the researcher, first hand. However, in contrast to when people are asked for factual responses (e.g., what treatment did you receive on admission?), only individuals themselves can offer a first-hand explanation about what is in their minds (e.g., how did you feel when you had to be admitted for treatment?). This manner of investigation for the purpose of eliciting interviewee's opinions becomes a first choice rather than a second option.

Skills of in-depth interviewing become those of good interpersonal communication since a dialogue is developed between interviewer and interviewee. Enabling a person to reveal deep and sometimes intimate parts of their personal values requires an atmosphere of trust much greater than when eliciting a series of factual short answers, as in undertaking conventional surveys. Adequate time must be allowed to establish this atmosphere before the main focus of the research can take place. Whatever the topic of the interview, it is essential that the questions are phrased in such an open-ended way as to elicit a response which takes the respondent's unique perspective and draws on his or her singular experience.

Patton suggests that there are three types of in-depth interview which result in qualitative data.[22] He terms these the informal conversational interview, the general interview guide approach, and the standardised open-ended interview. From a quantitative researcher's point of view, they would be valued in reverse sequence to the order in which Patton places them.

The standardised open-ended interview has always had a place alongside standardised closed questions. Here, as its name implies, exactly the same question is asked of all respondents but the open-ended phrasing allows for a free response. This form of interviewing is useful when there is limited time, and in instances where variations between interviewers needs to be minimised. A common usage is as part of a survey questionnaire where illumination of some aspects is sought when the researcher does not want to restrict the range of answers. In these instances, the answers are usually coded after collection, so they can be analysed numerically together with the rest of the quantitative data. In other instances, an entire interview can be conducted with standardised questions. Again, the benefit lies in the set structure, but the possible limitation of cutting off the respondent's train of thought can make the answers shallower than in less standardised questioning.

The general interview guide approach is the most commonly used of these three types in the area of health research. Here, the researcher sets out with the purpose of seeking answers to a series of questions during the course of the interview. However, the sequence and actual wording that will be used during the interview are very flexible and the interview guide takes the form of a checklist or reminder, rather than as a collection of questions set in rigid sequence. The resulting free dialogue between interviewer and interviewee allows the discussion to flow naturally, bringing an ability to focus on whatever relevant issues arise and to explore any new information that might not have been expected. This approach results in data in the form of flowing narrative, which can only be coded after the event.

The informal conversational interview, as its name implies, is a free dialogue between interviewer and interviewee where flexibility of content is the primary characteristic, and length and intensity of discussion are only loosely predetermined. The interviewer initiates the conversation in the direction chosen but is prepared for it to flow wherever the respondent takes it. This is the most common form of interviewing used in combination with participant observation, where questioning often evolves to enrich the observation findings. These evolving interviews may be short, to clarify and illuminate a single issue, or they may be built on and repeated over time as an investigation progresses. This form of interview has potential to provide the greatest richness but the breadth of flexibility makes analysis of data more difficult since each interview may range widely in its focus.

As health researchers recognise the need to focus on the social aspects of health and health care as well as the biomedical components, the value of exploring through open responses becomes more and more appreciated, and the inclusion of these forms of interviewing in health research becomes more commonplace.

Focus group interviews or discussions

Open responses are also of value when the exploration takes place with more than one interviewee at the one time. A particular form of group interview, which is becoming increasingly popular in health research, is the focus group interview. Here the interviewer asks a small group of people to focus on a topic of interest for a defined period usually between one to two hours. The popularity of this technique in market research over the past twenty years has been a strong impetus in health researchers recognising the applicability of focus group interviews to their work.[23] Here again the rationale for the use of focus group interviews is similar to that of in-depth individual interviews in that they are not an alternative to seeking factual information, but an appropriate way to elicit data about people's values, feelings, motivations and perceptions that are not able to be revealed in a survey approach.

What is valued and actually exploited in this technique is the tendency for people during social interaction to build on the comments of others. Whereas in individual interviews, respondents can become exhausted of ideas or only dwell on those aspects of highest relevance to themselves, in a focus group interview the answers of one participant may lead to an expansion of ideas subsequently being aired by the rest. Comments from others can raise unexpected issues, consider unanticipated options and generally enhance reflection to an extent rare in the single-person interview. This illumination can lead to a richness about the issue under focus that would be difficult to generate through any other mechanism.

There are some important issues concerning focus group discussions, which must be considered by health researchers if they are to conduct sound, credible studies using this approach. The first issue is one of definition. It has been the experience of the author to review grant applications, read research reports and, on more than one occasion, to accept an invitation to take part as a participant where what has been called a focus group discussion has had little in common with qualitative research techniques. There is a risk that the term can be applied loosely to any group discussion on a focused topic. If focus group interviews are to take their place rightly as legitimate qualitative research and not just ad hoc group meetings, then it is essential that they meet certain criteria, the most important of which are the following:

- As in any research, there must be a clear justification as to why this research method best meets the research question posed.[24]

- The selection of participants must follow a logical sampling structure.[25]
- An interview guide must be developed and if appropriate, trialled, in order to have some consistency across groups.
- The moderator must have high level interpersonal communication skills and have specific training in conducting this form of research.
- Supporting the moderator must be some form of substantial recording of the interaction which will vary depending on each situation, but which might include one or two observers/notetakers and/or audiotape or video recorders.
- There is a need to attain a balance between the moderator controlling the direction of the discussion and the participants being encouraged to discuss the topic openly and freely.
- Analysis mechanisms must be systematic and thorough, leaving a clear audit trail to verify the trustworthiness of the research.

A second issue of importance is that it is essential to recognise that the unit of research is the group as a whole, and not the individuals who separately make it up. A description of the interviewees will be about the make-up of the entire group itself rather than specific details of the actual group members. For example, it would be sound to state that eight groups were conducted with groups ranging in size from five to nine members, but not that 50 people were interviewed and gave their opinions. It would be sound to describe one group as being made up of females who were within an age range of 19 to 25 and who had attained a range of educational levels from year 10 schooling to tertiary qualifications, whereas it would be unsound to state that the group consisted of a female of 20 who had completed year 12, another of 22 who had a bachelor's degree and so on, detailing each person individually. By using the group as the research unit, the unique group characteristics are able to be drawn on, acknowledging that omitting or adding even just one member could substantially change the group's responses.

A third issue is the sampling and selection procedures used. These, of course, depend on the reason for the research. The researcher may want to explore opinions of a sample in a way that the results can be generalised to a wider population, but we know that without statistically based sampling procedures regarding appropriate size and randomness, we cannot draw inferences when there is little probability of this occurring in any other way but by chance. Thus, this limitation must be acknowledged from the start and some alternative approaches developed. The commonest alternative is to convene groups representing the characteristics important in the study. These may be age, education, gender, locality, ethnicity or experience, and so on. It is usual for groups to be homogeneous in some or a few of these characteristics. At least two homogeneous groups illustrating each characteristic should be convened. As an example, market research studies exploring the sales potential of a new children's breakfast cereal might possibly consider asking two groups of boys, two of girls, two of parents and two of retailers to get a picture of their product's acceptability. They may even break their target audiences up further, for instance in seeking to interview children in more affluent localities separately from those with fewer resources, or they may want the opinions of under ten-year-olds as compared with over tens. The researcher would seek to attain data saturation where no new ideas were emerging after eight or ten group interviews had been conducted. If however, one of those groups provided data that differed from the others, it would be most important to explore these differences by setting up further focus groups with participants holding similar characteristics to those in the one producing unusual results.

The results then would, of course, not be able to be generalised in a definitive manner, but they could be explained as indicative of other people's perception as well, and therefore as being worthy of consideration.

Another issue very important in enhancing the soundness of focus group interviews is dealing effectively with negative cases. Since the purpose of this form of research is to generate data about issues that may not be very clear to the researcher, it is important to explore and analyse both the data that build on what has gone before, echoing the direction and intensity of perceptions exposed, and the data that seem to be revealing the opposite. This negative case analysis has been described in an earlier section of this chapter since it has a valuable role to play in all qualitative research. However, the practice of using focus group interview findings alongside survey results to triangulate or enrich quantitative results makes it imperative to address the negative cases. With stringent analysis and cautious comparison, it is possible to consider to what extent these cases refute or amend the more constant emergent themes or patterns.[26]

Documents as data

Another form of collecting data in qualitative research is using written documents or text for analysis and interpretation in the search for meaning and experience. Text may take the shape of formal records such as legal contracts or deeds, or more personally composed items such as diaries and letters. It may be in the form of print media such as newspapers and magazines or in other forms of communication media such as graphic art, films and still photographs.

Analysis of written data in health research is increasing as the social considerations around health and health care are taking on greater significance. Although the various forms of written data could be analysed in a myriad of different ways, the health field has focused on four approaches. These are content analysis, discourse analysis, historical analysis and analysis of pictorial material.

Content analysis is a frequently used approach for exploring written content of newspaper or magazine articles through dissecting the content into smaller components and noting this breakdown.[27] For instance, interesting trends in the amount of newspaper space or the perspectives of coverage given to particular health issues over time are revealed in this way. More often this recording is by quantification, but it is also possible to analyse by theme in a more qualitative way.

Discourse analysis has a much greater qualitative emphasis in exploring the way language, images and symbols create meaning, and in investigating the political and cultural aspects that are revealed through written text. Discourse analysis particularly focuses on the style and the manner in which ideologies are represented, and reveals power relationships through the language used.[28] The analysis focuses not so much on the message per se, but the manner in which the message is conveyed. This form of qualitative research is valuable in exploring text which reveals relationships such as that between patient and practitioner, or the differences in the health beliefs around one issue held by various social groups.

Historical analysis offers to health and health care research the basic strategy of using both primary and secondary data derived from written documents in order to investigate the past to help understand the present.[29] Since the data are already on the page, the difference is in who does the interpretation. Primary sources of historical data are gleaned by the researcher who then critically and systematically interprets them him or herself. Secondary sources are equally important but the evidence is already collected and an interpretation is already at hand. A careful melding of both results in a richer story.

Analysis of pictorial data is a variation on participant observation where, instead of observing the actual situation in the field, the researcher uses the same kinds of qualitative observation methods to gain insights from a series of photographs. The photographer and the researcher may be one and the same person, but not necessarily so. In this type of study the photographer has actually already commenced the interpretation in choosing which scenes and perspectives to film and the sequence in which to present the photographs, and the researcher builds the analysis on this foundation.

Participant observation

Another valuable method of collecting data for health research is participant observation. This method follows the anthropologist's research model, in which the study of people in their natural settings is undertaken using a toolkit of observation techniques, with the researcher becoming immersed in the setting to a greater or lesser degree.[30] Whereas the traditional anthropologist concentrated on a single research setting over a prolonged period, often years, the technique of participant observation has more recently been adapted to be used over shorter time periods and sometimes to cover a number of settings. It is in this recent form that participant observation, or observation in the field, has taken its place in health research.[31]

The primary purpose of this research technique is to collect data in a way that systematically records observations of human behaviour as it occurs within its cultural, social and political context, and in relation to its physical surroundings. The technique allows particularly for documentation and analysis of process and of dynamic action. In most instances, participant observation is valued as a method of generating hypotheses, when little is understood about a particular phenomenon. The inclusion of the context is an essential part of the observation.

Choice can be made as to the degree to which the observer is separate from, or a component of, the natural setting. Observation involves primarily the visual sense but the information gleaned can be enhanced through feeling, smelling, tasting and especially hearing, with informal conversational interviews being commonly used to illuminate visual observations and to clarify meanings. Denzin and Lincoln describe a researcher of this type as a 'bricoleur',[32] one who uses whatever tools can best meet the need to answer the research question posed.

Collecting the data through observation is only one part of the technique. It is expected that interpretation of the data will occur concurrently from the moment the research starts, and is not restricted to a post-data collection analysis only. The documentation of the observation should be done in a way that allows this to occur. In writing up the observations, the researcher/observer may add comments and opinions in the margins, or as word processor memos, as they come to mind. This iterative use of observation and interpretation allows the research to focus on areas of interest that arise as the study progresses, and to actively influence the course of the study. Being open to attend to anything that occurs allows a rich, intense description to evolve.

Two important considerations must be kept in mind. The first is that researchers should interpret the data from their unique frames of reference, with subjectivity being welcomed. The researcher *is* the instrument. Anticipating this subjective view, researchers are expected to reveal 'up-front' the assumptions and perspectives brought to the research.[33] As a result, participant observation research reports usually include details of whether researchers are insiders or outsiders to the setting, and the relevant, existing assumptions they bring to the study. Second, the ethics of the observation must be addressed. Observations undertaken in private settings may require permission, but an unobtrusive observer in a public place may not. However, since many health behaviours such as sun protection practices or food choices are public activities, steps must be taken to retain trust.

Try the data collection exercise (exercise 9.1), either by yourself, or with a small group. This exercise gives you the opportunity to undertake a very short, focused, systematic, participant observation exercise, to start the process of understanding the contribution that this data collection method might make to your work in health. The exercise covers data collection only and does not address analysis.

Exercise 9.1 Participant observation

Seek out a place where people gather, where you can jot notes about what is happening without being conspicuous. Possible health settings include a clinic waiting room, a hospital ward, the playground of an early childhood centre or the gymnasium of a rehabilitation centre. You may wish to undertake a health-related observation outside a health setting, such as on the beach, observing sun protection behaviour, or in the park, watching levels of physical activity.

Take your pad and pen, choose a viewing spot and make a documented observation of these people, using the following guidelines:

- Write a research question on the top of the first page, so you can focus on a particular purpose in the observation. Examples might be: 'How do people fill their time in a clinic waiting room?' or 'What encourages sun-protection behaviour at the beach?'
- Draw a wide margin on your pad pages so you have room in the margin for comments you may add at any later time.
- Start timing your ten-minute observation.
- Commence writing, describing the site or setting before describing the people and their activities.
- Differentiate between factual description as opposed to interpretive description, but document both.

For example, you may want to describe an observed person's behaviour as 'angry'. However, 'angry' is your interpretation, so try to consider what were the more factual observations underneath, which led to an interpretation of anger. It may be that the person being observed spoke loudly using strong words; she may have used sudden, decisive arm movements and gestures; she may have clenched her jaw. The 'angry' person may not have been as revealing as the person to whom the anger was addressed—he may have cringed to the extent that discomfort was really evident. These are the more factual, objective observations which when taken together, can be interpreted as 'anger'. This differentiation is critical in cross-cultural studies as a simple gesture that has a very innocent meaning in one culture could be interpreted as an offensive gesture in another.

When you have completed the ten minutes of recording what you have observed, reflect on what you have done. Did you find it revealing that you saw so much more by being systematic? Did you feel uncomfortable? It can feel very rude to be looking at people and writing down things about them. (This brings in aspects of ethics in deciding when it is necessary to gain permission, and if by doing so you might cause those being observed to behave differently.) Did you feel it was impossible to write fast enough to get all the information on paper in a limited time? Finally, did you gain by endeavouring to separate the factual from the interpretive?

Qualitative data analysis

The social sciences have developed clear guidelines for analysis of qualitative data but these have rarely made their way into the journals or textbooks of health researchers since for so long the scientific method has held sway. From the start, the issues in analysis of qualitative data are two: first, to systematically organise and manage copious data in the form of words; and second, to make sense of the data in a way that is more than just intuitive ideas arising from anecdotal material.[34] A definitive aspect of qualitative research is its flexibility, so that when initial data analysis reveals certain patterns developing, it is likely that more data may be sought, or that a change in direction may occur. Hence, it is impossible to separate cleanly the sequence of method, findings (or results) and reflections on the findings (or discussion) since a well-executed study will revisit each of these steps iteratively.

Huberman and Miles have worked to systematise the processes of qualitative analysis.[35] Although they may be criticised for suggesting an approach that is so structured that it could mask creativity in dealing with the data, it is generally agreed they have added further respectability to qualitative methodology through the precision they advocate. They recommend that the process of analysis be divided into three parts: data reduction, data display and conclusion drawing or verification. By data reduction, Miles and Huberman refer to 'the process of selecting, focusing, simplifying, abstracting and transforming the "raw" data that appear in written-up field notes'.[36] They point out that the mass of words collected in a qualitative research study must be 'tidied up' so that it is accessible for analysis, but that whatever the manner the reduction occurs, it is important that this process never 'strips the data at hand from the contexts in which they occur'.[37] The essential component of this part of analysis is to revisit the research question and to reorganise the data in relation to this question. The importance of having the research question firmly in mind from the time the research is first planned, and then revisiting it continually throughout the analysis phase cannot be overemphasised. In this way, the issues arising from the data collected are always seen in relation to what the study is seeking to investigate.

Data display refers to some form of matrix, chart or concept map that reveals patterns that are arising from the data and that indicates relationships that can be seen to be developing. Conclusion drawing or verification is the process of gradually finding meaning from the mass of data. Initial conclusions may be tentative but these become more solid as further analysis confirms or refutes them. Miles and Huberman depict these three steps in an iterative way, indicating that they do not occur in a linear sequence, but each step is revisited as needed.

The precision sought by Miles and Huberman is counterbalanced by the writings of such authors as Janesick.[38] Here the creative and interpretive aspects of qualitative research are seen as the essential conditions through which findings are revealed. The lived experiences and personal meanings sought through these approaches require a degree of artistry and inventiveness in working towards their exposure. Rather than following a predetermined and structured process, Janesick suggests that good qualitative researchers use their artistic abilities to interpret the material that is before them. She points out that qualitative researchers expect and acknowledge that they will be bringing their own values and personal biases to the research, and they identify themselves and their ideological perspective clearly, as part of their introduction to the study or within their description of method. All analysis then proceeds with this knowledge in mind, so that the reader knows, for instance, whether female doctors have been interviewed by a male sociologist of similar age but with very different background, or whether a participant observation of a group of disabled persons has been undertaken by another disabled resident of the same group home. The revelation of whether the researcher is an insider bringing an emic view or an outsider bringing an etic perspective helps the meanings exposed in the findings retain their personalised and contextualised character.

As discussed earlier in this chapter, the use of inductive reasoning becomes central to the effort of searching for meanings in the data. The categories or codes into which we separate the mass of written material should ideally be chosen as the researcher becomes embedded in the data. The alternative of using predetermined categories is not wrong, but it would put the research back into the positivist paradigm. These categories can then be arranged and rearranged into a conceptual whole where the smaller categories can be clumped into themes, and the patterns of their relationships to each other indicated. The resulting conceptual map, which may be graphically depicted or may not have taken form outside the researcher's mind, then must be written in narrative form, with all pertinent findings supported by evidence documented in the field notes, transcriptions or other collected records. In other words, whereas in quantitative research the tables of numbers provide the evidence on which the research report builds a case, here the illustrative quotes are performing this same essential function. The quotes serve the purpose therefore not only of enriching the descriptive findings, but also of verifying the researcher's report and indicating how the findings have arisen from the data.

Computer-supported analysis

The bane of qualitative researchers' lives is the huge mass of data which emanates from the detailed observations and deep interviews. Setting up a way to manage such copious amounts of the written word can be daunting. Recent developments in the form of dedicated software programs, which aid in the management and analysis of the data collected, have brought about a revolution in the qualitative research arena. What is even better is that the earlier versions of these programs that were relatively time-demanding and somewhat tedious to use in the recent past are now being upgraded to be more user-friendly and faster. For instance, the Australian program NUD*IST has a new version in their series, entitled NVIVO, which was released in 1999 and which asserts that its best quality is its increased user-friendliness.[39] However, since everything to do with computers changes so quickly, this is not the place to assess the various programs or to make comparisons across the range available. Readers interested in making contact with such program suppliers can easily search the Web to gain appropriate information.

Basically, the merit of these programs is their ability to systematically store, code and retrieve chunks of written data in a way that allows precise and purposeful manipulation. The computer makes analysis easier because of its systematic operation around the data, but it must be emphasised that the actual analysis is still done by the researcher. As was made clear in the section above, the categorisation of data into meaningful themes and patterns is not a process chore but an artistic and creative venture. However, the viewing and reviewing of data which is an essential process in qualitative data analysis is made easy and inviting, and may therefore prevent creativity from being stalled in the face of too much material.

Research report

Once the analysis is well under way, the research report will then take form. As has been emphasised throughout this chapter, it is well worth keeping in mind that this form of research does not fit comfortably into quantitative research patterns, so that the usual section headings of introduction, literature review, method, results and discussion may not fit. Instead, the iterative nature of good qualitative studies means that these sections tend to run into each other and be revisited. For instance, sometimes the exploration of the literature may actually be a component of the investigation rather than a prior activity. Frequently, the procedures used change considerably as the research progresses, with the researcher choosing to change the original proposal to do more or fewer interviews, to seek different respondents from those originally nominated or to observe in further settings. Because a qualitative researcher is so often seeking the unanticipated and the unexpected, the interpretations of the researcher are revealed as the analysis is written up rather than at the end in the discussion.

Consequently, to account for these factors, slightly different section headings are recommended. The introduction comes closest to the quantitative pattern, although tight research objectives usually give way to more appropriate open research questions. The literature review section may become one entitled 'The evolution of the study', founding the study as much on local context as on global literature.[40] The method probably needs a preliminary section justifying the use of qualitative methods in the anticipation that the reader will need more description here than would be needed in a conventional research design. The results sections usually becomes 'Findings', so that the inclusion of the researcher's interpretations can accompany the analysis results as they are revealed. Discussion may become 'Reflection' to indicate the overall reviewing undertaken at this stage. Finally, attention to the article or report title is important. Readers may like to explore the frequency with which headings given to qualitative study reports are drawn from quotes from research participants, and the consequent punch that this inclusion brings with it. (However, overly clever titles, using quotes, may not reveal the actual subject of the research sufficiently well—and could mean that future researchers disregard the article even if search facilities bring it up because of relevant keywords.)

Strategies of inquiry in health research that lend themselves to qualitative methods

In order to make more sense of the value of qualitative methods to health research, this section will briefly discuss some recent applications of these methods with which the author has been associated. An attempt has been made to illustrate how different research questions within health and health care can be addressed appropriately.

Assessing community health needs

In recent years, health care with a community focus has moved from being a reaction to individual patients' needs to being proactive, intervening sooner in the natural progression of disease. Prior to this development, the dominant form of community health care had been on a one-to-one basis between practitioner and patient, and the resulting health care intervention had been in response to the condition that brought the patient to the practitioner. Recent movements towards population health have emphasised the value of regarding the community as a whole and implementing health promotion, health protection and disease prevention programs to enhance the health of the community earlier. When the community is regarded as a whole instead of as a collection of separate individuals, an important step in promotion and prevention programs is to assess the community's health needs before planning and implementing strategies to counter the health problems.

In these circumstances, the voice of community members must be heard and understood. Moreover, community members must be given the opportunity to identify the health concerns as they see them rather than as the authorities see them, and to suggest ways that these concerns can be addressed. As a result, qualitative methods are frequently used to tap community perspectives.[41]

The author has recently been involved in seeking the perceptions of Spanish-speaking women, in a metropolitan area health service in Australia, regarding their beliefs about menopause, their understanding of the role of hormone replacement therapy and their relationship with the medical fraternity in seeking good health care.[42] The overall research question asked was: What are the experiences of South American-born women regarding menopause? Focus group interviews were the method of choice since the purpose of the research was to gain deeper understanding about the needs of this group of women. Additionally, focus groups were chosen because the group situation was felt to be less threatening to those who may fear interrogation. Findings revealed that in the case of these women, the health professionals who serve them have a way to go to really understand how best to support them at this stage of their lives. However, an unanticipated finding was that these women felt that the opportunity to address issues of concern in this type of friendly forum was empowering for them. As a sequence to this research activity, some of the women have organised to continue to meet regularly to enhance their capacity to cope with issues of this nature.

Understanding patients' health-related perceptions

A similar issue to assessing health needs is to explore why some unexplained health-related behaviours occur. Unless we understand what motivates people to do what they do, we are not in a position to help change to more positive behaviours. Motivation is a poorly understood aspect of people's ways of addressing the world, and is usually highly individualised. The author was involved in a recent study that took account of these factors in a paediatric emergency department in a teaching hospital.[43] The general research question was: Why do so many parents utilise the emergency department for non-emergency situations with their children? A previous quantitative investigation had indicated clearly, in number terms, that emergency department visits were being used for non-emergency situations, but not the reason. The qualitative investigation was undertaken using in-depth individual interviews with twenty-five parents in the waiting room of the emergency department, and analysed inductively through searching for emergent themes. Of the dominant themes identified, the primary one of interest in this study was the new understanding that parental triage was based on definite but different criteria from those used by health professionals in triaging patients according to the urgency of care required. This new understanding was allowed to emerge through the openness of the research procedures used, which offered opportunities for respondents to discuss issues not anticipated by the researchers. Further research is needed to test the hypotheses generated since the findings have quite important implications for health service planning.

Exploring health professional practice

It is not only the motivations of patients that need to be explored. Another valuable use of qualitative research methods in health is in investigating perceptions and perspectives held by health professionals regarding their practice. A recent study was undertaken to examine the role of prevention in the practice of rural community nurses.[44] The basic research question posed was: What is the lived experience of rural community nurses of including prevention in their practice? To address this question, four rural nurses were invited to participate in long, detailed, in-depth interviews. The findings were fascinating in that they raised aspects of rural nursing competencies not previously adequately considered in preparing these staff for their job roles. Nurses discussed how they felt they had to respond to a demand to move between two models of practice: a valued one of clinical care and a much less valued one of prevention. Whereas it had been expected that the preventive/promotive role could be integrated into their regular work, the study revealed that in the practice of these four nurses, the integration did not happen. These findings may have major implications for those attempting to build the capacity of any and all health workers to include health promotion in their work, since the assumption of health service decision-makers that integration is straightforward and simple is not supported in these four instances. Further studies are now needed to test these new observations.

Another study of professional practice was recently undertaken where the research question was: What makes one physiotherapist better than another?[45] In particular, the research asked: How do clinical experts in rheumatology-physiotherapy approach a clinical problem? The study sought to investigate whether there were common patterns in the cognitive processes, knowledge structure and artistry of seven identified 'experts'. Each was presented with the same hypothetical case and asked individually at interview to think-aloud how they would manage this case. The analysis revealed that these seven physiotherapists did not follow a consistent cognitive process in their clinical management and no formula on the processes leading to expert decision-making could be elicited from this exploration. However, in these seven cases, consideration of context and content were seen to be far more important in this decision-making than the literature currently implies.

Revealing the meanings behind cultural practices

An essential prerequisite to working with any peoples whose health is a concern is to have some understanding of how they view the world and what prompts them to have the beliefs they hold dear. This is difficult enough when health professionals and community members or patients have the same social and ethnic backgrounds, but it becomes exceedingly problematic when different traditional cultural beliefs and practices are the dominant determinant of behaviour for people in a community. Here, qualitative research methods are being used increasingly to determine the meaning behind traditional cultural practices, in order that they can be harnessed, rather than confronted, in the quest for better health. An in-depth ethnographic study was conducted in Cambodia with traditional healers, with the overall research question posed being: What is the meaning behind current beliefs held by Cambodians and their traditional healers which lead to current practices in child rearing?[46]

Close to a thousand traditional healers from all provinces in Cambodia were involved, resulting in a rich understanding of many previously misunderstood practices. There are immense implications in this new understanding, which can lead to better support for Cambodians when they are confronted with the Western medical system, both in their own country and as migrants outside it.

Making observations of a case

Qualitative research methods have also proved to be very valuable in case studies undertaken usually through participant observation, although interviewing and perusal of textual material are also appropriate methods of collecting data. Just as the term 'case history' in the health disciplines refers to documented observations by a health professional of a patient, so the term 'case study' can apply to the documented observations of individuals, whether patients or practitioners, of groups or of settings or systems. Stake suggests that 'Case study is not a methodological choice but the choice of object to be studied'.[47] Whether exploring one phenomenon or several, the case study is the classic qualitative approach to sampling for understanding rather than representativeness. An example illustrating this form of research was undertaken by Kavanagh when she researched nursing functions in respect of discharge planning.[48] Her research questions were two: What functions are common to nurse discharge planners across a variety of specialty areas of care? What expertise is required for nurse discharge planners to fulfil these functions? Kavanagh's primary finding was that the context of practice shaped what the nurses did much more than what was written regarding their role definition. Her findings have implications for the need for education of nurse discharge planners to be more flexible and visionary.

Participatory action research as evaluation of health-related practice in a community context

Participatory action research (PAR) refers more to an approach for knowledge development than to a method in itself. Based on an ideological foundation of researching *with* rather than *on* people, PAR is a form of qualitative research where the purpose is to explore 'what should be' more than 'what is', where participants are co-researchers in decisions regarding the way the research progresses and where action and investigation occur concurrently.[49] Given that health promotion practice, to be effective, seems to need to be multistrategic and multifaceted, and to actively place itself within a specific context, evaluation of community-based health projects in conventional ways that seek to evaluate a single variable in a controlled context are bound to produce inconsequential findings.[50] PAR has recently attracted attention as a means of evaluating projects in a way that focuses on the dynamics of the process and is consumer driven. Additionally, this form of research coupled with action is a most appropriate way to translate to implementation the recent emphasis on promoting the health of less-advantaged groups.

The author had the opportunity of co-researching with 40 blue-collar workers in a steelworks to answer the general research question: To what extent can blast furnace workers take control of addressing their identified health concerns in a way that optimises their current and future health? The PAR process proceeded in a series of spirals of four sequential steps: raising issues, making plans, implementing action, and lastly, reflecting on the outcome. Each spiral led into the next, thus strengthening the capacity of participants to make decisions regarding their health. In general the outcomes of each spiral were positive and the workers achieved some very constructive changes primarily in the workplace environment and minimally in personal behaviours. However, participants doubted they could sustain the process after the withdrawal of the initiating researcher at the end of the allocated time.[51]

To explore a similar process with another relatively voiceless group, the author was part of a PAR approach with older persons who are residents of three urban retirement villages.[52] The same four-part process was initiated with surprisingly high participation of village residents. As with the steelworkers, the entry phase was very important in allowing rapport and trust to develop between the initiating researcher and the participants as co-researchers. Once a firm relationship had been established, the process was straightforward and the residents in each retirement village were proud to influence changes addressing many of their health concerns.

The contribution of qualitative research to evidence-based practice

The recent focus on evidence-based practice that has swept through the health disciplines has brought conventional scientific method back into the limelight.[53] This is so, as described earlier in this chapter, because only research in the positivist paradigm is able to predict outcomes, and can show a linear relationship between cause and effect.

However, this pronounced emphasis on scientific method risks reducing consideration of the humanistic aspects. Within the realm of health care, there is a marked difference between seeking an objective research outcome and pursuing an individual clinical care outcome. As Cox has written so succinctly: 'Scientific method focuses on one variable at a time across a hundred identical animals to extract a single, generalisable 'proof' or piece of 'truth'. Clinical practice deals with a hundred variables at a time within one animal ... in order to optimise a mix of outcomes intended to satisfy the particular animal's current needs and desires.'[54]

Without input that allows the people involved to reveal their experiences, perceptions, beliefs and opinions, a real gap remains in our understanding. It is not useful to the health disciplines to know that theoretically a course of treatment is likely to produce effective results if people are not complying with that treatment. It appears that the error lies in a narrow definition of the term 'evidence'.

Evidence-based practice in health care, prevention and health promotion must draw its evidence from two dimensions, both the more objective, technical research results and the more subjective, personal perspectives, as experienced by those who are recipients of these interventions. The challenge lies in investigating and documenting the latter form of evidence in a manner that meets the criteria expected of good research.[55]

Here is one example of response to such a challenge to traditional 'evidence' summary, as might be posed to physiotherapists: 'How do adolescents with asthma interpret their peak flow readings to make decisions about school sport involvement?' This entails a continuing process of inquiry, perhaps beginning with a detailed qualitative exploration of the adolescents' behaviour, either by observation or interview. The answers elicited by a qualitative study of this nature might reveal patterns of behaviour which subsequently could be subjected to a conventional quantitative study to test the relationships so revealed.[56]

The richness of understanding that qualitative methods can bring cannot be underestimated. The incorporation of qualitative research methods in the total picture of evidence-based practice can only enrich and enhance the research process and lead to fuller knowledge development.

10
Quality and quantity

DEBORAH SALTMAN AND NATALIE O'DEA

The aim of this chapter is to assist researchers to decide which research technique, qualitative or quantitative, will best answer their questions. Through a series of tables and figures, this chapter provides a quick reference to a range of issues that affect the choice of technique. The continuum of research will also be covered, including ways in which both qualitative and quantitative research can be applied consecutively to research themes over time. An example of application of both types of methods in a single study is explained, and the reasoning behind method choice in different health contexts is explored. Basic concepts of qualitative and quantitative research are revisited, so that this chapter may be read on its own.

As you read, you should note that these authors routinely use qualitative techniques as an adjunct to a more quantitative approach. The alternative, to emphasise qualitative approaches, is best illustrated in Jan Ritchie's chapter 9. Combining the methods often highlights a researcher's preferred paradigm as the dominant feature in the research.

What is qualitative and quantitative research?

The two main research techniques that dominate health research are qualitative and quantitative work. To some researchers the terms 'qualitative' and 'quantitative' refer to methodological approaches, while to others, the terms describe paradigms which are fundamentally different, encompassing a different view of the world. For example, qualitative research is contextual and driven by the environment of the research, whereas quantitative research is grounded in scientific method and empiricism. The philosophies behind these research styles have been explored in more detail in previous chapters. The reader could revisit chapters 4 and 9 in particular to consider the underpinnings of the different research approaches. This chapter is more concerned with the application of these techniques in the health arena.

Qualitative research

Qualitative research is any kind of research that produces findings not arrived at by means of quantification.[1] Themes for qualitative inquiry usually focus on an in-depth study of real world situations over time without manipulating them.[2] Qualitative research emphasises processes and meanings rather than specific measurement. Qualitative questions may begin with the words 'how', 'what', 'who' and 'why'. The research questions are usually open-ended and the answer is longer than 'yes' or 'no'. The data used to answer such broad questions are usually obtained from in depth interviews or through observation. The key features of qualitative research include capturing the individual's point of view, examining aspects of every day life and ensuring that the ensuing descriptions are full of detail. The depth of qualitative research makes it difficult to reproduce.

Quantitative research

The scientific method which is the basis of quantitative research requires that a researcher proposes a theory and subjects that theory to empirical testing. The conduct of quantitative research is concerned with applying theories and techniques (both descriptive and inferential) to assist in the manipulation of the data.[3] The capacity to count and aggregate data with precise methods is the basic principle underlying quantitative research.

The reproducibility of quantitative research is enhanced by its adherence to the scientific method. In quantitative research, a series of questions are posed that can be answered numerically, in a graded fashion or by 'yes' and 'no'. One of the features of quantitative research is the reliance on statistics. Statistics can be used in many ways.[4] Chapters 5, 6 and 7 describe statistical analyses in some detail.

Table 10.1 What are the benefits and limitations of each research technique?

Qualitative	Quantitative
Benefits	*Benefits*
The ability to examine situations in depth with open-ended questions.	The capacity to capture a breadth of information within a closed answer format.
The capacity to explore complex questions.	The ability to provide a simple answer.
A research framework with flexibility to respond to the needs of participants.	A research framework which is reliable and reproducible.
The capacity to provide explanations for quantitative findings.	The capacity to quantify a qualitative finding.
The ability to produce meaningful results from a small population study.	The capacity to deal with a large study population.
The potential to assist in the development of quantitative projects.	The acceptance of secondary analysis of data to provide further information.
Limitations	*Limitations*
The intrusiveness of the researcher with probing questions.	The necessity to confine questions that can only be answered numerically, in a graded fashion or by 'yes' or 'no'.
Rigour on its own merit, but often limited statistical validity and reliability in quantitative terms.	The tendency to use a large sample size to allow for statistically significant results on analysis of many factors at one time.
Varied interpretations of recollections.	The constraints of reproducibility.
The lack of transportability of findings.	Detailed knowledge of statistical methods.
The potential to identify symptoms only for small populations and not core problems.	The need for a large or complex sample if the result is to be generalised to a population.
The lack of recognition of this technique by quantitative researchers.	The need for representativeness, which may be technically difficult.

Table 10.1 outlines the benefits and limitations of each research technique, from a researcher's perspective.

In choosing a research technique to commence or continue research, the two most important questions we need to ask are: 'What type of research does the topic lend itself to?', and, 'What style of research is appropriate for the current phase of the research?' The questions that we ask are best phrased in a way that is parsimonious enough to allow us to complete the research task within whatever budgetary and time constraints exist, and yet broad enough to ensure that we will have a meaningful answer at the end. The following series of questions may help you to choose the technique that best suits your research needs.

What am I looking for?

The formulation of a specific research question must relate to the topic chosen. In general, research helps us to explore a new topic, describe the world and/or explain why something occurred. When you phrase your research question, it is important to work out what you would like to know. For example, when a well-defined answer is not expected, a qualitative method may be more appropriate.

Conversely, when an answer may be well defined and categorised, a quantitative methodology may be more effective.

Qualitative and quantitative research questions are quite different. Qualitative studies usually look for meaning by exploring breadth or depth of an issue. The open-ended nature of qualitative questions are useful to review topic areas where there is some complexity that cannot be simplified into a 'yes' or 'no' answer. For example, a qualitative question might be: 'What are patients feeling about the type of health care they receive and how do these feeling impact on their care?'. Not all qualitative research begins with a clearly defined research question. Qualitative research may begin with a series of observations, such as looking at the way a group of health professionals work together on a mental health program.

A quantitative research question is more confining and defining. A quantitative question demands an answer. Therefore the broader the quantitative question, the less likely it will be able to provide an answer. For example, the question 'Does a particular anti hypertensive drug lower blood pressure?' can be answered with a simple 'yes' or 'no'.

While the quantitative question appears straightforward, it is quite narrow in what it tells us. If the answer to the above question is 'no', then all we know is that the particular medication in question does not lower blood pressure. We do not know if the medication raises blood pressure or keeps blood pressure the same or what else the medication does. This type of unidirectional hypothesis is very resource intensive and often frustrating as the question is quite specific and the answer quite narrow.

A more effective way of using hypotheses in quantitative research is to employ the null hypothesis. With the null hypothesis, we postulate the lack of a relationship between two variables. Thus, our question, or exploration, about blood pressure now becomes: 'There is no relationship between a particular anti hypertensive and subsequent blood pressure.' It is easier to prove this question false than it is to prove the previous question correct.

If you are exploring a new topic, a qualitative question may be more useful. It does not confine your thoughts, but rather allows you to cast your net as broadly as possible over a broad range of issues. Some refining is necessary to shape the idea into a topic that is researchable. Pilot studies using focus groups or individual interviews can help a researcher narrow down a project to a manageable question. While qualitative research may be useful in the initial stages, once some clear research questions have been teased out, it may be useful to undertake some quantitative work to provide more concrete and specific answers. Thus, a qualitative study has led to a quantitative one.

Sometimes, these answers are unexpected or do not explain the issues we sought to look at in the first place. In such cases, the quantitative research may be followed up with some qualitative research to explore the meaning behind the facts. This qualitative–quantitative–qualitative cycle is the traditional relationship

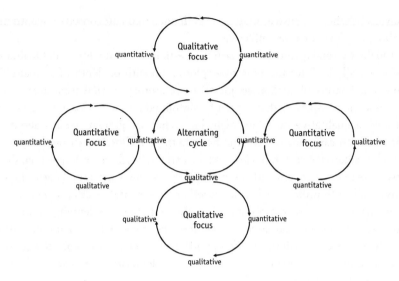

Figure 10.1 Aleternating cycle of research methods

between qualitative and quantitative research. When these methodologies are alternately sequenced, it may be described as an alternating cycle, as in figure 10.1.

Not all studies start with a qualitative focus. Sometimes data have been collected for one purpose, such as census data. These data are then available to a researcher for secondary analysis. Such a project may commence with a quantitative focus. Often the topic under research lends itself to a continuous process with one project leading on to the next. Following an initial qualitative or quantitative phase, ensuing questions may lend themselves to either methodology.

While the research process can be seen as a continuum of different components that require a variety of methodologies over time, particular topics may lend themselves to different methodologies or research sequences. For example, social sciences, sociology and anthropology have embraced qualitative methods, whereas public health has adopted a more quantitative framework.

Other relationships between qualitative and quantitative enquiry are also possible. A case study of how research questions and methodologies interdigitate around a central theme of aged care is shown diagrammatically in figure 10.2 below. In this case study, certain questions in aged care lent themselves to qualitative analysis—as illustrated in the questions: 'What do elderly patients want to know about their functioning?' and 'What do they make of this information?'. Other questions in the study were best answered by quantitative techniques—as demonstrated in the questions: 'Does functioning relate to service provision?' and 'Can functioning predict costs?'.

In answering the qualitative question 'what is functioning in the elderly?', a focus group could be convened by the local University of the Third Age. A facilitator might ask the group to describe what functioning means to them. This

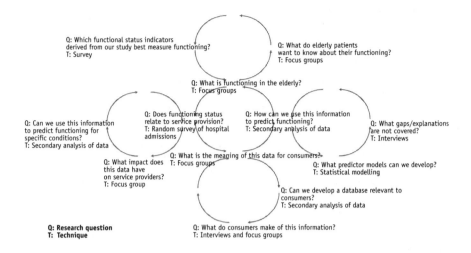

Q: Which functional status indicators
derived from our study best measure functioning?
T: Survey

Q: What do elderly patients
want to know about their functioning?
T: Focus groups

Q: What is functioning in the elderly?
T: Focus groups

Q: Can we use this information
to predict functioning for
specific conditions?
T: Secondary analysis of data

Q: Does functioning status
relate to service provision?
T: Random survey of hospital
admissions

Q: How can we use this information
to predict functioning?
T: Secondary analysis of data

Q: What gaps/explanations
are not covered?
T: Interviews

Q: What is the meaning of this data for consumers?
T: Focus groups

Q: What impact does
this data have
on service providers?
T: Focus group

Q: What predictor models can we develop?
T: Statistical modelling

Q: Can we develop a database relevant to
consumers?
T: Secondary analysis of data

Q: **Research question**
T: **Technique**

Q: What do consumers make of this information?
T: Interviews and focus groups

Figure 10.2   Alternating cycle: An aged care case study

discussion would be transcribed and analysed for themes. In such a study, the older persons identified a range of activities and states of mental health that they associated with optimal functioning.[5] The analysis here was qualitative and involved reviewing the data and analysing complex issues and themes which could not be dichotomised.

To assess how the perception of older persons' functioning relates in a clinical setting, the themes identified in the focus groups could form the basis of a survey of general practitioner attitudes to functioning in the elderly. A random sample of general practitioners might be surveyed with a questionnaire to assess how their perceptions of the views of older persons matched the data obtained from the focus groups. The analysis here would be a quantitative one.

How flexible do I want my study?

Flexibility in a research study is a factor of the capacity of the institution, the researchers and the research design. The capacity for an institution to change research direction mid stream may be low or high. For example, a laboratory that is set up to conduct genetic testing would be highly specialised, and therefore projects involved in the laboratory would be well defined before the research commences. Similarly, the capacity of an institution to conduct qualitative or quantitative research may determine its flexibility with either type of research.

While superficially, qualitative research appears to be more flexible in that it requires less institutional infrastructure, there may be other areas of inflexibility. For example, reference groups and consumer involvement in qualitative studies

Table 10.2   Design flexibility

Technique		Research facility size	Available technology	Consumer involvement	Community/ institution	Change resulting from study
Qualitative						
	Observational studies	Small	Simple	Low	Both	Minimal/long term
	Focus groups	Small	Simple	Medium/ high	Both (better in community)	Local/long term
	Personal interview	Small	Simple	High/ individual	Both (better in community)	Minimal/long term
	Telephone interviews	Small	Simple	Low	Community	Minimal/long term
Qualitative or quantitative						
	Mail surveys	Large	Complex	Low	Community	High/medium term
Quantitative						
	Telephone surveys	Large	Complex	Low	Community	High/short term
	Written unstructured feedback	Large	Simple	High/ individual	Both	Minimal/long term
	Randomised controlled trials	Large	Complex	Low	Both (better in institution)	High/short term
	Cohort studies	Large	Complex	Low	Both(better in institution)	High/medium term
	Analysis of secondary data	Small	Variable	Minimal/ none	Institution	Medium/long term

take some time to acclimatise and therefore also require some time to work with changed directions.

The type of outcome required from a study may also determine its flexibility. A quantitative study designed to look at the health of a population over a number of years, such as the Framingham study, must be relatively inflexible so that the data collected during the study period is comparable.[6] Conversely, a qualitative study conducted as a quality assurance initiative looking at work practices within a hospital has as its focus short-term changes, or a study of attitudes of consumers to mental health providers may be seeking to inform long-term change, and therefore may be more flexible within the study design.[7] Table 10.2 summarises some of the features which affect design flexibility.

The choice of methodology should not take away the creativity and innovation that encouraged research to be undertaken in the first place. Making choices between methodologies can be exciting. It often involves a degree of self-reflection ('What type of project do I have the skills and energy to complete?') and corporate analysis ('What resources are available to complete this project?').

What resources do I need to conduct my research?

Qualitative and quantitative research require different sets of resources. Qualitative research is usually more manageable by an individual or small team. An individual can conduct a qualitative project with little assistance as long as they are trained appropriately. Labour and opportunity cost are the major drains on resources in this type of research. Qualitative research requires a range of expertise: skills in undertaking interviews and focus groups and analysing the data obtained are important.

Conducting research in environments where part of the process involves developing relationships with the participants can be very time consuming. Also, once this type of data is collected, the analysis requires even more energy. Transcription of interviews and focus group proceedings for example, can take longer than originally anticipated. As a rule of thumb, one hour of taped interviews takes three hours to transcribe and approximately twenty hours to analyse. For researchers not skilled in transcription, a dedicated transcriber may be necessary. This person needs to have not only typing and transcribing skills but a high level of accuracy in picking up and incorporating other verbal cues such as silences and encouragers. Maintaining the anonymity of data may also be an issue in qualitative studies. The researchers will need to be sure that the transcriber does not recognise any of the voices on the tape.

In quantitative research, a wide range of resources are often required over long periods of time. In the beginning, much planning is needed to develop a project that is designed to collect large amounts of data to be analysed. Forming a research team is an integral part of this early planning. The research team will need to include a competent biostatistician to advise on research design and analysis, someone familiar with quantitative research methodologies, a group of field researchers, someone capable of data entry and analysis, and finally, someone skilled in the writing up of quantitative research projects. In well-established teams, these roles may overlap.

To enrol enough people in a study to attain statistical significance, it is often necessary to conduct research over a number of sites. Multicentre research trials require additional resources. Much more co-ordination and a spread of resources over geographically separate locations are required for a successful multicentre trial. These activities can add exponentially to the cost of a project.

In summary, the major differences between qualitative and quantitative research in terms of resources is the type of resources needed, for example, expertise in social science methodology (qualitative research) or expertise in statistical methods (quantitative research). Qualitative research can often be conducted in one geographic location which keeps expenses down. Also, an experienced qualitative researcher can often perform many of the roles required in the team. Qualitative research is more labour-intensive of the individual researcher, whereas quantitative research requires a larger team.

Table 10.3   Comparison of qualitative techniques used in service locations

Technique	Benefits	Limitations
Participant observation	Minimal inconvenience to participant Opportunity for detailed feedback Identifies systemic or sequential problems	Researcher may be intrusive Limited statistical validity and reliability Requires trained observers Observers unfamiliar with setting Participant reluctance to identify problems if still using service
Action research	Participants involved in all aspects Information volunteered Minimal inconvenience to participants Empowerment improves morale Feedback can be detailed	Objective observation requires specialised training Participant reluctance to identify problems if still using service May not be useful for other settings
Focus groups	Feedback can be detailed Helps focus on problem areas Allows new problems to surface Shows service interest in clients	Requires trained facilitator Limited statistical validity, reliability May identify only symptoms, not core problems Feedback limited to small group Recollection of specific problems may be lost Group member dominance of the discussion

Can research techniques be used to assess health services?

With a greater emphasis on providing quality services, the health sector is increasingly reviewing itself. Qualitative research techniques are used to review practices. It is not just empirical research but rather applied. As a management tool, qualitative inquiry has many benefits for both the investigators and the participants. The key benefits are set out in table 10.3, along with some of the limitations associated with introducing qualitative research as a management instrument into a service institution.

Health care research is constantly changing and evolving. Not only are health researchers developing statistical and interviewing techniques, but also researchers from other disciplines are adapting their methodologies to the health care setting. For example, economic analyses increasingly are finding their way into health research studies. In pharmacoeconomic studies, a mixture of quantitative and qualitative techniques are used. Table 10.4 describes the features and suggested uses of four different pharmacoeconomic analyses in the health care setting: cost–benefit; cost-effectiveness; cost utility and cost identification.

Generally, economic analyses use a mixture of qualitative and quantitative techniques. In some techniques, a particular paradigm dominates. For example, cost-identification studies have a quantitative focus and cost–benefit analyses have a large qualitative component.

Table 10.4 Pharmacoeconomic analysis

	Cost–benefit	Cost-effectiveness	Cost utility	Cost identification
Definition	Cost of an intervention compared with benefit	Monetary cost of an intervention compared with its effectiveness in clinical terms	Monetary cost of an intervention compared with value patients gain from intervention	Enumerates costs involved, ignores outcomes
Comparisons	Total costs and total benefits of different interventions. Incremental costs and incremental benefits of new interventions over conventional approaches	Total costs and total benefits of different interventions. Incremental costs and incremental benefits of new interventions over conventional approaches	Total/incremental costs against patient values as measured by quantitative means (e.g., QALYS) or qualitative means (for example, standard gamble time track off, interviews)	No comparison, rather cost/unit service
Challenges	Comparisons must be in monetary units. Health outcomes difficult to measure in monetary terms	Health outcomes difficult to measure in monetary terms	Society must develop a utility value. Measures must be able to elicit preferences under conditions of uncertainty	
Use	Best for determining new health care investments	Best when clinical focus required, for example $/year of life saved	Best when patient/consumer focus required	Best when outcomes are already known to be equivalent

What is my research time frame?

Time is a critical dimension in all research. Time can refer not only to the time taken from commencement to completion of a project, but also to the time span in which the research question or topic is viewed.

Traditionally, quantitative research designs have provided a snapshot in time, as in for example cross-sectional studies. A questionnaire administered on one day, and analysed subsequently, provides information only about the moment in time at which the questionnaire is administered. Some quantitative researchers have undertaken longitudinal studies. Such studies follow a cohort of people and record sequential snapshots over a period of time. Two examples of this longitudinal approach are the Busselton study,[8] and the Whitehall study.[9] While longitudinal quantitative design methods allow us to look at changes over time, they still only provide a window of concrete answers ascertained at particular moments. Also, longitudinal cohort studies suffer from the problems of attrition and on-going expense.

Qualitative research can also provide snapshot and longitudinal perspectives. These views are elicited more by the nature of the question than by the time frame of the research. For example, an open-ended question such as: 'Tell me about your health over the last five years' allows the qualitative researcher to gain a detailed analysis of an individual's health over time.

While the capacity to access longitudinal issues with just one question is elegant and cost-effective, there are problems with such an approach. Some of the major problems are recall and bias. Obtaining a longitudinal view of an issue by asking participants to remember previous events is subject to the capacity and willingness of the subjects to remember facts.

The impact of time can also be felt in the development of research questions. In the quantitative research paradigm where precision is essential, it may take years of analysing the literature, conducting qualitative research and designing survey instruments before a research question that is answerable can be defined. In qualitative research, the identification of a research question may not be the defining step. Rather, it may be understanding the social processes that led us to ask the question that takes a long time.

Depending on the type of research, the time taken to conduct the research can vary. Organisationally, more time is often required to establish a quantitative research program. However in a qualitative program, more individual time is required by researchers in forming relationships with participants in the study.

Quantitative research is usually conducted over a longer period of time than qualitative research. The latter usually requires a short period of intense effort to collect data once recruitment is completed.

The final time limiter is of course funding. The available funding to conduct a research project will always limit the amount of time spent on the project.

Who and how many subjects will I recruit?

Recruitment may be a major factor in influencing the selection of a research technique. In qualitative studies, numbers are fewer than in quantitative studies, and involvement in the study is more of a personal nature. Quantitative studies can be conducted with small samples, which are thoughtfully drawn from the relevant population. In studies which tease out many factors, large numbers of observations are usually made to ensure that the statistical results are valid and could not have been achieved by chance. The numbers in such quantitative studies become large because the more statistical tests run, the greater the chance of concluding significance mistakenly with a small sample. A thorough description of the study population is essential for both research designs.

The recruitment of a large number of subjects in a quantitative research project is often difficult. Geographical isolation and small sized populations may make not only recruitment but also randomisation difficult. The gold standard of quantitative research designs, a randomised controlled study, requires a large enough study population to have an intervention group and a control group. This may not be possible, for example in rural and remote areas.

Selection bias is also an issue for quantitative studies that seek to prove that the observed findings did not occur by chance. Randomisation is the best way to ensure that the study population is representative. Where it may be difficult to recruit subjects for study in a random fashion—for example, for a study of intravenous drug users—a qualitative approach may be the only one practical. Similarly, large databases that can ensure that findings did not occur by chance (e.g., the National Health Survey) are unsuitable for conducting an interview-based piece of research and therefore a qualitative approach may be the practical approach.

The deviance of a study population from the reference group is defined as selection bias. In a quantitative study, such bias is important to clarify or control for. Sometimes in quantitative studies the inherent exclusion biases may not even be mentioned or controlled for. Messing, in her article on women and occupational health, concludes that women may be excluded without mention from quantitative studies concerning occupational health by limiting inclusion criteria. Pregnant women, for example, are quite often excluded from studies of industrial toxins and new pharmaceutical products.[10]

The effect of gender is explored differently in qualitative and quantitative studies. There has been a tendency for quantitative studies to control for gender or avoid the issue altogether.[11] Qualitative studies may be used to redress this imbalance.

Methodological features that are seen as a weakness in one style of research may be a strength in another. Randomisation and representativeness are rarely issues for qualitative research designs. Qualitative studies seek to highlight differences and not similarities, which is the complete opposite from the notion of randomisation.

When recruiting subjects, response rates need to be taken into consideration. Response rates to studies vary according to the nature of the topic studies and the study design. For example, mail surveys have response rates of 80 to 90 per cent when associated with reminder letters and telephone calls.[12] In certain populations that are traditionally oversurveyed, for example general practitioners, response rates to mail-out questionnaires can drop as low as 30 per cent. In qualitative studies, exploration of sensitive topic may inhibit recruitment or retention. Poor response rates can be improved with attention to study design. For example, in questionnaire design, attention to the length of the questionnaire and its face validity can enhance the response rate. With focus groups, careful explanation of the purpose of the study and the mechanisms in place to maintain anonymity may help. The researcher also needs to recruit enough subjects to account for the anticipated attrition rate in the study.

What sort of analysis will my data require?

The analysis of qualitative and quantitative data is markedly different. Qualitative analysis has traditionally been less reliant on computers. The original methods for analysing interviews and focus group feedback relied on reading and re-reading the written data and analysing it for themes. Often this was performed by 'cutting and pasting' pieces of text by hand.

Randomised controlled trials (RCTs) remain the gold standard of quantitative research designs. The data collected in these trials are appropriate to complex statistically analyses. Once they have been conducted on a particular topic, the same study is rarely undertaken again. To overcome the practical difficulties of RCTs and to utilise existing data, two less expensive derivatives have emerged: secondary analysis of data and meta-analysis. A comparison of the three techniques in terms of cost, sample size, data collection, reproducibility and limitations is shown in table 10.5.

In contrast, the data obtained in qualitative research is unique to the researcher and study population. It is the product of their interaction and does not lend itself to re analysis by others.

Over the last two decades a number of computer programs have become available to assist in codifying qualitative data, for example NUD*IST[13] and Ethnograph.[14] The packages require some training and data entry. These packages have benefits and limitations. While making manipulation of large pieces of text easy, they force the qualitative researcher into a particular way of viewing the data. For example, searching for specific nouns or phrases in order to categorise the data is accomplished in a particular way in each package. These kinds of searches may inhibit the intuitive flow of ideas between researchers and their subjects. While the use of computerised packages in data analysis is viewed critically in qualitative studies, the same cannot be said for quantitative studies.

Table 10.5 Comparison of major types of quantitative techniques

	RCTs	Secondary analysis of data	Meta-analysis
Cost	Expensive	Cheap	Cheap
Sample size	Significant	Variable, usually significant	Additive from smaller studies
Data collection	Well described	Defined by previous study	May not be clear from original studies
Reproducibility	Yes (rarely done)	Usually unique set of primary data	No (but primary data may be reviewed)
Limitations	Funding, recruitment, co-ordination, heterogeneity, heteroskedacity	No checks on original study: • data collection • storage • registration • missing data Recording errors specific for original, e.g. different classification	Can lead to conclusions which cannot be substantiated in RCTs Research questions limited by those asked in contributing studies

Quantitative data usually require a certain degree of statistical sophistication for proper analysis. The most important features of quantitative analyses of data are ensuring that the statistical methods that are chosen are correct and applied correctly and that the inferences obtained are right. As the research area of biostatistics increases in sophistication, the techniques are becoming more complex.

Many computer programs exist to assist in the analysis of quantitative data, for example, SPSS[15] and STATA.[16] The use of these programs is highly specialised. Quantitative analysis should not be undertaken without the assistance of an experienced statistician to provide advice not only on how to use these packages, but also on how to interpret the results.

In both qualitative and quantitative studies, data analysis tends to take much longer than expected. In qualitative studies, data analysis is prolonged by the transcribing process, and by the need to set aside thoughts and ideas for a period of time and then come back to them. Breaks between viewing the data allow for synthesising and processing some of the messages in the text.

In quantitative studies, the checking and cleaning of data is quite time consuming, as is the performing of particular analyses. For example, establishing the representativeness of a sample against a recognised data set may result in one line of a final publication but require many hours of statistical analysis.

The role of the literature review in the analysis of qualitative and quantitative data also differs. In qualitative research, the literature often helps us to formulate our ideas, models and themes while we are working with our data. It is not unusual with qualitative research to halt analysis while reviewing what other people have written on the topic. This process can add some considerable time to the analysis. In quantitative work the literature contextualises our questions and helps to place our results within a research framework.

How will I present my findings?

There are a variety of ways in which qualitative and quantitative works can be presented to audiences. The process for presenting quantitative research projects is well defined. It is based on the IMRAD format. IMRAD is an acronym for Introduction, Methods, Results And Discussion. In the 'Introduction', the researchers must identify the reasons for conducting their study and their research hypotheses. In the 'Methods' section, what was done needs to be outlined. The findings are shown in text and graphically in the 'Results' section. Finally, the 'Discussion' section should synthesise the key findings, show how they are different from previous studies, and suggest directions for future research. The length of articles describing quantitative research is also prescribed, usually by the journal publishing the work. In quantitative studies, quite often graphs and tables are used. They can occupy much space. Thus written articles are usually limited to between 1500 and

3000 words and fewer than five graphs or tables. These issues are explored further in chapter 14, 'Writing and publishing'.

The presentation of qualitative research is far more flexible. It usually involves a detailed description of the study population and the underlying theoretical frameworks on which the work is based, for example positivist, postmodern. The development of themes is usually supported by direct quotations which can take up much space.

Typical displays of the findings include: clusters, themes, theoretical definitions, narratives, typologies, taxonomies, straight and analytic descriptions.[17] The final analysis, unlike the discussion or conclusion for quantitative studies, is not designed to show completion of an idea. Due to the use of quotations and complex theoretical concepts, written qualitative work is usually much longer than its quantitative counterpart (usually in excess of 5000 words).

Who is my audience? Where do I want my research results published?

Experienced researchers will understand the value of disseminating ideas. Less experienced researchers may find this process too daunting or undervalue their work to such an extent that they do not think it is worth publishing. In quantitative publications, accuracy and statistical reproducibility are defining steps. Also, where collaborative teams are involved in the research, such as multicentred trials, achieving consensus may take some time. The combination of these factors means that quantitative papers are usually slow to get to the stage when they are ready to be sent off to a journal.

In contrast, qualitative studies usually raise new ideas. For example, studies that use grounded theory lend themselves to early reporting because the analyses begin at the outset of projects. The final work, however, may take some time.

Apart from academic motivation to peer-review publication, the drivers behind disseminating work can come from a variety of sources. Where the work is commissioned, for example by government agency or an employer, the dissemination may be limited by the commissioning group. Many quality assurance activities are qualitative research projects that may be more relevant to a specific rather than general audience.

The greater the generalisability of quantitative data, the more likely it is to be published. For qualitative data, publication is more likely to be related to the cohesion of the conceptual framework and its application to the empirical data.

What are the impediments to completing my research?

Energy levels of researchers may vary due to external conditions but there is also a natural history of any research endeavour, which is described pictorially in figure

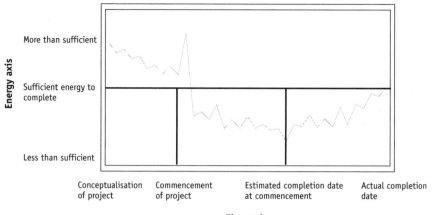

Figure 10.3 Project energies

10.3. It is important to realise the ebb and flow of energy and resources for any project. Energies are highest at project commencement, but usually slide to below sustainable levels due to the inevitable range of setbacks and draining of resources that occurs with many projects. Near completion of the project there is usually a surge of energy that is required to finalise the task.

Factors influencing the successful completion of any project are often unique. However, certain features of qualitative and quantitative methodologies can stall the pathway to completion.

With qualitative projects, ethical considerations may arise from within the participant group that may slow or halt the project. For example, the disclosure of notifiable activities such as HIV status to a researcher may uncover ethical concerns that need to be dealt with. The research process may also be stalled by incomplete recording or lack of funds or time for transcription. Feedback of the analysed data to reference groups and participants may take too long so that collective memory of the research may be lost. The focus of dissemination may not be unified. For example, researchers may want to share their ideas in a research forum and work towards a peer-reviewed publication, whereas policy planners may want to disseminate the information quickly to their constituents.

In quantitative methodologies data collection may be delayed or incomplete. The ensuing analyses may prove too complex for the skills of the research team and finding specialised statistical support may be difficult. When researchers from different disciplines are involved, there may be varying opinions as to where to publish the finalised paper for maximum effect. A summary of key inhibitors to project completion by research methodology appears in table 10.6.

When selecting a research method, it is important to remember that there is no one right way to explore a research question. Often it is not appropriate to select only one technique. Sometimes a variety of techniques need to be used to

Table 10.6 Inhibitors to project completion

Quantitative	Both	Qualitative
	Delayed data collection	
Missing data		Transcription difficulties
	Complicated analyses	
Lack of appropriated statistical support		Coding problems
	Timing	
Data out of date		Work superseded by new theoretical frameworks Delayed responses from participants
	Researcher differences Authorship problems	
Lack of unified approach to target audience		Lack of definition of target population for dissemination

obtain the answer the researcher is seeking. In many situations, qualitative and quantitative research can complement each other over time in a research project.

The choice of qualitative or quantitative methodology is quite complex and depends on a number of features that range from topic selection to the position a particular piece of research has in the sequence of a research plan.

11

Assistants and mentors

ALIX MAGNEY, ELIZABETH O'BRIEN, AND VANESSA TRAYNOR

This chapter has been written by three research assistants. They represent the diversity of health researchers. One is trained in nursing and public health, one in sociology, with a focus on health issues, and one is trained in community health and the social sciences. All work in health research. They talk about how they gained confidence in research, the tasks they commonly tackle, and how they like to be briefed when starting on a project. This chapter will be very useful for other budding researchers, and also for the people who will need to mentor them as they learn about the practicalities of conducting research.

It is not uncommon in handbooks of health care research to find a plethora of information on how to design research. Indeed, many of these issues have been raised in earlier chapters of this book. By contrast, information on those who carry out research is relatively harder to find. The role of research assistants and mentors in the research process has been largely forgotten in the wider literature on research methods and processes. Research manuals tell us how to construct a survey, or design a focus group, and how to identify a sample of participants. Yet, they tell us little about the practicalities of the day-to-day running of a research program, either from the assistant's or the chief investigator's or mentor's point of view.

This chapter covers some of the practicalities associated with being a research assistant, including professional background and skill, common research tasks and career development. It addresses two issues of particular importance to the progress of research: briefing sessions and research assistant resources. Mentors and their central place in the research process and impact on the career development of the assistant are discussed in detail. Finally, the various experiences and aspirations of the chapter's authors are described. Throughout the chapter, brief tips are presented to highlight key points.

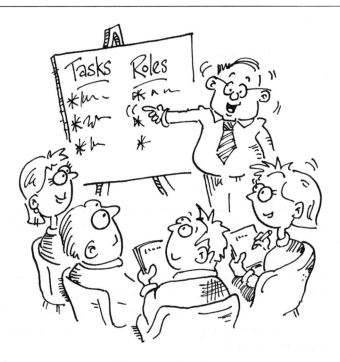

Professional backgrounds and skills of research assistants

Research assistants can be many things to many people. Defining what they do and who they are is therefore a difficult task. In some cases, research assistants are employed on a consultancy-like basis to perform single tasks such as collecting and collating literature. In other instances, they play a broader role in research, being responsible for all aspects of the day-to-day running of an ongoing project. Whatever the task, and wherever the setting, a research assistant can offer valuable assistance to a research team.

Most commonly, assistants in health sciences research have degree-level qualifications. While a background in a health-related field can be advantageous, it is not always necessary. Indeed, research assistants within the health sector come from a variety of backgrounds and disciplines, including:

- the social sciences
- the behavioural sciences
- clinical medicine
- the natural sciences
- nursing, and
- allied health (e.g., physiotherapists and occupational therapists).

Given such a variety of backgrounds, it is not surprising that the tasks undertaken by research assistants and the skills they possess are also wide-ranging. In the following sections we will explore some of the more common tasks and skills required of the research assistant.

Tip: Look for graduates or those with equivalent experience. In many cases a university education will have equipped graduates with at least some basic research skills, particularly in information retrieval, analysis, and writing.

Core skills versus desirable skills

The most commonly needed skills and attributes in research assistants correspond to what happens after research is planned. Planning is usually undertaken by the chief investigators. The investigators then require research assistance for the conduct of that planned research process. The common tasks in research are: collecting and reviewing literature; recruiting participants; coordinating different parts of the research team, and different health care professionals; collecting, storing, entering and analysing data; administration; and preparing reports, articles or conference presentations. The practicalities of these tasks is covered within this chapter. The responsibility for these tasks can be essential within different contexts, but it is rare that all will be required of the research assistant in any one project. Often the nature and scope of the research will define which skills are necessary and how well developed they need to be. It is often useful to develop some criteria by which you can decide which are core skills for the research assistant and which are desirable. In order to pinpoint the specific skills needed for the particular context it can be helpful to look to the research plan. Just as the *research question* helps to guide the project design, the *research plan* helps to determine the tasks and skills required. There are also some key questions investigators might ask when attempting to choose the best person for the job. These include:

- What (if any) input will the research assistant have in the design of the study?
- What type of data or information will be collected?
- How will the data/information be managed (collection and storage)?
- How will the data/information be analysed?

- How much involvement will the research assistant have in writing and presenting findings?
- How many research assistants can the project employ?

A note about personal attributes

Skills are not the only important consideration for research assistants and their potential employers. There are a number of key personal attributes that make for a good research assistant, such as:

- flexibility and adaptability to change
- personal initiative
- friendliness and openness
- ability to work within a team
- self-motivation
- commitment
- being organised and systematic
- capacity for reflective thought, and
- thirst for learning.

All of the above attributes are beneficial to a project. A thirst for learning, and commitment to the research process are the more important. Across most research settings, it is these attributes that can most ensure a long and fruitful career in research.

The briefing session

The success of a research project depends on the time and resources put into 'preparing the way'. There are many aspects to good preparation; however, a particularly central one for the research assistant is the briefing session. Generally, a briefing session is used to provide the research assistant with key information about the project, and to explain the research plan and design in detail. This discussion needs to be to a level of specificity that is useful to a research assistant: what is to be done, by whom, when, where, why and how.

The briefing session

The briefing session should cover:

- the background to the project (i.e., the nature and scope of the research)
- the research plan (and rationale)

- the expectations of team members of the research assistant and vice versa
- a review of the job description for any points that might need clarification and a discussion of roles and responsibilities
- the availability of resources and equipment
- timelines and deadlines, including a regular meeting time for the investigator and the research assistant, and
- identification of important contacts and networks.

The time should also be used to allow the assistant to ask questions and to provide copies of any appropriately helpful material including background briefing papers, relevant contact lists to the assistant. The session should be held as soon as possible, either before or closely following the commencement of the assistant's appointment to the research team.

In addition to the briefing session, the research assistant needs time to do some reflective background reading. In many cases, the newly appointed assistant will need to become oriented to the particular field, and so will need to become familiar with a range of relevant literature. Even when the assistant is familiar with the field, this time could be used to reflect upon the background materials (such as the project submission), establish networks and organise a range of administrative details such as establishing e-mail accounts, etc. If the assistant has adequate preparation in the initial stages of the project, difficulties may be avoided later on.

Tip: Don't rush the briefing session. Set aside sufficient time, so that both the briefer and the assistant get as much from the session as possible. Short, hurried briefing sessions can lead to confusion and problems further down the track.

The tasks

There are numerous tasks that a research assistant may be expected to carry out, from initial recruitment of participants to writing the final report. The range of tasks will depend on the nature and setting of the research, as well as the resources available. A number of health care settings and institutes in which health and medical research takes place have limited resources, both financial and personnel. A research assistant in this type of environment may be responsible for all project tasks and management. In a larger better-resourced environment, such as a pharmaceutical company, there may be a number of research assistants, each with their own particular set of tasks. Whatever the setting, there are some broad roles which can be identified. These are outlined below.

Collecting and reviewing the literature

Literature collection and review is an essential component of most research methodologies. In conjunction with the research proposal, the literature review helps to prepare the way and set the scene for a study. A well-conducted literature review provides the basis from which the researcher can start to conceptualise the place of the study in the broader literature, as well as guiding the theoretical development of the research. Literature reviewing is an ongoing process, important across all phases of the project. It should not be thought of as a separate phase of the study, as the published results of others help not only with the planning of the study, but also with interpretation of the findings.[1] The research assistant therefore must be reliable and thorough with the ongoing literature review. This is especially important if the research leader relies on the assistant to keep them informed of important published findings.

The initial grant submission, which will probably contain a short literature, is a good starting point. The references from here can be used to start developing a more comprehensive framework for the literature search. Key words and other relevant search terms (including key authors and journals) need to be identified so relevant research and literature databases can be explored. There are a number of such databases available, both in CD Rom and Internet formats, including:

- Medline
- Core Biomedical Collection
- CINAHL
- Current Contents
- Psychlit
- Sociofile.

Many of the above will be available from a local university library. If you do not have immediate access to a university library, the closest university library will be able to describe the range of options available. In Australia, a large number of universities have a significant presence on the World Wide Web, something which has made remote access to information services much easier. For example, some university library web sites now offer you the option of searching their databases via CD-ROM or the Internet. In addition to university library collections, hospitals, health departments and state and national libraries can prove useful. Discussion between the research supervisor and the research assistant will ensure that the initial reference list is appropriate.

Tip: Make friends with your librarian. We cannot stress enough how important librarians are in helping the research assistant in information and literature retrieval tasks. They can provide important details on which databases to use, organise inter-library loans, search for obscure literature on your behalf, and make use of networks of contacts that the rest of us only dream of.

Once on the right track, you need to collect the literature. Getting the information off the shelves and photocopied will take a number of days of work in the library. Most university libraries have staff (and public) photocopying and borrowing facilities for this purpose. Be prepared to go beyond your original reference collection list. Some of the most interesting articles can often be found by spending some time leafing through journals on the shelf. While this can be time-consuming, it can be ultimately worth the effort. Though the library may be the main source of literature, there are other avenues which you can use to collect information. In recent years, there has been a proliferation of what are referred to as electronic or e journals. E journals can be electronic versions of published journals, with access to content varying from full electronic copy to titles and abstracts. Most of those professional journals still require subscription, by the library usually, before you can gain access to full electronic content. Be warned, however, that much of the information on the Internet is not in a peer-reviewed journal equivalent and is not vetted in any way. If you do use material from the Internet, you must ensure it is from a reputable source and clearly reference it as being from the Internet.

When you have a substantial collection together, spend some time organising it into meaningful categories, either alphabetically or by subject matter. If available, a reference database, such as Bibliograph or Reference Manager, can be helpful in storing and organising your collection. It is important at this stage to scan all the articles to ensure that all relevant subjects have been canvassed and to check for irrelevant articles which can be put aside. Ideally, you should write a short summary of each article. This will help organise and summarise the data as well as draw out commonalties and differences.

Tip: Never throw an article out, even if it appears irrelevant to the review. You never know when it could come in handy later.

As the literature review is an ongoing process, it is important to keep an eye out for new research and information. There are a number of tools now available which can help with this task. One of the most useful is the journal e-mail notification system. Many journals will advise you of new journal content by e-mailing a regular monthly table of contents. In addition, you can use an automated search service offered by an increasing number of university libraries. The library will set up an automated search according to your specifications as denoted by a range of key words and subject headings. The searches can be as simple or as complex as you require. Talk to your librarian about the availability of this service.

Recruiting participants

Like the literature review, participant recruitment is often an essential task in research, no matter what the research process or method. Effective recruitment requires good communication, persistence and patience. The aim is to achieve optimal response rates, so you can expect to ring participants a number of times before you talk to potential participants or receive a final answer on participation from each person on your contact list. It is sometimes useful to set a limit on call-backs, and while the actual limit will depend on the importance of achieving high versus medium response rates, for most studies you can expect to do at least three call-backs. Use a 'call sheet' to keep track of where you are up to with recruitment, listing contact details and allocating space for call-back times and general observations. For the first round of recruitment, it is important to try to get through the entire contact list in one go, even if it is over a number of consecutive days. Some people prefer to allocate recruitment time each day—however, this can easily be put off in favour of other tasks. It is much better to at least have made initial contact with all potential participants (even if it is just to know when to call them back) within the first couple of days or weeks and then allocate specific call-back times later on.

Tip: Collecting brief information about non-participants, such as reason for refusal and demographic characteristics, can be useful. Comparisons of participants with non-participants not only enriches the final results, it helps determine whether any differences between the groups exist or not. This is an issue of external validity.

Be flexible and realistic. Expecting to achieve a high response rate with all target groups is not realistic. Some groups are notoriously difficult to recruit, and despite all efforts the best response rate you can expect might be 65 per cent. This is not an excuse to be lax in your recruitment efforts, indeed such groups often need more intensively planned recruitment. What is important is the extent to which you can establish that reasonable means to recruit participants have been planned and used. For example, if recruiting busy physicians for a telephone survey does not seem feasible, options that do not take up their work time might be, like a brief mail-out survey. If your target group of single mothers cannot attend the focus group, think about offering to organise child care and transport. Being open to the unexpected can mean the difference between a return rate of 45 per cent and one of 65 per cent. You should always clear any changes to the research protocol with your team leaders, and possibly the ethics committee.

Tip: Approach potential research subjects at an appropriate time, in a space in which they are comfortable, be aware of potential vulnerabilities and give them plenty of opportunity to ask questions and time to reflect upon your proposition. Be careful not to coerce or offer undue inducement, as participation must be voluntary.

Effective communication is another important aspect of recruitment. Whether face-to-face or over-the-telephone surveying is being used, establishing rapport with potential participants can help significantly in optimising the response rate. Good communication and rapport in the context of research, however, should not be confused with excellent grammar and an impeccable dress sense. You should dress neatly, but not overdress or underdress in comparison to your target population. You should always be polite. How you recruit participants will vary according to your target group. The methods that you use to recruit a sample of elderly nursing home patients for a study on dementia will be different from the methods that you use to recruit street kids for a study of youth homelessness. While both might be carried out face to face, rather than over the telephone, details such as how you communicate both verbally and physically will vary.

However you recruit potential participants, ethical issues, such as informed and voluntary consent and maintaining privacy and confidentiality, should be considered at all times. In Australia, the National Health and Medical Research Council (NHMRC) provides ethical guidelines for recruitment of research participants, and these were updated in 1999.[2] These are clear statements of what is expected of researchers when dealing with human subjects, and include issues pertaining to patient informed consent, voluntariness, confidentiality, privacy, and anonymity. These are the gold standard for all medical and health research in Australia and essential reading for any research assistant. It is essential that researchers are up to date on these guidelines. More information about ethical issues can be found in chapter 12 of this book.

Tip: Check with your research office (or a similar committee/group in settings other than universities) for appropriate research ethics guidelines.

Communicating and coordinating

A research assistant with good communication skills will benefit the project from start to finish. In the recruitment phase of the study, a research assistant who can develop a good rapport with prospective participants will be a great advantage to the study and will also help in terms of retaining participants for future follow-up. In qualitative research or studies utilising survey methods, a person able to facilitate fruitful interaction between members of a group, or encourage individuals to 'open up' in an interview is desirable. Communication skills are also important within the research team itself, which is often multidisciplinary and may even be multicentred. The research assistant may be the project coordinator or manager and will therefore be the focal point for communication. Liaison and networking skills can add significant value to the project, by bringing in expert opinions or experience.

Collecting the data

Collecting the data is perhaps the core task of the research assistant. How one goes about it depends on the orientation of the research. If the research is of a qualitative design, then the tasks might centre around conducting focus groups or interviews, observing study participants or collecting case study material. If the research is primarily quantitative, the tasks involved might include the implementation of surveys or the conduct of clinically based experiments. Increasingly, researchers in the health field are developing multidisciplinary and multiple method approaches. The implication of this is that research assistants may be expected to undertake a combination of the above tasks. Explaining the trend of combining methods is a feature of this text. In some instances, research assistants will be required not only to implement research instruments and protocols (such as surveys and interview guides), but also to design them.

The data collection skills that are needed will depend on the particular data to be collected. The research assistant may be involved in the design of a questionnaire and so should have some experience with this. Experience with interviewing or surveying may be required. A clinical background may be necessary for the collection of clinical readings or specimens. An understanding of medical terminology may be required for a medical record audit. Experience with facilitating focus groups or discussion groups may be necessary for a qualitative study. The research assistant may need to videotape interviews or observations, and experience with the use of such equipment would be advantageous. Whichever data are collected, the research assistant needs to have consistent collection methods to ensure the reliability of the data. If more than one assistant is collecting data, checks should be made to ensure they are collected or measured in the same way by each assistant. Issues concerning reliability and rigour are discussed earlier in this book, particularly in chapters 4 and 9.

Storing the data

Whether the data or information is numerical, textual, visual or auditory, it must be stored in a safe and accessible system. Back-up copies should be made and all original information must be kept in a system that is well organised and secure. Numerical or quantifiable information should be transferred to a suitable computer program to enable it to be both stored and analysed. The research assistant should be able to code data for these purposes. Competency with the use of database systems for statistical analysis such as SPSS,[3] SAS,[4] or at least, the spreadsheet packages is desirable.

Tip: Establish codification of survey or questionnaire information prior to its collection. Have the codes on the questionnaires to enable efficient storage after collection. This is called a 'coding master'. Take care with Y2K (year 2000) issues, so that dates and years have four digit fields. If you plan to compare data over a number of years, double check that the year codes will be accurate.

The assistant might be expected to transcribe qualitative information into a word processing program or into a program for qualitative analysis such as NUD*IST.[5] Transcribing such information is often time-consuming and requires patience. However the data are stored, the assistant must be aware of the importance of maintaining the privacy and confidentiality of study participants.

Entering the data

While it is not uncommon in large-scale studies to have the data entry step carried out by a specialist data entry organisation, in smaller studies, in-house data entry is more common. In this case, assistants may be expected to enter both quantitative and qualitative data. Set aside a regular time for data entry each day or each week, depending on how much data are coming in. A backlog of data is harder to deal with and more mistakes are made when sitting for hours.

Tip: Using two people, one for reading out the data, and one for typing it in, helps prevent mistakes. No matter how you enter it, it should be double-checked.

Analysing the data

Like data collection, analysing the data is another central task of the research assistant in most research studies. While many research studies employ the services of a statistician for detailed statistical analysis, this is not always possible (particularly on a long-term basis). Research assistants may be expected to undertake various analytical tasks, ranging from reviews of the literature to statistical analysis or in-depth content analysis. They should always refer back to the research question when undertaking that analysis.

In many quantitative studies, the input of a biostatistician is sought to help plan the statistical analysis and to offer guidance on sampling and methodology. In some studies such expert input may be ongoing, in others it may only be available in the initial planning stages. It is important for the chief investigator or team to choose their research assistant after determining the level of expert input throughout the project. If the research assistant is to carry out the analysis without further support of a statistician, then the assistant's level of statistical competency should be high. However, some projects may have additional funding for consultation with a statistician to help the assistant with the analysis. In this case, a good understanding of statistics may be enough. In either case, the research assistant must be familiar with the particular statistical computing program the project intends to use. In some projects, research assistants may not be required to carry out the analysis themselves. However, they should have enough of an understanding to enable them to interpret the findings.

Tip: Do not start with complex analysis until you have a 'feel' for the data. This involves taking a broad look for trends or divergences in the data to begin with. Most statistical software packages such as SPSS and Epi Info have data summarisation options. Print these out and look for where to go next.

Once the 'raw' data have been examined, begin to think about the research question and the statistical tests that might be useful for answering the question. From this point on it may be necessary to group or re-code the data to enable particular tests to be carried out. The data will no longer be in their raw form. However, a copy of the raw data must always be kept for further reference and perhaps for different methods of coding and analysis. Then it is time to run the appropriate tests. This must be done in a methodical manner and printouts of each test should be kept for later reference.

The analytical skills required for qualitative studies are very different from those required in quantitative studies. Again, the advice of an expert in qualitative methods and analysis should be sought in the planning stage. Just as in quantitative analysis, qualitative analysis requires a high degree of skill. It is time-consuming, involving the organising, shaping, summarising and explanation of the information gathered.[6] The research assistant may be experienced and able to manage this task unassisted, or may have recourse to an expert. Even where expert input is available it is advisable for the assistant to do some background reading of their own. An earlier chapter in this text gives an overview of qualitative research methods. Finally, while it is not essential, familiarity with relevant qualitative data analysis software programs such as NUD*IST can be advantageous.

Tip: The primary data should always be 'backed up'. That is, they should be duplicated and stored in another location. For interviews and focus groups, always use a second method for recording the information as well (e.g., tape, scribing, etc.). Back-ups can be life savers in case of technical disasters.

Administration

Research often involves a number of mundane tasks such as filing questionnaires and other documentation, writing correspondence to participants, photocopying various materials and arranging meetings and interviews. The importance of such tasks should not be underestimated. Administrative and organisational systems are central to the effectiveness and efficiency of the research.

In many cases, a research assistant will responsible for all aspects of the day-to-day running of the project. Therefore administration and organisational skills are essential. Tasks such as letter writing, filing, photocopying, and arranging meetings are often included as part of the job. Maintaining a safe and well-organised storage system for information gathered from study participants, backing up computer files and hard copies of data and results are also tasks for the research assistant. A research assistant will therefore need to be an organised person with a systematic approach. Assistants will also need to be willing to learn new organisational skills. Talking to others will help assistants form better information management and administrative practices.

Confidentiality is crucial across most aspects of research. Filing of data, whether stored on tape, disk or paper needs to be managed in a confidential and secure manner. Research materials must not be left in public view. Locking filing cabinets or offices and restricting access to those directly involved may be required. Particularly sensitive material may need to be handled in the privacy of a secure office.

Writing the report

Report writing refers not only to writing up the final research report, but also to writing progress reports during the course of the study. While it is uncommon for research assistants to be expected to take sole responsibility for writing the final research report, they should have some role in writing up those aspects with which they were involved most closely. This will ensure accuracy of reporting, as well as giving the research assistant valuable experience and insight into the whole research process.

Tip: Don't leave writing the report to the last minute. Use the original grant submission as your starting point, incorporating and building upon what is there, particularly in the aims, background and methodology sections. Offer to be involved in the writing process if you have not already been asked.

Preparing articles and presentations

At the heart of much research is the way and extent to which the findings are disseminated to the wider research community and the public. Journal publications and conference presentations are central to this dissemination. In this context the research assistant, given the opportunity, can begin to develop a career in research. Presenting at your first conference or seminar can be a daunting experience. Nerves have a way of hijacking even the most prepared and experienced speaker. Practise your talk well beforehand with the audio-visual aids that you intend to use on the day. Using your colleagues as a sounding board can help put you at ease in a familiar environment and identify any problems with the presentation early on. Go through the talk as many times as necessary, until you feel confident and comfortable with the subject, and remember to time the presentation. If using slides or colour overheads, plan your presentation at least six weeks in advance to ensure that you can get them done in time. Finally, always have a back-up copy of your slides on paper.

Tip: If, on the day, the slide projector does not work, you lose your place, or someone interjects with a difficult question that you cannot answer, don't panic. Take a moment to collect your thoughts and then keep going from where you left off.

Writing skills are important in their own right. A research assistant with well-developed writing skills will be of benefit throughout the project. In addition to the final research report, regular progress reports must be submitted as a requirement of funding of some projects. Another important aspect of writing and presentation skills is preparation of journal publications. When preparing a journal publication, it is important to write the article in the style preferred by the particular journal. The style guides will tell you which referencing system to use, the preferred length of articles, formatting details and, in some cases, subheadings to use. They will also tell you how the editors prefer the final manuscript to be delivered (e.g., in multiple hard copies or on disk or both). As with preparing for conference presentations, use your colleagues as a sounding board. It is useful to leaf through past copies of the journal that you intend to publish in to get an idea of the writing style used by past authors.

Tip: Everyone starts somewhere. It is unlikely that you will be asked to write an original research article for journal publication on your first project. An ideal way to start publishing is to submit a letter to the editor or a short research notice. If you have not been asked to write, offer to write and let your team know that you want to start to learn about the writing process.

Resources

Like most people, research assistants require adequate resources to carry out their task effectively and efficiently. How you determine what is adequate will largely depend on the nature and setting of the research. In some instances, it may be possible and desirable to ensure that the assistant has their own office and the latest computer technology, but in others, where funds are limited, the ideal might not be possible. Whatever the scenario, it is important to consider resource availability early on, before employing staff who you subsequently find cannot be accommodated. To guide you in this process, we have listed some key resource considerations below.

Space requirements

What kind of space requirements the assistant might have will be influenced by whether the position is permanent or temporary, whether a private office space is required for conducting confidential interviews, and whether the research takes place on- or off-site. With many short-term projects, tasks are sometimes carried out either off-site or from a shared office space. Remember, however, that research undertaken off-site brings its own set of problems, particularly in accessing a library, photocopying, and using the telephone, facsimile and e-mail facilities. Such issues need to be discussed early on in the project and, if necessary, it should be explicitly stated in the contract as to whose equipment is being used.

E-mail and Internet access

E-mail and Internet access is an important consideration in today's increasingly computer literate research environments. Establishing networks of contacts for research can be greatly aided by access to e-mail, electronic discussion forums and news groups. Equally useful is the Internet, which is fast becoming an essential research tool in its own right. Such tools are particularly useful for research which is carried out off-site.

Computer equipment

Good computers are essential. Outdated computer equipment can be a source of ongoing problems and difficulties for many researchers. An assistant who spends the majority of his or her time trying to deal with computer break-downs will be neither efficient nor effective. While there might not always be a need for the latest in computer technology, sound equipment is, in most cases, essential. The other important consideration here is access to ongoing computing support.

Access to photocopying, facsimile and telephone facilities

In most research projects, particularly in long-term contracts, it is essential that assistants have access to photocopying, printing, facsimile and telephone facilities. While shared access to such resources is acceptable with photocopying, printing and facsimile facilities, shared telephone access can be more complicated. In projects in which telephone contact with participants (both in terms of recruitment and interviewing) is an ongoing task, the need for a dedicated phone line is important.

Access to the research team

Access to the research team is also an important resource consideration. Regular team meetings should be organised so that the assistant can report progress and the research supervisors can identify problems or difficulties routinely. This also helps to ensure that the project remains on track.

Whatever the resources available, there needs to be ongoing support and discussion about issues as they arise. This will help to ensure a smooth running project, and in most cases, a happy assistant.

Tip: If it has not already been done, introduce yourself to key administrative and support personnel. They can often help in arranging photocopying access, library cards, use of car if necessary, travel, expenses, etc.

Developing career paths in research

An important aspect of being a research assistant is the extent to which you are prepared to extend your own skills and learning to pursue a career in research. This requires dedication and commitment. There are a number of aspects to making the transition from assistant to researcher, including a commitment to:

- developing your own area of research expertise
- attending meetings and conferences to present your work
- publishing material widely through journals, and
- volunteering for representation on key bodies and organisations.

While not instantaneous, such a transition is ultimately worthwhile. Mentors can help research assistants greatly in this respect. They can help get you started with publishing work, something which is a particularly important aspect of developing a career in research. Publishing careers often begin as co-authorship on papers emanating from research projects. Offering co-authorship is recognition of the research assistant's commitment and effort to the project. Publications mark the author's professional growth and are crucial to any future job application. One of us explains the transition from assistant to researcher later in this chapter, and highlights the role played by her mentors in this process.

Tip: Encouragement is the key. Remember to express confidence in your research assistants' abilities and confide stories of your own experiences (good and bad ones!) so that they can learn from you.

Authorship and the research assistant

Increasingly, research assistants within the health sciences are involved in writing articles for publication, as well as being an integral part of the research process. Publication is seen to be the key to success for an academic career.[7] However, authorship is a sometimes contentious issue. Criteria for authorship has been developed by the International Committee of Medical Journal Editors.[8]

The criteria state that authorship should be based only on a substantial contribution to:

(a) conception and design or analysis and interpretation of the data *and*
(b) drafting the article or revising it critically for important intellectual content *and*
(c) giving final approval of the version to be published.

All authors become publicly accountable for the published work, and research process. It has been argued that these criteria do not give enough weight to those who contribute substantially to the project in a practical sense (such as research assistants) and that it would be unethical to exclude them as key contributors. Co-authors include those who conceptualised the study as well as those who gathered the data. Whichever process you prefer, authorship criteria should be agreed early on in the project to avoid later disputes and problems.

Mentors

A review of the literature relating to mentoring shows a surprising deficit of information about the role of the mentor in research settings, particularly the implications of the mentor–protégé relationship to career paths of health researchers. Despite this paucity, mentoring is an important aspect of the research process, particularly in relation to the development of career paths for research assistants. Mentors can provide assistants with valuable insight and experience, and can facilitate access to networks of contacts, encourage publication and conference presentation, encourage further education and training, and provide a link to further job opportunities. In this section we will outline what a mentor is, lessons to be learnt from mentoring programs in other sectors, the relationship between mentors and their protégés and the importance of mentors for enhancing the career paths of assistants. Readers should note that this discussion focuses on the relationship between mentor and protégé as practised in office-based (as opposed to laboratory) research in universities and hospitals.

The *Australian Concise Oxford Dictionary* defines a mentor as a 'wise or trusted adviser or guide'.[9] Mentoring is carried out in diverse settings such as corporations, schools, universities and research institutions. Other forms of mentoring include apprenticeships in trades, noviciates in religious orders, trainees in business and amateurs in theatre. Broadly, the aim of the relationship between a mentor and their protégé is to encourage and guide the protégé to learn through experience. Trust, confidentiality and intuitive supervision are some of the aspects of a healthy mentoring relationship and the nature of the relationship is pivotal to the protégé's experience. Traditional notions comply with the idea of patronage, in which the mentor plays the role of detached overseer. Contemporary expressions, by contrast, include mentors themselves in the learning process, by virtue of the nature of the relationship and the sharing of experiences.

Mentoring programs in other sectors

Mentoring has increasingly become a focus of the corporate sector, primarily as a business tool providing benefits for individuals and companies alike. A review of the personnel management and human resources literature showed that the corporate world is a keen proponent of mentoring, developing programs designed to facilitate the smooth running of the company. Many businesses in the United States and United Kingdom have implemented such programs, and a significant amount of money is being spent on devising and assessing the impact of these programs. Mentor programs have provided opportunities for new employees to learn about company policy and practice quickly and effectively. [10] Messmer points out that such programs and practices have had positive results for corporations through higher new employee retention rates and improved company productivity. [11]

Mentoring is also popular within the educational literature where some authors have highlighted the impact of implementing peer-mentoring schemes for academic staff.[12] Others, focusing on the mentoring programs for doctoral and post-doctoral students, have explored methods for matching supervisors with students.[13] While these studies are important, they are generally written from the point of view of the mentors with regard to achieving satisfactory outcomes, rather than from the protégé's point of view.

Mentoring in the research setting

Mentoring, and the relationship between mentor and protégé, can be established under formal guidelines, but more probably in a research setting is impromptu. For the most part, mentoring is not explicitly sought. Rather, it develops out of shared interests. In universities and clinical settings particularly, there is an expectation that research mentoring will just occur through these shared interests. In clinical settings, a clinical supervisor is usually assigned, and other people in the field can be looked up to as senior mentors. Those with research interests seek each other out. In universities, senior students seek out supervisors, and the supervisor can then decide whether or not to take the student on. Some of the most productive mentoring relationships develop out of networking. Contact is often made indirectly through a colleague of a colleague. Interested parties are free to meet and see if their interests coincide. Another way of establishing this relationship is through the workplace, when a junior researcher becomes the specific protégé of a more senior employee.

There are advantages in coming to the relationship in a less formal manner, not the least of which is common interest. If the mentoring process goes well then the protégé can expect to be part of a trusting, cooperative, career-enhancing relationship. If things go wrong, then neither party benefits from the process. As such mentors and their protégés should continuously reflect on the process and relationship. Protégés should also be encouraged to voice their concerns. It can be extremely difficult for the more junior party to extricate herself or himself from an unsatisfactory partnership.

Understanding each other's expectations is a key element to making mentoring work. The relationship is dynamic and will necessarily change over time as the research assistant's skills and confidence increase. Regular reviews are essential. Eventually protégés will want the opportunity to attend conferences, co-author papers and present seminars. Mentors must be both academically generous and sensitive to providing such opportunities.

Tip: Encourage research assistants to attempt new challenges and responsibilities such as attending important meetings or conferences on your behalf.

To avoid incorrect matching of mentors and protégés, mentoring programs in corporations asked for matched expectations with formal written agreements.[14] Writing down expectations not only formally recognises them, it also helps both parties focus on the similarities and differences. At the least, an open discussion of expectations is needed. For junior researchers this can be a daunting task and one that they will need to re-work as they learn more about the job and its possibilities. A good idea is to put assistants in contact with each other and encourage their own mentoring program. Less experienced employees often benefit from networking and communication with their own peers.

The core quality in the relationship between mentor and protégé is trust. As McDougall and Beattie point out 'such relationships tend to be built on a combination of differences and similarities'.[15] They go on to state: '[i]mportant similarities included sharing a common philosophy or values, while key differences included offering another perspective or having contrasting ideas, backgrounds or experiences'.[16] It follows that trust is the crucial element. Inherent in trust is confidentiality, a belief in the other person and interdependence between the parties. Therefore honesty and openness are also important elements. Ritchie, writing about his mentor Ray Miles, reflected upon their first meeting when they discovered shared personal interests and common experiences in growing up.[17] Ritchie's account is of a particularly intimate mentoring relationship. Even in less intimate relationships, sharing some mutual philosophies and values is helpful.

As Deborah Roesler has said, one of the qualities of being a good mentor is to 'listen and coach rather than jump in and solve problems'.[18] Ritchie points out that his mentor was able to show confidence and conviction in his (the protégé's) abilities. He could 'demonstrate and coach the skill needed...[and was]...also open to critical feedback himself...He listened, developed, taught and provided feedback.'[19] Mentoring is about guiding the protégé and encouraging that person to gain experience by actually doing an activity. Good mentors stand back and allow the protégé the opportunity to experience for themselves, in an environment of trust, free from harsh judgment. They are ready to offer practical help, and be a safeguard for difficult issues.

One of the most difficult aspects of mentoring can be finding time to spend together. Since much of the mentoring in research projects happens on the job, scheduling specific time may not always be crucial. However, there will be occasions when more focused appraisal is necessary. Mentors and their protégés might make use of more relaxed meetings, taking time before work or during lunch breaks. When and how meetings take place should be organised beforehand as regular contact and dedicated meeting times are important to maintaining a close and productive alliance.

Tip: Set aside a time for a meeting at least once a week. This time can be used to develop understanding of the research at hand, as well as gauging your assistant's progress, level of confidence, satisfaction in the job.

Experiences

The accounts that follow record some of our experiences in the research world. It is hoped that the stories give an insight into the variety of backgrounds that research assistants can come from and the different directions that they can follow. It is also hoped that readers understand not only the diversity of experience but also the enjoyment of being able to work in such a dynamic and challenging field.

Research assistant as freelance consultant

By the time I began working as a research assistant in health research, I already had years of experience in the field of public relations, special events management and corporate videos, both as a consultant and as a hands-on production assistant. Many of the basic skills required for my new career as a researcher were well entrenched before my first job. Organisational ability, attention to detail and an acute awareness of deadlines combined with what I had learned as a mature-age university student such as analysis, synthesis, creative thinking, and dogged determination, to form many of the skills needed as a research assistant. My first research job came just as I was finishing my undergraduate degree.

Generally, I accept short-term projects of a qualitative nature and work only with the research supervisor. These suit my commitments to study and family and I find my background is ideally suited for the constraints of this type of work. These include tight deadlines, limited time with research supervisors, and being able to work without dedicated office space and support.

My motto has always been to accept the job and learn very quickly how to do it. This means accepting a project that complements my existing skills and talents but also not being afraid to learn on the job. For one particular project, I facilitated a series of focus groups with medical students. I met with them at the beginning and end of session to see if the introduction of a new learning format affected their way of studying. While I had no formal experience in group facilitation, I had run tutorials and felt that the skills required for a tutor would be similar to that required for a facilitator.

I feel that one of the keys to being effective is being able to ask questions and finding out whom to ask. A lot of knowledge is travelling around in other people's heads and if you don't ask them they will never tell you. Interacting with people gives an insight into their talents and skills. For example, librarians are a magical and wonderful source of information, not only about the libraries in which they work but systems of accessing vast arrays of information. One project on blood-borne viruses and institutional policies required that I retrieve articles from a number of discrete professional libraries all over the metropolitan area. It was a fabulous insight into the wealth of information stored in speciality libraries, curated by such knowledgeable librarians.

Another vital element to being a good researcher is flexibility. Often the scope of the brief shifts. For example, the topic for the literature search refines as the search begins to unfold, or it may become apparent that certain questions forming an ad hoc telephone poll elicit responses that require further evaluation. The other important aspect is being critically aware of the project, making time to reflect, and having the courage to offer ideas on how the project is progressing. Usually I work alone for busy people, which means that I am the only one working at the coalface. My reflections upon the project provide supervisors with feedback which they usually do not have time to glean for themselves. Therefore, it is important that my feedback is well considered and generative to the project.

Research work is challenging and rewarding and. above all, it is a partnership in which it is essential for both parties to be amenable to learning from others and to be academically generous. Open, communicative and mutually satisfying working relationships produce the best results all round.

By the middle of 1998 I had completed my Honours degree, and I am currently on a scholarship, undertaking my PhD at the University of New South Wales within the School of Sociology.

From clinical practice to research

After thirteen years working as a Registered Nurse, I decided to alter my career path by becoming involved in research. While working in both hospital and community settings was immensely challenging, I wanted to be involved in the 'bigger picture' of health care. This desire led me to complete a Masters in Public Health degree, in which research methodology and practice was a major focus. This work effectively became the bridge between my clinical and research careers.

My first job as a research assistant was a relatively long-term contract (two years) on a project about hospital and community health services with a group of elderly patients. As with many research projects in the health sector, research assistants are employed for the funded period of the project, and the time period varies considerably depending on the type of project and how much money is granted to pay for the research assistant. Others, such as staff members or associates, may be involved on a more permanent basis. It is also quite common, as occurred in my case, that ongoing work would continue beyond the official funded period.

Coming into research from a nursing background with experience in hospitals, the community, and management was a wonderful way to 'round out' my skills as a health worker. Research involves many of the skills I already possessed, including working within a multidisciplinary team, organisational skills and observation. However, it was a very steep learning curve to apply those skills systematically, as putting theory into practice often is.

From the chief investigator's perspective, having a research assistant with years of experience working in the health system was an advantage for the project. I was able to contribute to the ongoing adaptation of the project as required because of my understanding of the health system and of people's roles within it. I found it easy to liaise with hospital staff and talk with patients involved in the study. Medical terminology was part of my language.

From my experience, a number of skills are essential when working as a research assistant. Writing skills, adaptability, initiative and communication skills are important. Ability to work alone is important. Building relationships with experts in the field who can help out with technical or other information is very important. Knowing when to ask for help or voice concerns is essential. Accessing and keeping up to date with other research and information is also important.

Having hands-on research experience is invaluable as a health care professional. Research is becoming an integral part of clinical practice for all health professionals as it is important to have evidence of the efficiency and efficacy of the care and programs provided to patients. Working as a research assistant has been a challenging and enlightening experience. Using both quantitative and qualitative research skills has also been very rewarding, as they complement each other, providing a real understanding of the issues under investigation.

The assistant–mentor relationship

I began my career in research in 1990, as a junior research assistant working on a large-scale National Health and Medical Research Council (NHMRC) funded project investigating morbidity and treatment in Australian general practice.[20] I had just completed a degree in social sciences. Since this time I have worked on a wide variety of research programs undertaking a range of tasks from data entry to preparing funding submissions. I have gained experience in a number of different settings and methods, and established a wide range of contacts and friendships with everyone from academics to general practitioners. For the most part, my career has developed within the area of general practice research. In the nine years since I started in research, I have gone from being a junior assistant with limited experience to a fully fledged 'researcher' with my own research interests and a clear career path. And while I have had immense encouragement from a variety of people along the way (not least of whom were my colleagues from my first research job, to whom I owe an immense debt of gratitude for inducting me into the trade), it is perhaps in the last three years that I have felt that my career in research has really taken off. This has been fostered, to a large degree, by the presence of two very committed and supportive mentors.

My relationship with my mentors began after being employed on a study exploring ethical issues in general practice.[21] While I came to the project half-way through, I felt an immediate affinity not only with the research area, but also with many of those working on the research team. Our team meetings became philosophical discussions as much as discussions about the practicalities of running a research program. What united us was a shared commitment to the particular area of research and a valuing of everyone's contribution. Such valuing is one of the key facilitators of a successful mentor–protégé relationship. The fact that team members respected my opinions and contribution was rewarding and gave me the confidence to explore things on my own.

Through the support and encouragement of my mentors I have been able to submit articles for journal publication as well as present papers at a range of conferences and seminars. They have also played a central role in fostering my interest in the areas of bioethics and qualitative research methodology. Indeed, through their encouragement and support I am now undertaking my major project as part of a Masters of Community Health on these very areas. Not surprisingly they are my supervisors and mentors in this work too. I have also been able to explore other professional avenues, such as tutoring work in bioethics, which is something I enjoy immensely.

As much as anything else, and maybe this is what has ensured the success of this particular mentoring relationship, I have gained two friends whom I respect and admire greatly, both as professionals and as people. Without them I may never have contributed to this book.

12
Ethics as part of research

CATHERINE BERGLUND

This chapter overviews ethics in research. A simple checklist of issues to be aware of is offered, and a way of finding out more about ethics for particular types of methodologies is covered. Key issues for quantitative and qualitative research with people are explained. The Australian institutional ethics committee system is described, and up-to-date information on submitting research proposals for approval is referred to. These issues should not be added on to research at the last minute. They are part of planning. The way the ethics issues were part of each chapter of this research text is highlighted, as a review of research options in the planning, conduct and analysis process. This chapter introduces common ethical concepts and issues in research involving humans. It makes specific reference to the general ethics principles in the National Health and Medical Research Council's (NHMRC) *National Statement on Ethical Conduct in Research Involving Humans*,[1] and offers explanations for why these principles are concerns of ethics.

Research deserving ethical reflection

Research involving humans is notoriously difficult to define, and is usually defined broadly by process as well as objective. In the *National Statement*, human research activity is stated to be that which 'involves human participation or definable human involvement and has a purpose of establishing facts, principles or knowledge or of obtaining or confirming knowledge' (p. 7).

Throughout this text, you have seen many examples of information gathered in the pursuit of knowledge and understanding. Most of that information came in some way from human participants. The aim of the research, the collection of information, the analysis and interpretation of the information, and the communication of research findings all have an ethical dimension. Sorting out what is the ethical issue, and why, is the object of this chapter.

The process of information collection in human research can range from accessing previously gathered information such as medical records, to asking questions in an interview or questionnaire, observing people, or doing a physical examination, performing a blood test or taking or using tissue samples, giving an experimental treatment or intervention and observing results, or doing an experimental operation and observing the results. Research with humans is both health and social research, and spans a wide range of methodological constructs.[2]

There is a growing literature on practical ways to tackle ethics reflection on the endeavour of human research. One way of making a start is to use agreed ethics tools, to summarise issues of concern. The principles of beneficence, respect for persons and justice are an established set of ethics tools for considering research. They were coined in the Belmont Report, over twenty years ago, and have been referred to ever since as research ethics principles, and are called the Belmont principles.[3] They were agreed on as useful tools by ethicists who preferred different ethical frameworks, hence their broad application.

The Belmont principles are defined in this excerpt:

> Issues involving assessment of the risks and benefits to individuals can be thought of as coming under the principle of beneficence; issues surrounding personal autonomy as being under the principle of respect for persons; and issues of the benefits and burdens of society in general as coming under the principle of justice ... The principles should all be considered in any research situation. That is because some issues relate to more than one principle— there can be conflicting ethical concerns in research practice, as in any health practice.[4]

The Belmont principles are not principles in the sense of mandating certain actions. Rather, they are useful shorthand terms for a cluster of concerns in research ethics. The concerns under the principles often conflict, and a balance of issues under the principles is usually weighed up, with the aid of an ethics theory or framework, to resolve dilemmas on what should or should not be done in research contexts. The Belmont principles are increasingly referred to as 'values' so as to avoid the misinterpretation of them as overarching obligating principles.

It is stressed that the Belmont principles will aid in a listing and consideration of research ethics issues, but understanding how conflicting issues can be resolved requires upper level theoretical reasoning. The two most widely applied ethics theories or frameworks are utilitarianism, and deontology. Both identify care and benefit for others, and the minimisation of harm, as important. Both identify autonomy and individual exercise of choice as important. Yet, the balance of these issues can be different under the different reasoning. While utilitarians emphasise outcome in their ethical reasoning, deontologists emphasise process.[5] As one example, Kant's approach is to support the individual pursuit of morality, with individual freedom necessary for that pursuit. Respect for others is supported not only as part of freedom, but also so that each person may safeguard their own well-being. Put simply, individuals should not be treated as means to ends. Alternatively, J.S. Mill's utilitarian approach is to champion maximum benefit and minimum harm for a society, with each person allowed to pursue their own happiness, providing it does not infringe on other's similar liberties, or threaten the fabric of society.[6] The implications of these differing frameworks for dilemmas in health care have been the subject of considerable philosophical reflection and writing.[7]

The NHMRC's latest research statement, the *National Statement on Ethical Conduct in Research Involving Humans*, was issued in 1999 and largely replaces the previous version (*NHMRC Statement on Human Experimentation and Supplementary Notes*). The *National Statement* applies to all research with human participants. The statement adds 'integrity' as a value of ethical conduct to the list of respect for persons, beneficence and justice. The value of integrity is to be considered by researchers in designing and conducting their research. Principle 1.1 reads: 'The guiding value for researchers is integrity, which is expressed in a commitment to the search for knowledge, to recognised principles of research conduct and in honest and ethical conduct of research and dissemination and communication of results' (p. 11). So, integrity is applied as researchers actively reflect on their research aims and process. This is to state the key notion of ethics—reflection on actions and thoughts and striving to act ethically—as an obligation.

Each principle and value is considered by the human research ethics committees (HRECs), previously known as institutional ethics committees (IECs), as they make decisions on the ethical acceptability of proposed research with human participants.

Beneficence

The principle of beneficence encompasses caring for others. Care has two aspects. The first is actively doing good for each person. The second is preventing or minimising harm to each person. This second aspect is sometimes thought of as a principle of non-maleficence, a duty not to cause harm intentionally, as in Beauchamp and Childress's formulation of bioethics principles.[8] When beneficence was described under the Belmont Report, it was also thought to include the maximisation of potential benefit to society.

The natural starting point for consideration under the umbrella of beneficence concerns is the aim of the research, and its justification, and the appropriateness of the nominated researcher to pursue this aim. The central concern in this assessment is at the level of what the individual research participant, or potential research participant, may experience by way of benefit or harm in the research process.

Research aim and justification

The research aim and justification is partly about conforming to general moral and scientific principles, as set out in relevant international and national covenants and declarations. These are explicitly required to be followed in the NHMRC's *National Statement.*

General moral principles as expressed in such guidelines are about the basic obligations we have towards each other, in a world community sense. If research aims contravene notions of basic human dignity, respect and fairness, it would be very difficult to find research compatible with societal aims, or palatable to communities within that society. This means that research acceptability should be considered for each specific community. Tolerance of research, and research process, including ownership of the research process, may vary for indigenous populations, for instance.

General scientific principles may be found in each researcher's professional codes, or through mentoring and peer reference, espoused as reputable and expected professional conduct. Professionals are trusted by the public to abide by recognised peer standards. These peer standards are assumed to set a reasonable and safe level of practice. That is why reference to such scientific and professionally relevant principles of conduct is vital.

The research aim and justification is also dependent on a demonstrated need for the research. Any input of resources, or involvement of research participants, would be difficult to justify in the absence of a considered case for the research need, and likely contribution to knowledge. To avoid duplication of research effort, and to avoid research proceeding with humans prematurely, the researcher is also advised to find out about prior research, and to ensure that appropriate laboratory or animal model experiments have already been conducted (if appropriate), and that they support the planned research with human participants.

However, there is an exception. That exception is if prior research was not conducted ethically. There is now strong international pressure to give the findings from such research no credence. To build on previously unethical research would be regarded as a tainted process.

Duplication of acceptable research, or premature research, would needlessly involve human participants for little relative gain in knowledge and understanding. Unless research has been planned with care and considerable thought, it would be viewed as being premature. As Jeanette Ward and D'Arcy Holman emphasised in their chapter 'Who needs to plan?', the reliance on meaningful results is only possible with careful planning of the research design and practicalities of the research process.

The message on duplication is that each researcher should not have to conduct each experiment or research process to be able to rely on results. Researchers should be able to access peer-reviewed knowledge, or results of prior research, assess its weight in terms of their existing professional knowledge, and make a reasoned decision on research direction.

Peer-reviewed publication adds significantly to the safeguard of avoiding needless involvement of human participants. A researcher therefore needs to be able to access relevant literature, and also eventually to contribute to that literature. This is expressed as an obligation of researchers once they have completed their research to offer their research for publication, and to their peers for relevant professional assessment of its worth.

All researchers thus effectively have an ethical obligation to publish what has been completed, so that it is available to others, and an ethical obligation to access the published literature in the planning phases of their studies. The chapter on 'Writing and publishing' encourages you to view publishing and dissemination of your research findings as part of the research endeavour. As in situations requiring informed consent, or reasoned informed decision-making, unless information is available, reasoned decisions on future research or clinical directions cannot be made.

The NHMRC *National Statement* has as its principle 1.13, 'Every research proposal must demonstrate that the research is justifiable in terms of its potential contribution to knowledge and is based on a thorough study of current literature as well as prior observation, approved previous studies, and where relevant, laboratory and animal studies' (p. 13).

And in relation to peer review and publication, the NHMRC *National Statement* has as its principle 1.18, 'The results of research (whether publicly or privately funded) and the methods used should normally be published in ways which permit scrutiny and contribute to public knowledge. Normally, research results should be made available to research participants' (p. 13).

Clearly, the process of research is viewed as a discipline which is embedded in the skill of the profession to which the researcher belongs. Difference in research methods is tolerated, but support for an approach depends on solid reference to an accepted body of knowledge among a researcher's peers. This is the

reasoning behind competitive peer review of research proposals prior to allocation of funds as well.

Researcher

The skill of the professional is a primary issue in considering likely harm or benefit for a research participant. Professionals are highly trained in particular skills,
which they offer in service of the community. By definition, there are limits to
their skill. Considering what they can do proficiently, and therefore effectively and
safely, is a natural starting point for ethics reflection.[9] The background, and pre-
paredness of the researcher to undertake their chosen research process, is an essential ethics consideration. Unless each researcher is properly prepared, and
equipped, the consideration of possible benefit or risk for the potential participant
is purely hypothetical, and at best, very difficult to estimate. Further, to go outside
one's own skill may in itself be unethical. That would be like holding oneself out
to be a trained professional in another field, or in a specialty, when the requisite
training had not been acquired. There are risks that the job might not be done well
if that were the case, even apart from possible increased risk of harm, and
decreased probability of benefit for the participant. There is a tendency to err on
the side of caution in relation to professional skill in research, because by definition, research may not hold out probability of benefit to any research participants.
The NHMRC *National Statement* principle 1.15, states: 'Research must be conducted or supervised only by persons or teams with experience, qualifications and
competence appropriate to the research. Research must only be conducted using
facilities appropriate for the research and where there are appropriate skills and
resources for dealing with any contingencies that may affect participants' (p. 13).

The researcher is best placed to use his or her skill, and to assess the process
objectively, if free of potential conflict or interest. If there is possible conflict of
interest, it should be disclosed. This information serves to trigger an added peer
review at the time of research proposal, and journal consideration of the reporting of results.

The researcher's background and skill enables each researcher to make a
unique contribution to research. This was illustrated in chapter 1, 'Beginning the
quest', in which a research problem was brainstormed, and then different research
questions formulated by different skill groups. In Phillip Godwin's chapter also,
the clinical skill and insight of the practitioner was discussed. It is sometimes the
practical insights which highlight useful research questions.

Risks and benefits

Once the general aim of the research and the preparation of the researcher has
been considered to be satisfactory, the key concern is what will happen to the

participants if they take part. By definition, it is impossible to know exactly what will happen to research participants, and what the effect of their participation will be, because that is the nature of research. Research is about finding things out, exploring issues, and seeing the effect of interventions. Good estimates though, and more specifically, probable risks and probable benefits, are ethically relevant to the overall ethical acceptability of proposed research.

Risk is not just tangible physical risk. A potential for causing harm to participants is defined in the NHMRC *National Statement* as causing 'harm to the well-being of participant, whether physically, psychologically, spiritually or emotionally; or in the exploitation of cultural knowledge and/or property, where their involvement, or the use of their personal or community-based information, has a potential for infringement of their privacy or of the confidentiality or ownership that attaches to that information; or where their involvement imposes burdens with little benefits' (p. 8).

Generally, the more risk with less benefit which is likely to befall a participant, the less acceptable the research would be. That is because the central issue in beneficence is to do no harm, and to promote benefit. If risk is entailed in the pursuit of benefit, it is a little more difficult to draw the ethically acceptable line on amount of risk that research participants can be exposed to.

Therapeutic and non-therapeutic distinctions are important in balancing acceptable risks and benefits. This distinction is whether a process is likely or not to bring benefit to the person taking part in the research. In some guidelines, therapeutic benefit is interpreted very broadly, as being therapeutic benefit to the class of persons to which the research participant belongs. You may like to follow the early debate on this topic in writings by Levine, Nicholson, and Capron.[10] The broad community therapeutic benefit is not the interpretation of therapeutic benefit adopted by the NHMRC. The wording stipulates therapeutic benefit to the participant. The limit on risk of harm in non-therapeutic research is 'the absence of intended benefits to a participant should justly be balanced by the absence of all but minimal risk', as stated in the NHMRC *National Statement* at principle 1.6 (p. 12). This is supported also by principle 1.3, in which the individual effect takes priority over community benefit: 'Each research protocol must be designed to ensure that respect for the dignity and well being of the participants in research takes precedence over the expected benefits to knowledge' (p. 11).

The distinction between benefit for an individual and benefit for the community is particularly relevant when people with diminished capacity to exercise their autonomy are being asked to take part in research. In research involving children, for instance, there is a tendency for greater caution.[11] The research question should be important 'to the health and well-being of children and young people', and their participation needed, with the research question unable to be answered another way. The child is afforded greater decision-making input in the revised *National Statement*. There is increased importance placed on children considering whether or not to participate, and their refusal is respected, even if their parents think that they could take part (p. 25).

The nature of risks and benefits are different issues to the probability of those risks and benefits occurring. This distinction can be highly relevant to deciding the acceptability, on balance of the research, and to individuals subsequently weighing up whether they will take part in any process. In recent informed consent guidelines, the probability of side effects is thought to be relevant in deciding what information should be given to patients by their doctors, as well as the detail of what the side effects are.[12] The NHMRC guidelines on providing information to patients state: 'Known risks should be disclosed when an adverse outcome is common even though the detriment is slight, or when an adverse outcome is severe even though its occurrence is rare.'[13] It is also a common ethically informed social judgment for us to impose restrictions on public risks, if they are serious and imminent. This wording is informed by J.S. Mill's writing, in which individual liberty may be restricted in circumstances of serious and imminent risk posed to others.

It could be argued that only prospective research participants can decide if what will happen in research is acceptable or not. That position would elevate autonomy to an extreme position of importance. Generally, though, a prior decision is made by ethics committees about whether the planned process is acceptable. Then, all participants must also decide if they find the process acceptable for them.

In instances where all other medical avenues have been tried and have failed, more of the decision of acceptability has been left up to the prospective research participant. Such instances are fairly rare, and occur most commonly in life-threatening conditions for which there is no recognised cure. Some interesting debates occurred on this balance of what research subjects should be allowed to decide in relation to HIV and AIDS research, particularly in drug trials, in the early 1990s.[14]

If at any time, there is actual harm in research or increased probability of it in relation to the benefit, or decreased likelihood of benefit, the researcher has a responsibility to minimise further relative harm. This is stated in the NHMRC *National Statement* at principle 1.7: 'A researcher must suspend or modify any research in which the risks to participants are found to be disproportionate to the benefits and stop any involvement of any participant if continuation of the research may be harmful to that person' (p. 13).

As part of the overall minimisation of inconvenience and harm in the process of research, only the number of people required to gain meaningful results should be included. To continue to include people when their numbers add nothing more to the reliability, or depth of the information, would be to impose undue burden.

Ongoing assessment of the research process, by the researcher, is the key safeguard to finding an acceptable balance between benefit and harm once the research is in train. This ongoing reflection is the integrity value in action.

Respect for persons

Individuals choose to live their lives in very different ways. The principle of respect for persons is about respecting individual differences, and choices about individual actions. When groups of people adopt certain ways of living, respect for each person becomes cultural respect.

The NHMRC *National Statement* holds the issue of respect for persons as a cultural as well as individual issue of respect, at principle 1.2: 'When conducting research involving humans, the guiding ethical principle for researchers is respect for persons which is expressed as regard for the welfare, rights, beliefs, perceptions, customs and cultural heritage, both individual and collective, of persons involved in research' (p. 11). Thus, different research processes may be appropriate, and even essential, in different communities, as highlighted in Jan Ritchie's chapter on qualitative research methods, 'Not everything can be reduced to numbers'.

Consent

Respect for persons concerns an obligation to uphold the autonomy of individuals. Autonomy is literally self-rule. The capacity to make one's own decisions is a central issue in autonomy. Also, encouraging people to put their capacity for decision-making into practice is a central ethics concern. That is why both allowing an individual to make a decision and maximising the factors in decision-making, such as provision of information, are given such prominence in the NHMRC's *National Statement*. Equally, any hindering of a person in making a decision about research participation would be viewed with concern. Some of the principles in the NHMRC statement are safeguards against this occurring.

The concern with the process of consent is evidenced in the NHMRC *National Statement*, by the sheer number of principles which are about the decision-making process, and the exercise of individual choice. For instance, principle 1.7:

Before research is undertaken, whether involving individuals or collectivities, the consent of the participants must be obtained...

The ethical and legal requirements of consent have two aspects: the provision of information and the capacity to make a voluntary choice. So as to conform with ethical and legal requirements, obtaining consent should involve:

(a) provision to participants, at their level of comprehension, of material information about the purpose, methods, demands, risks, inconveniences and discomforts of the study. Consent should be obtained in writing unless there are good reasons to the contrary. If consent is not obtained in writing, the circumstances under which it is obtained should be recorded; and

(b) the exercise by participants of a voluntary choice to participate.

Where a participant lacks competence to consent, a person with lawful authority to decide for that participant must be provided with that information and exercise that choice. (p.12)

The research assistants who contributed the chapter 'Assistants and mentors' were very conscious of these ethical requirements. Research assistants are quite often the ones who approach potential participants, to explain the project, and to seek their consent. It is vital that research assistants are briefed on the ethical importance of this process, so that the project is conducted at the level of accepted standards.

The elements of informed decision-making, information, competence, understanding, and voluntariness, are crucial to understanding the consent process.[15] These elements are apparent in the NHMRC *National Statement* principles, as set out above. There is new emphasis in the revised statement for information not only being provided, but also being provided in as accessible form as possible, that is packaged in a way that will suit the participants on an individual basis. This is consistent with the emphasis in decision-making in health contexts. Information on process and risk that is material to the individual, explained in a way that can be best understood by the patient, is increasingly being adopted as preferable practice by health care professionals. It is a practical way of maximising autonomy.

The caution in relation to intervention in the health of individuals, in balancing risk and benefit is also evident in the NHMRC guidelines on providing information to patients, which states: 'Complex interventions require more information, as do interventions where the patient has no illness'.[16] Health volunteers need to weigh up any risks in participating in research carefully, as they do not face other adverse health risks. In complex interventions, the risks are likely to be more numerous. There is a balance to strike between the purpose of the intervention and the information needed to make an informed decision about whether to participate.

Continuing autonomy also means that participants can withdraw their participation. They are without obligation to the research or to the researcher— principle 1.12 of the NHMRC *National Statement*: 'A participant must be free at any time to withdraw consent to further involvement in the research.' Further, if there would be consequences of withdrawal, such as may occur in access to innovative treatment regimens in clinical trials, the information should be available to participants before they begin involvement (p. 13).

Vulnerable and incompetent subjects

The detail of principle 1.7 in the NHMRC *National Statement* is concerned with provision of information in an accessible form, so that an informed decision can be made. This repackaging of information applies to groups such as children, and to the elderly. It is part of an assessment of competency and capacity to make decisions. Generally, if information delivery can be enhanced, then decision-making capacity can also be enhanced.

Decision-making capacity in elderly people has been neatly summarised by Finucane, Myser and Ticehurst.[17] The social context and delivery of information are equally important in enhancing decision capacity, and in assessing whether a decision can be made competently at any point in time.

The increased emphasis on children being part of decisions on their own participation in research is noted above. It is ethically significant that this emphasis is on dissent (refusal) as well as assent, even before a child may be thought mature enough to give legal consent. This is consistent with the ethical notion of developing autonomy even if full competency to make all decisions has not yet been attained.

Dependency

Sometimes, a potential participant is at a risk of being dependent on either the research, the researcher, or the institution in which the research is conducted. Examples include patients, when their clinician or affiliated clinical team may be involved in research programs; children and elderly, who are regarded as being dependent on others more than able adults; and students in tertiary institutions that have research recruitment drives. A risk of dependency creates a risk of feeling of coerciveness in the decision to participate, and so calls for safeguards and checks that free consent is given by participants. There may even be circumstances in which the risk of feeling coerced remains, and either the researchers or the ethics committee may decide that the research cannot be conducted with a satisfactory transparency of informed consent processes.

The issues of process of recruitment and what happens after a participant withdraws from the research have been studied with the aim to maximise the free choice of the potentially dependent participant.[18] One practical step is to separate the clinical care, or teaching, and research recruitment processes. Another is to remind potential participants of their option not to take part, and to withdraw at any time. A 100 per cent participation rate is not the norm in any research program, and a high participation rate would be regarded with suspicion in circumstances of dependency.

The guiding principle in the NHMRC *National Statement* is principle 1.10: 'The consent of a person to participate in research must not be subject to any coercion, or to any inducement or influence which could impair its voluntary character' (p. 12).

Payment

Money can act as an inducement to participate, and alter a decision on whether a person would take part. In its stead, adequate recompense for inconvenience is often substituted, like a lunch voucher, or a taxi cab charge to cover transport. As a general guide, it should be smaller recompense than would induce a decision to participate for that 'reward'.

Privacy and confidentiality

Decisions about what happens to one's own body, or active participation in research, is fairly obviously an issue of autonomy. The concern also extends to information that is collected about individuals.

The terms privacy and confidentiality can be defined as follows: 'The issue common to both privacy and confidentiality is respect for an individual's control over his or her personal information. Information privacy issues centre on control of access to personal information. Confidentiality issues are derived from privacy; confidentiality relates to control over the use or further disclosure of that information.'[19]

Personal information is identified or identifiable information. It could be identified with either individuals, or groups. Researchers are well used to deidentifying, or code numbering, research participants and their data, so that the identify of participants is not on documents which may come into view by others than the research team. Identifiable information is kept in locked filing cabinets. Practical ideas for data storage are in the chapter 'Assistants and mentors'.

Caution in handling participant data is also required in the reporting of small cell data, as there is greater risk of identifying individuals in those categories. Researchers who work with categorical data, such as described by Mary Phipps and Dusan Hadzi-Pavlovic in their chapter 'Meaningful categories', are conscious of their obligation to safeguard the identifiable information, and are reluctant to report data with cell frequencies less than 5.

In qualitative research, the very reporting of results raises issues of confidentiality. In qualitative work, it is common to ask the participants to describe their own experiences and feelings, and then to report that information as an illustration of interesting themes that were found. By virtue of the personal nature of experiential information, researchers need to carefully consider whether the distribution of the results could identify the participants. If there is a real possibility of individuals being identified, then participants should know that before they agree to take part.

The privilege of being granted access to sensitive information becomes a responsibility to use that information with care, and to safeguard further unintended distribution of each individual's personal information. The trust in that safeguard ensures the continued cooperation by individuals and collectivities in research.

The NHMRC *National Statement* states in principle 1.19: 'Where personal information about research participants or a collectivity is collected, stored, accessed, used, or disposed of, researchers must strive to ensure that the privacy, confidentiality and cultural sensitivities of the participants and/or the collectivity are respected. Any specific agreements made with the participants or the collectivity are to be fulfilled' (p. 13).

Privacy issues are covered in a NHMRC information paper on medical records and privacy.[20] That paper is intended to work in concert with the Commonwealth *Privacy Act 1988*. In short, there is a balance to strike over access to information in the public interest, and the public interests in privacy. The preferable course is to ask for consent of individuals for use of their personal information in research. If consent would be impossible or very difficult to obtain, a HREC has discretion to decide if the public interest in the research substantially outweighs the public interest in privacy. This standard was developed for the *Privacy Act* exception, but it has been increasingly applied outside the Commonwealth jurisdiction.

Further information papers and guidelines on use of personal information in business and private health industry contexts are being developed.[21] Each researcher will need to consider the relevant guidelines, paying special attention to the context in which information was sought for the research, and the expectations that people had for the use of that information when they provided it.

Justice

Fair distribution of benefits and burdens

Having identified the likely benefits and burdens of a research process, the researcher then is able to consider how the benefits and burdens can be shared. Fair distribution is the core concern of the principle of justice, and this consideration is assisted by models of justice. The main models of distribution: justice as fairness (in which equality or restoration from unlucky burden is pursued); comparative justice (in which need is the primary distinction); and distributive justice (in which need and socially distinguishing factors can be combined), can be applied for specific 'goods' when thinking about the group which is planned to take part in the research, and the broader community group which may benefit from the research.[22]

The common issue in justice models is the consideration of due benefit and burden, and conversely, unfair benefit and burden. Institutions, and institutional ethics committees, are able to implement justice models differently.

If there are probable goods or bads (benefits or risks) in a research protocol, the selection of the sample participants is also a justice issue. By their selection, participants are given access to probable benefit, or exposure to possible harm.

Vulnerable subject population

The selection of research participants, and what they are asked to do for the research, is relative to the use to which the research will be put in the future. Beyond the research process, once the knowledge from the process is available, its use and application to comparable or different groups from those of research participants should be considered. There has been comment about the ethics of conducting drug trials on poorer communities, who may not be able to afford to buy the drug if it is proven effective. Equally, there has been considerable comment on the ethics of conducting research with institutionalised, and accessible research participants, such as in schools, or living facilities, or hospitals, or prisons, when that research is generally applicable to the broader community, and could have been conducted on participants drawn from the broader community.

The NHMRC *National Statement* notes the importance of considering whether the burden of research participation should be placed on vulnerable groups. The same question could be asked of groups which are researched repeatedly. If burden is placed on one group, but the benefit yielded to another group, there would be concern.

The NHMRC *National Statement* principle 1.5 states:

a researcher must:

(c) avoid imposing on particular groups, who are likely to be subject to overresearching, an unfair burden of participation in research;

(d) design research so that the selection, recruitment, exclusion and inclusion of research participants is fair; and

(e) not discriminate in the selection and recruitment of actual and future participants by including or excluding them on the grounds of race, age, sex, disability or religious or spiritual beliefs except where the exclusion or inclusion of particular groups is essential to the purpose of the research. (p. 11).

Analysis and reporting

Accurate analysis and careful interpretation of research findings are part of the honest pursuit of research. This is tested when the analysis raises unexpected findings, or is almost, but not quite, significant. Deborah Black, Andrew Grulich, Dusan Hadzi-Pavlovic and Mary Phipps all comment on statistical options, and the appropriate use of those data manipulations, in the statistics chapters. Jan Ritchie comments on the process of drawing interpretations from qualitative information. Each is concerned with the process of crystalising results. In ethical terms, this is an important process. Unless accurate and honest analysis and interpretation are made, the research burden has been to no real purpose. It will have been unethical to have conducted the research at all, as the balance of benefit and burden becomes unacceptable.

The obligation to publish findings, as noted above, is part of the research endeavour and provides information for future researchers and practising fellow professionals. The participants, or the groups to which they belong, may also find it useful for understanding their health and condition. The findings can be required by communities, as a condition of taking part in the research process.

Ethics committee review

Human research ethics committees (HRECs) are the institutional forum for ethical review of research plans. Each institution that conducts research with humans and wishes to be eligible for government funds must have an ethics committee, and must review all research proposals, regardless of the proposed funding source for the project. Researchers submit protocols for review and may not start the research process in so far as it involves humans without committee approval.

The new name for the committees is contained in the NHMRC's 1999 *National Statement on Ethical Conduct in Research Involving Humans*, as are the new required committee operating proceedures. Previously, the Australian committees were named institutional ethics committees (IECs). Their equivalent are known as institutional review boards (IRBs) in the United States, and research ethics committees (RECs) in other countries.

The issues in this chapter should all be thought about before submitting a research proposal to the human research ethics committee for approval. You can use the submission checklist as a running guide to reflect on the issues in your research before writing an ethics committee submission.

The committees are intended to serve both a monitoring and an educative function. The process of review is a prompt for researchers to consider the ethical implications of their own research, and to continue to reflect on their research as they conduct it. The committees also serve a gatekeeping role, so that research that may pose an undue burden on potential participants can be stopped before participants are exposed to that burden.

The human research ethics committees are composed of, as a minimum, people in the following seven categories:

(a) a chairperson
(b) at least two members who are lay people, one man and one woman, who have no affiliation with the institution or organisation, are not currently involved in medical, scientific, or legal work, and who are preferably from the community in which the institution or organisation is located;
(c) at least one member with knowledge of, and current experience in, the areas of research that are regularly considered by the HREC (eg. Health, medical, social, psychological, epidemiological, as appropriate);
(d) at least one member with knowledge of, and current experience in, the professional care, counselling or treatment of people (eg. Medical practitioner, clinical psychologist, social worker, nurse, as appropriate);
(e) at least one member who is a minister of religion, or a person who performs a similar role in a community such as an Aboriginal elder; and
(f) at least one member who is a lawyer. (p. 16)

Well-established meeting and working procedures and recording of decisions, and a responsibility to monitor the research which is conducted, are outlined in

Submission checklist

Beneficence
- reasoned and well-researched basis of research
- assessment of the benefits of the research
- assessment of the risks of the research
- weighing risk against benefit
- skill of the researcher
- resources available to the researcher

Respect for persons
- respect for personal and cultural values within the research process
- informed consent from research participants
- participants being free to withdraw from research
- additional provision for vulnerable or dependent participants
- confidentiality
- payment/compensation to participants

Justice
- advancement of understanding
- assessment of distribution of burden
- assessment of distribution of benefit
- fair balance of burden and benefit in research process
- honest and accurate analysis and interpretation of results
- sharing of knowledge and dissemination of results

the NHMRC *National Statement*, to which the committees must conform as of 1 January 2000 (pp. 17–20). The detailed section on committee processes in the *National Statement* illustrates the importance of effective committee consideration as an ethical safeguard in human research. Expedited review is available for research of minimal risk, and multicentre research in which another HREC has fully considered the protocol.

Many committees have standard forms which must be completed by researchers before they submit their research proposal for ethics committee review. If you are submitting a proposal, first contact your ethics committee and ask:

- Is there a pro-forma for submission?
- When does the committee meet?
- What is the deadline for your submission to be included in the agenda for the next meeting?
- How many copies of the proposal would the committee like?

Asking these simple administrative questions can save you time and frustration so that you understand the working schedule of the committee which must consider your proposal. Bear in mind also that there are extremely busy times of the year for these committees—just before funding application deadlines, for instance, when the committees are stretched to absolute capacity. The people on the committees are committed and hard-working people who have taken an interest in ethics. For the most part, they are unpaid for that committee work. Their reflection on your research process is invaluable, and like any reflective process, it takes some time. In much the same way as a research team can formulate a better research plan than one person alone, and a reading group can help with the process of your writing, an ethics committee can help to highlight potential concerns in the process of your research. Far better that they be raised before your research is conducted than after the ethical risk becomes real.

Once you have ethics approval, the process of ethics reflection should continue. The following questions to ask yourself may help in that process. The questions can be expressed in the past tense when reflecting on the full course of completed research, or put into the present or future tense, as a starting point in thinking about a research protocol and its ethical implications.

- What was your research about?
- Were you skilled enough to undertake the research?
- Where did your research subjects come from?
- What did you ask your research subjects to do?
- How did the participants consent to the research?
- How was your research used?
- Was the process worth it, given the results?[23]

An ongoing reflection process is the key to ethics guidelines working well in the process of research. The researcher is closest to her or his own professional skill and own research process. The researcher is best placed to actively reflect on a process and its implications, and the researcher is also in the best position to bring ethical reflection into practice. Striving for ethical reflection is a professional responsibility.

In the NHMRC's *National Statement on Ethical Conduct in Research Involving Humans,* the preamble contains this statement on ethical and legal considerations: 'Ethical guidelines have the objective of defining standards of behaviour to which researchers should adhere. Where the guidelines prescribe a standard that exceeds that required by the law, then researchers should apply this higher standard' (p. 5). The key is in identifying aspirations and obligations, and maintaining self-reflection, coupled with reference to peer and external perspectives.

Try exercise 12.1 as a review of this chapter.

Exercise 12.1

Take a published piece of health research from one of the journals relevant to your profession. Apply the ethics checklist in this chapter to that research, and make a summary of what you would change if you were to conduct that research so that it met your own optimal ethics standards.

Your changes may in part reflect your profession's stated values, and your own value judgments of the relative importance of the ethics concerns of beneficence, non-maleficence, respect for persons and justice.

Look back over your changes, and make a note about which of the ethics concerns you have emphasised. Try and explain your concerns to another person or a group.

13

Disciplines and boundaries

JOHN DEVEREUX

Legal boundaries for research are defined by professional discipline, statutory and common law, administrative guidelines, and community expectations. When researchers work across disciplines, they need to consider the boundaries of each discipline.

It is important for researchers to consider ethical obligations established by their own profession. Written professional guidelines express the expected standards. Codes of ethics of nurses and doctors are an example of a written expression of expected standards in clinical practice. The codes emphasise duties to care for the patient. Professionals are expected to fulfil their duty of care, by virtue of being professional, and being charged with particular skills and responsibilities. Codes of ethics also emphasise the careful conduct of research in furthering knowledge. It is expected that duties to care for the participant will take precedence over the conduct of the research.

Many legal issues in the conduct of research overlap with ethics considerations. The latter are covered in chapter 12, 'Ethics as part of research'. This chapter does not repeat those fundamental issues, but does note their legal importance. Their importance arises partly because they are covered by the administrative regulations that researchers are required to consult and abide by in the conduct of their research. In Australia, the key administrative guideline of this type is the National Health and Medical Research Council's

National Statement on Ethical Conduct in Research Involving Humans.[1] This statement has been referred to in detail in chapter 12. An important reference for researchers in reflecting on their responsibilities under the *National Statement,* which also explains some of the legal aspects of research issues, is the operations manual for human research ethics committees.[2]

Law, like any other discipline has its own unique discourse, style and technique. It also has its own research tools. The purpose of this chapter is to try to de-mystify some of the intricacies of legal research. A secondary purpose of the chapter is to identify some legal considerations which researchers should bear in mind when conducting research.

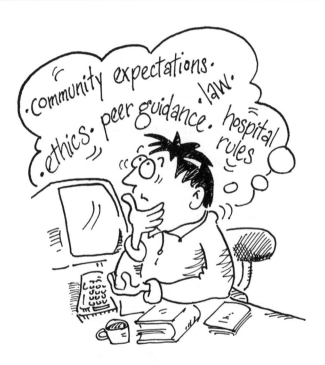

The genesis of legal research

A law library is to a lawyer what a laboratory is to a scientist: the basic tool of research. Within the depths of the law library, information can be found that allows lawyers to find out about a general area of law, update their knowledge on a particular area of law, or frame an argument that a particular legal case should no longer be regarded as being good law.

Legal research methodology is generally said to have 6 steps.[3]

1   Assemble the relevant facts
2   Identify relevant areas of law, jurisdictions (for instance, state) and time frame
3   Background reading—searching for secondary sources of law
4   Locating relevant authorities—searching for primary sources of law
5   Analyse the law and apply it to the facts identified in step 1
6   Draw conclusions

On the assumption that a researcher has identified steps 1 and 2, we can move straight to step 3.

Outlining the general area of law

As a researcher, you need to familiarise yourself with the general area of law. There are various ways of doing this. One is to examine a recent textbook on the area under consideration. If you are researching into the law which governs a person suing another person for doing harm to him or her (called torts), you may, for example wish to consult Balkin and Davis *The Law of Torts*.[4] A less detailed book (though not any less useful) would be McGlone and Gardiner's *An Introduction to the Law of Torts*.[5] A good introduction to Queensland or Western Australian criminal law may be found in Kenny *Criminal Law in Queensland and Western Australia*,[6] and there are comparable texts for other jurisdictions.

Textbooks sometimes have to be approached with caution. It is important to note, as Enright points out, that a legal textbook does more than simply state the law: 'Textbooks summarise the law, and in the process will usually organise and analyse it. They may also explain, amplify and even criticise the law, and they may go to the outside world and look at the law in some wider social, philosophical or historical way'.[7]

Another approach may be use a legal encyclopaedia. *Halsbury's Laws of Australia* (produced by Butterworths) and *The Laws of Australia* (produced by the Law Book Company) are both to be found in regularly updated loose-leaf volumes and on CD-ROM. These services aim to produce concise statements of the law, free from academic criticism, philosophical debate or commentary.

CCH publishers produce a number of loose-leaf services which give a good overview of various areas. 'Typically a loose leaf publication will include an outline or summary of the law, the full text of relevant statutes and delegated legislation'.[8] Health law researchers may find *The Australian Health and Medical Law Reporter* to be of most benefit, though the *Social Security Reporter* or *Torts Reporter* may also be of interest.

A lesser known source of useful summaries of general areas of the law is reports of the various law reform commissions. The Queensland, New South Wales and Victorian law reform commissions have been particularly active in health law research. (The latter body has now been disbanded, though reports of its work should still be in the law library.)

When you read through a summary of the law in the particular field of interest, you may find certain terms used that are unclear. Osborne's *Legal Dictionary* provides a clear summary of legal terms, as does Butterworth's *Australian Legal Dictionary*.

Locating relevant authorities

Having perused one or more of the above sources, you will notice that lawyers quote an authority for each principle of law which they state. The authority will either be a case name or a section of an act of Parliament (the latter referred to often as a section of an Act).

You may be interested in reading the relevant case authority or section of the Act. Cases are bound into volumes which may be easily found in the library—provided you understand the rules of legal citation. Citation of legal cases takes the form: *Smith v. Bloggs* (1998) 148 ALR 466. The first named part is the plaintiff: the person who brought the legal action to sue the other party. If the cases reported is an appeal to a higher court, against the order of another judge, then the first named party is the appellant, i.e. the person who is appealing against the judgment.

Note: The term 'v.' is pronounced (in Australia) as 'and', except in criminal cases where it is pronounced as 'against'. The party named after the 'v' is the defendant: the person who is being sued; or, in the case of an appeal, the person is the respondent (the person responding to the appeal). The year in brackets is the year the case was reported in the law reports. The next number is the volume number of the reports. Not all law reports have volume numbers. 'ALR' is the series of reports in which the case was reported. ALR stands for Australian Law Reports. The last number is the page number at which the case is reported.

A full list of abbreviations of report series may be found in Osborne's *Legal Dictionary*. Below is a list of some common report series and their abbreviations:

ALR	Australian Law Reports
CLR	Commonwealth Law Reports
QdR	Queensland Reports
NSWLR	New South Wales Law Reports
SASR	South Australian State Reports
VR	Victorian Reports
WAR	Western Australian Reports
AC	Appeal Cases

QB   Queens Bench
WLR   Weekly Law Reports
All ER   All England Reports

Statutes are referred to by their name (usually the short title), the year they were passed by parliament (referred to as the year of enactment) and the jurisdiction. For example: *The Prevention of Toads Act 1956* (Qld).

If you wish to find out whether there have been any acts of Parliament which impact on your field of research there are various tools which vary according to the state in which you are searching. A good guide to these tools (and how to use them) is to be found in Cook et al. *Laying Down the Law*.[9] Cook's book also contains useful information on the use of statutory annotators which are research tools which allow you to check for any amendments to an act of Parliament which you may be examining.

You may have the name of a relevant case on an area, but need to find out if there have been any more recent cases on the topic. There are various research tools you can use, again dependent upon the state whose cases you are researching. See the chapter in Cook's book on research. It is important to remember that, in addition to paper-based services, on-line and CD-ROM products are available. Two of the more important sources are AUSTLII (Australian Legal Information Institute) and LEXIS. AUSTLII has its own web page with links to other legal sites. It has on-line copies of case reports from most of the Australian jurisdictions, as well as selected articles. Access to AUSTLII is free.

LEXIS is a service for which payment is necessary, but it is an incredibly versatile on-line service. LEXIS allows you to search for and download Commonwealth, English and American cases, American journals and some Commonwealth journals. It is especially useful for access to cases which are not reported elsewhere.

Selected legal aspects of research

A researcher who is not vigilant can easily fall into error. Legal errors can be costly and are best avoided. It is not possible, in a chapter of this size, to outline all relevant legal considerations, nor to give legal advice. The purpose of this part of the chapter is to highlight some matters that may be of concern and that have direct consequences under law. If you are in any doubt at all, you should seek professional legal advice.

Intellectual property

An old joke has it that to copy from one person is plagiarism, to copy from many is research. Irrespective of the accuracy of that position, copying from one or many is an infringement of that other's intellectual property rights. The rationale for such rights may easily be stated: 'The law recognises that original and creative work will not be encouraged if the product of an inventor or author may be used or exploited by those who have put neither effort nor resources into the work of creation or development.'[10]

There are three main statutes to be aware of. The first, the *Copyright Act 1968* (Cwlth) grants an exclusive right of reproduction in a material form of the expression of an original literary, musical, dramatic or artistic work. The *Designs Act 1906* (Cwlth) provides for a sixteen-year monopoly over the commercial exploitation of certain industrial designs. The *Patents Act 1900* (Cwlth) provides for a monopoly of up to twenty years of the commercial exploitation of an invention.

Describing all of these rights in detail is beyond the scope of this work. The intellectual property right which is most in question in research is copyright.[11] Copyright is not so much a protection of ideas as of their expression in a material form. It protects against someone else reproducing the work. Reproduction includes publishing, reproducing, performing or transmitting a literary, dramatic or artistic work. The phrase literary work in the Act is apt to mislead. Nothing special is required; a list or a sequence of numbers has been held to be a literary work.

It is important to note that copyright can exist separately to ownership of a work. Thus, for example, a person may buy a textbook, but not own the copyright of the information contained in the text. It is also possible for copyright to be assigned, sold, or a licence given to reproduce work, which, without the licence, would be a breach of copyright.

Generally speaking, the author of any work is the owner of any copyright subsisting in that work.[12] There is no need to register copyright with any body, nor to use the now familiar © sign at the beginning or end of the text. An important exception to the rule outlined above is that where a work is produced by an author pursuant to his terms of employment, then copyright in the work vests in the employer.[13] It is possible to make an agreement between employer and employee to the contrary, and researchers would be well advised to check their terms and conditions of employment.

It is possible that a researcher who uses copyrighted material belonging to another may escape liability for breaching copyright if he has done so for the purpose of 'fair dealing'. The difficulty is that exactly what amounts to fair dealing is unclear. In *Hubbard v. Vosper*,[14] the English Court of Appeal held that fair comment is a matter of impression and degree. Fair dealing for the purpose of research or study does not infringe copyright. Section 40 of the Copyright Act specifies that, in assessing the defence of fair comment in respect of research or study regard must be had to:

- the purpose and character of the dealing
- the nature of the work or adaptation
- the possibility of obtaining the work or adaptation within a reasonable time at an ordinary commercial price

- the effect of the dealing upon the potential market for, or value of, the work or adaptation, and
- in a case where only part of the work or adaptation is copied, the amount and substantiality of the part copied taken in relation to the whole work or adaptation.

It should be noted also that fair dealing for the purpose of criticism or review is exempted, provided that an acknowledgment is made of the work.

Many journals require, as a condition of publishing an article, an assignment of copyright in that article to the journal. Authors should be aware, that, once they have assigned copyright in the article in this way then, subject to the exceptions noted in the Copyright Act, an attempt to reproduce the article or parts of it elsewhere, would be an infringement of copyright.

Research into illegal activities

A researcher conducting studies of illegal activities faces two legal issues. The first is that it is imperative that the researcher avoids becoming party to an illegal activity. A researcher must avoid two separate ways in which he or she could become a party to an offence.

The first way that a researcher may become a party is by counselling or procuring the commission of an offence. At common law this is referred to as being an accessory before the fact. The law governing accessories before the fact is well summarised by Kenny:

> A person counsels or procures the commission of an offence if he/she advises, urges or solicits the commission of the offence or conspires with another in its commission: see *Stuart* (1974) 134 CLR 426 at 445, *Oberbillig* [1989] 1 Qd R 342 at 345, *Calhaem* [1985] 1 QB 808 at 813 and *Hutton* (1991) 56 A Crim R 211 at 217, 220. Additionally, the accessory may have procured, in the sense of 'produced by endeavour', the commission of the offence: see *A-G's Reference (No 1 of 1975)* [1975] 1 QB 773, *Solomon* [1959] Qd R 123 at 129 and *Menitti* [1985] 1 Qd R 520 at 532.[15]

It is one thing for a researcher to watch, or silently observe behaviour which is being carried out by a third party. It is completely another for the researcher to suggest or encourage the commission of an offence, even if the latter is done in the name of science.

The second way a researcher could become a party to an offence is by aiding or abetting the commission of an offence. At common law, this is referred to as being a principal in the second degree. The concept of aiding is fairly well understood: assisting another to do something. Note that it not necessary before liability can arise for the accused to desire that the person aided actually commits the offence.

> Although the accessory must knowingly aid, counsel or procure, it is not necessary that the accessory desired or intended that the crime of the perpetrator be committed and a conviction

may arise even where the accessory is indifferent to the commission of the offence. Such was the case in *Lynch v DPP for Northern Ireland* [1975] AC 653 at 678, where the accessory was held to have aided a murder by driving the murderer to the scene, even though there may have been evidence that the accessory regretted the crime or was horrified by it: see also *National Coal Board v Gamble* [1959] 1 QB 11 at 23 and *Beck* [1990] 1 Qd R 30 at 35, 38, 41, 47.[16]

In some circumstances, a researcher's approval of a research subject's criminal act will amount to aiding and abetting. In Coney's case, Hawkins LJ noted:

> In my opinion, to constitute an aider and abettor, some active steps must be taken by word, or action, with the intent to instigate the principal, or principals. Encouragement does not of necessity amount to aiding and abetting, it may be intentional or unintentional, a man may unwittingly encourage another in fact by his presence, by misinterpreted words, or gestures, or by his silence, or non-interference, or he may encourage intentionally by expressions, gestures, or actions intended to signify approval. In the latter case he aids and abets, in the former he does not. It is no criminal offence to stand by, a mere passive spectator of a crime, even of a murder. Non-interference to prevent a crime is not itself a crime.[17]

The second area in which researchers are in peril is in respect of confidentiality. A researcher conducting research into illegal activities may wish to give what has been described as 'an absolute assurance of confidentiality'.[18] It is important to note that, notwithstanding any ethical obligations of confidentiality which may bind a researcher (for instance, a medical practitioner's duty of confidence in respect of information gained from a patient), such duties must give way to overriding legal duties. In particular, a researcher must divulge information in response to an appropriate subpoena or question from a court. It is no defence that such information was obtained in confidence.

The one exception to this rule is any study conducted pursuant to the *Commonwealth Epidemiological Studies (Confidentiality) Act 1981* (Cwlth) or the *Epidemiological Studies (Confidentiality Act) 1992* (ACT).[19] These acts guarantee confidentiality of information gained from a prescribed study. To date, very few research projects have been prescribed studies under the Commonwealth Act. Epidemiological studies into the impact of Agent Orange on Vietnam veterans, radiation effects on Commonwealth personnel at Maralinga, and certain studies of illegal drug use have been prescribed.

Seeking further advice

This chapter has briefly outlined some legal research tools as well as some legal pitfalls a researcher may encounter in the conduct of research. It is important to remember that this chapter is not meant as a substitute for professional advice. If a researcher has any doubts, he or she should seek professional advice as a matter of course.

14
Writing and publishing

CATHERINE BERGLUND

Researchers at some stage need to write up their work, either for internal reporting, funding body reporting, thesis examination, peer-reviewed journals, or for presenting at conferences. Some practical steps in this process are addressed. Writing up is suggested as part of the research process, which could include the researchers' own observations on their project and on their area of interest as the research idea develops and as the research itself is conducted. The practical suggestions throughout the text encourage researchers to jot down relevant background material in an area of interest, and to keep notes on the research choices they make for their own research.

Learning to write and reading

Learning to write begins with learning to read. A love of reading brings the experience of having heard the stories of others, and the experience of seeing different ways of communicating those stories in written form. It is sometimes a factual and sometimes an emotional journey. Reading in your own field will develop and maintain the specialised language that you need to continually hone to communicate effectively within your own profession. Reading more widely, and reading for pleasure, will expand your experience of language, and will place different styles before you. All reading experiences help prepare you for writing. Quite simply, the more you read, the more writing options are known to you, and the more naturally writing options and language styles will come to you. Having a book on your bedside table is a way to start to read more. The book can just as usefully be a novel as something more relevant to your field.

When you conduct research, it is usual to read about others' research in the area. As you read, you will notice not only common themes and research methods that are used by others, but also how they write their research experiences up. You can learn how to communicate your research findings from the writings of others. As you read others' research reports, you will notice that they have also read widely.

An introduction in a research report or paper commonly contains a review of relevant literature. This is a considered and critical summary of the work in your area of research, and an interpretation of how relevant it is to your further work in that area.

As you read, summarise and critically analyse others' work, you are preparing to write about your own work. This draws on the skills of analysis and synthesis, which pervade the research process. It is no more difficult than synthesising the reason for pursuing a research topic, and deciding the best way to go about it, having learnt about how others have previously tried. Critical analysis exercises have been a feature of this book, because the analytical skill is the hallmark of a researcher. The introduction is the starting point for you to communicate what your research is about, and what triggered you to undertake the research, and it is useful to write at least a draft of the introduction at the beginning stage of your research. It is then that the relevant literature will be uppermost in your mind, and it is then that the reason you want to pursue the topic is clear. Capturing that drive, reasoning, and critical overview of research to date is often best done at the beginning of the research process. As your research progresses, and as the relevant literature in the field continues to expand, you will make changes to your introduction. In some research processes, the scope of the topic and the rationale for the research can even change, which would mean significant changes to the explanation of research topic and focus.

The introduction section requires you to be a reader, a critic, and a writer, all at the same time. If you think about those three roles, the introduction will be relatively straightforward to write. You will start to read with an expectation that you will summarise and critically analyse others' work, and with an expectation that you will write your appraisal down. So you can start to write almost at the same time as you start to read the relevant material.

Critical appraisal of literature and previous studies can include the following:

- purpose of the research and the research methods used,
- motivation of the researchers,
- what themes and major concepts were in operation in those studies,
- how the studies were conducted,
- what populations, in what contexts, at what time were included in the studies,
- findings or observations from those different populations or contexts of study,
- discrepancies between studies' findings,
- interpretations that the researchers placed on their findings, and
- the interpretations you would make giving their study concept, sample, context and stated findings.

In brief, this is the how, what, where, when, who, and why of the other studies.

A critical appraisal of literature is described by Lee Cuba for students of social sciences as starting with a summary, but then concentrating on interesting themes and concepts, which can be compared between studies. The reason for choosing the themes, and your critical approach, should be disclosed to the reader in an early 'thesis' type statement.[1] Comparative and critical analysis is a basic building block of many research traditions. A review of previous studies in patient populations is always undertaken in clinical health research so that the new research approach is informed by results with other patients, and so that the limits of others' findings are understood. It is drawn on in meta-analysis, so that the findings from different studies can be compared or pooled in meaningful ways.

Describing what someone did and what they said they found is not enough in any description of past studies. Your critical appraisal of the detail of their research process, findings and interpretation is central to any reasoned decision about further research directions.

A rule of thumb: do not include things in the introduction that have little relevance to the topic, and if you do mention previous research, offer a critical appraisal of it and an interpretation of what it could mean for the area of your interest.

Another rule of thumb: in your introduction, you should canvass all literature that is referred to in your discussion section.

Then, the next step can be to write how you will undertake your research process, to a level of detail that it could be replicated by another researcher. This is the method section. It includes the planning detail, and a summary of how the method was applied, or how the research experience progressed. Theoretical choices and practical application of research methods should be documented.

The planned process of your research is usually documented in detail before you start the research, because you need that level of detail on paper to gain funding and ethics committee approval. The start is a good time to get both the introduction and method sections of your research writing drafted. The detail of the method should be documented as the work progresses as well, because even the best planned method will be changed slightly when the real project begins. Leaving the writing of the whole planning and conduct of the research to the end is inviting disaster in terms of energy level to complete the whole writing task. Perhaps more importantly, some detail of the process can be lost to memory.

Writing to learn and writing for others to read

Writing to learn techniques are gaining recognition in academic contexts as a tool to aid critical appraisal, deep conceptual understanding, and memory retention of complex issues. They feature discovery thinking, as in personal journals and notes.[2] Under these techniques, a student would rarely experience or read something without writing a summary about it, and making notes on it as they wonder about it, and interpret it. The notes are usually for themselves, so they are written in a personal way. The experience of learning is the subject of writing as much as the substance or content of learning.

Writing to learn techniques can be combined with writing to communicate techniques, so that critical analysis and effective written communication skills are developed to a level that is suitable for publication. A training process in writing to learn and writing to communicate for undergraduate nursing students is described by Paula Broussard and Melinda Oberleitner. They have achieved considerable success with the program, with many undergraduate nursing students having manuscripts accepted for publication in peer-reviewed journals.

In their program, the skill of writing and publishing is developed in stages. In first year, in a class orientation exercise, students answer short questions about what they hope to achieve in the class and how they like to learn. The exercise involves reflection and communication skills. Further reflective thought is developed when students write about what job they hope to be doing in five years time. Contextual appraisal and conceptual analysis is added to the reflection process in two further exercises. Students write a letter (unsent) to an author suggesting how they might more accurately portray a character who is a nurse. Students also exchange a written question with a classmate on a topic of discussion in a class, and answer each other's questions.[3] These exercises could be adapted to your professional group quite easily. Notice that none of the tasks is overwhelming, and that each skill is developed and practised slowly. It does not matter that the pieces are short. One of the more difficult skills to learn is to write with accuracy and be concise. If students begin to develop their writing skills at the start of their course, writing is less frightening.

In upper level subjects, the nursing students write a piece and offer it to local newspapers, so that information on a topic is conveyed to the public. Midwifery students write on topics like prenatal care, breastfeeding, car restraints, adolescent pregnancy, and their piece is written for a reading age of 12–14 years. Fourth year students describe their clinical experiences as students, and work with a faculty mentor to prepare a manuscript for professional journal publication.[4] These writing to communicate exercises require critical analysis and conceptual skill, and the development of particular writing styles. According to Broussard and Oberleitner, the last publication task involves diagnostic reasoning, and a greater level of objective analysis.

The lessons to be learnt from this successful program are that writing needs to be taught alongside critical analysis and that steps in the writing and analysis processes need to be included throughout a whole undergraduate course.

Research framework and writing variations

The writing process can vary depending on the research framework that you are using. Susan Peck MacDonald has discussed variations in academic writing, and named them as extending across the spectrum from science to social sciences and humanities. These distinctions are similar to the spectrum described in chapter 1, from positivistic sciences to relativism. The spectrums suggested by MacDonald as characterising differences in writings in the science, social sciences, and humanities fields are: '(1) variations from compactness to diffuseness, (2) variations in explanatory versus interpretive goals, (3) variations from conceptually driven to text driven in the relation between generalization and particular, and (4) variations in the degrees of epistemic self-consciousness that are explicit in texts.'[5] The way writing varies, according to MacDonald, can be understood in the purpose of undertaking the writing. Researchers write as part of the problem solving and 'knowledge making' of their field, so they apply the problem-solving approaches that they know from their field to that writing.

Findings and interpretation

Howard Becker, an eminent sociologist, sees the research process as having web-like stages. The stages are: having images to study, developing ideas about what to study, and choosing samples (of people or subject matter), applying concepts to analysis, and applying the analysis to the cases under study in a logical manner.

These are not necessarily sequenced in a formal order, and there is continual inter-pretation from the researcher and from people within the field of study. The inter-pretation becomes the writing material as much as the fact or observation.[6] In this style of research then, the process of exploration and interpretation is the essence of the writing process. A journal of research process and interpretation, and writ-ing as the research develops, is therefore essential.

Exercise 14.1

Try keeping a journal over a period of time, say a week, on a concept that is part of your normal life. As you write each day about the issue, you could make notes about the context you are in as much as the issue itself. The interpretations around the events involving your concept are as important as the occurrences, if not more so.

When you attempt exercise 14.1 or any other writing project, you will soon realise that you will become hazy about past details and interpretations, so you need to learn to write whenever you can. Each little bit written also saves a huge task at the end of the time period. The issues of keeping notes within a qualitative research process has been covered earlier, in Jan Ritchie's chapter 'Not everything can be reduced to numbers'. You may like to read that chapter again before you begin the writing exercise.

Remember also Howard Becker's advice that: it isn't true that nothing is hap-pening. 'Something is always happening, it just doesn't seem worth remarking on.'[7] Part of the skill of the researcher is to develop an ability to 'notice' things that have become so seemingly mundane and routine that we fail to consciously notice them, much less interpret them. Developing an ability to document small details is the stuff of breakthrough research.

The gradual interpretation of information in context in the social sciences is not unlike the gradual interpretation that can take place in any process of data gathering, and assimilation. As you work with your data, you may have occasional insights and interpretations that make sense of what you are finding. Writing them down at the time you think of them will save you enormous effort and energy, compared to what is required if you leave all the interpretation to the time when you write the findings and interpretation, or discussion section, of your paper or report. Having a rough template of your report, designating a discussion section, and placing dot point paragraphs in it as you think of interesting issues and inter-pretations is a useful way to encourage yourself to write your flashes of insight down somewhere. A pen and paper beside the bed for the most absorbed researchers is an age-old technique too. This is for when you wake up having realised something, but fear that it may be lost again by morning.

Humanities-based and qualitative researchers usually write up research in an introduction, methods (or process), findings and interpretations format. Often the results are presented so that the experiences involving certain concepts are explored in detail, and are highlighted with selected quotes from those who helped the researchers to understand the concepts. Lengthy quotes or explanations from those participants are frequently included. Generally, it is the perspective and experiences of the participants that are valued, and the participants' interpretations of issues, as much as the researchers, that are documented.

Sciences-based and quantitative researchers usually write their results and discussion up separately, so that the data are presented in full in a sequence of tables, or in prose form, with detail of the results of statistical manipulation. The interpretation of that data is dealt with in a discussion section.

In both formats and approaches, the interpretation of a research process and observations from that process are related to previous work in the area, and reference to studies which were mentioned in the introduction is included. Researchers working between these frameworks, and combining methods, generally choose one of those accepted formats, depending on which method was primary in their project.

Teaming up to read and write

Review of others' work involves reading and detailed critical examination. Your work needs to be ready for that scrutiny. It should be a piece of clear and effective communication, and should stand up to critical review. You can prepare for that in corresponding phases of the writing process: drafting and critical appraisal. The appraisal leads to editing and further writing and critical appraisal and so on. It is a continuing process.

Whether you are a beginner or you have some experience writing, a writing group is invaluable for both parts of the writing process. Your writing group may be one person or a small group of people who are willing to read your early stages of writing and make some constructive but critical comments. The group will shape your writing, and encourage you to produce something.

Tip: If writing seems too hard, give yourself a deadline, and make it real by asking someone to read your draft. Let them know when you will give them your draft as your deadline.

Don't try to do both the writing and critical appraisal of your writing alone. Writing is about being able to convey issues, meanings, and feelings to others. You will not know if you have succeeded until others have been able to read your work, and let you know what they thought about it. In many cases, you will be able to achieve some critical appraisal of your own work. Putting it away for a couple of weeks, and then looking at it fresh is a good idea. The time gives you some distance and objectivity, so that when you return to the piece of work, you are less protective and unwilling to change it. Of course, other people, especially those who have not seen the writing in progress, are valuable because of their distance from the process that you have immersed yourself in. They are already standing back with a fresh eye on your work.

Tip: Always thank people for reviewing your writing. Even if you don't agree with their comments, remember that they have taken time to look at your work, and that the most helpful comments are usually ones that you don't agree with. Those comments that make you feel uncomfortable challenge you either to develop your own line of argument, or to question whether you have missed some key issues or assumptions.

It is usually easier to start publishing in teams, particularly when the team has some experienced and published writers and researchers. They can mentor you about the process of drafting, submission to an appropriate and realistic forum, redrafting, responding to comments from the peer-review process, and checking documents as they approach publication. Some people also prefer to write in teams. If you do write in teams, make sure that people understand what portion of the report or paper they are responsible for, that the workload is shared fairly, and that you have an agreed format or style you will write to. If you are writing as a group, set a deadline for when you will give each other something to read.

There are requirements for authorship on joint papers. They are designed to ensure that each named author is publicly responsible for the work which they are presenting. In brief, the main internationally accepted authorship requirements are that: 'Authorship credit should be based only on substantial contributions to

(a) conception and design, or analysis and interpretation of data; and
(b) drafting the article or revising it critically for important intellectual content; and or
(c) final approval of the version to be published.'

Further: 'Participation solely in the acquisition of funding or the collection of data does not justify authorship. General supervision of the research group is not sufficient for authorship. Any part of an article critical to its main conclusions must be the responsibility of at least one author. Editors may ask authors to describe what each contributed; this information may be published.'[8]

Each author and each researcher should be conscious of these requirements.

Publication and presentation forums

Reports

A full write-up of the research background, rationale, process and results is part of the normal research program. In some cases, these are required by funding bodies, or for internal reporting. If a report is required, the institution normally has a set format for the report, and the report should be written with those requirements in mind.

In general, a report is a full record of the research, and includes a level of detail that is more complete than in journal articles or conference papers. For example research tools like surveys and full tables of results, even before statistical manipulation, are included as appendices. All of those who were part of the research process should take part in some way in writing up the full research report.

Reports commonly include:

- title page, with the research project title, author and funding support details
- acknowledgments, usually on a separate page, so that people who made significant input are publicly acknowledged; supporting organisations can be acknowledged too—their permission should be sought to be acknowledged for their part in the process; it is not unusual to include a note of thanks to research participants here too
- an executive summary, in which the process and results and interpretation are summarised in one or two pages; this can replace the abstract, which would provide a brief outline of the research rationale and process
- glossary of terms, which is words, names of organisations and acronyms or abbreviations that are used within the body of the report
- sections on the background, rationale, and process of the research (traditionally termed Introduction and Method sections)
- sections on the findings and interpretations gleaned from the research (traditionally termed Results and Discussion sections)
- concluding remarks on the implications of the research, and suggestions for future research directions
- references or bibliography list
- appendices, which include full results, such as interview transcripts and statistical summaries, as well as the full results of any analysis or statistical manipulations of that data; appendices also include the basic tools which were used for collection of information, and copies of consent forms.

The funding for the project, institutional requirements, and any agreement which was made with participants will determine whether the report can be made public, or whether parts of the research can be written up for professional and public dissemination.

Conferences

Conference forums are an excellent way to start to present your work. Conferences are a meeting point for professional groups and for interest areas which span different professions. Generally, conferences are organised by professional associations or institutions on a broad topic or theme of interest to those in the organisation or institution. They are ahead of journals in being up to date, partly because researchers often present their formative findings at conferences before their completed research is ready for journal publication, and partly because they can be arranged quickly around contemporary issues. You do not usually need to be a member of the body to go to the conference, or to offer to present a paper at the conference.

When a topic for a conference is set, there is usually a 'call for papers', an invitation for people to submit an abstract of what they would like to present. The 'call for papers' is often made through the professional body's newsletter, or by letter or e-mail to members, or by advertisement placed in other forum leaflets or journals, so being aware of those information channels is important if you wish to find out what conferences are on, where, and when. You do not need to be asked individually to offer a paper. When submissions are received, the conference convenors decide which papers would be suitable for the conference, in a brief peer-review type process.

Occasionally, the full paper needs to be submitted at this stage for the process of culling and review, but usually, an abstract is sufficient. The 'call for papers' gives details about what to put in your submission, and who to send it to. Conferences usually try to encourage more junior people to present work as well as the more established names, so that all members of the profession (and interested others) take part in the forum. It is part of most professions' approach also that interested people are mentored in presentation, so even inexperienced presenters should not feel intimidated by making a start on the public presentation of their work.

An abstract is a brief paragraph of what the paper you want to present is about, and is normally about 300 to 500 words. For research papers, it is a snapshot of the rationale for the research, and a summary of the process of the research. The results can either be mentioned in the abstract, or held until the actual presentation. Abstracts in response to the call for papers are somewhat different from abstracts for journal articles, in which a brief summary from each of the sections of your research process—introduction, methods, results and interpretation or discussion—is always included.

Once you have heard that your submission has been successful, you can plan how to present your paper on the day you have been allocated. Writing out what you want to say is part of that process, and often conferences will ask for your full written version of the paper as a record of the conference, and perhaps to reproduce as part of the proceedings.

Visual aids, like overhead transparencies, slides, or computer-aided summary headings, as in Powerpoint, are useful, and you will need to find out what audiovisual facilities will be available before you present. The research assistants who contributed to chapter 11, 'Assistants and mentors', had some very useful tips on presentation preparation and conference paper delivery. Generally, visuals should aid, but not dominate, your presentation.

Sometimes, conferences also invite poster presentations. These are useful as publication forums as well. A summary of research can be written on a few pages, and arranged on a poster, with visuals if you like, so that people can read what you have done and what you have found. If you want to give a poster presentation, you are normally required to be present to answer questions on your material at designated times throughout the conference.

Journals

Journals represent the cutting edge of health care and health research. They are usually peer reviewed, so the information in them has stood up to peer assessment of credibility, rigour, and reliability. Professionals report to their peers through the journals. They report interesting cases, ideas for advances, comparisons, data on new assessment, treatment or management regimens, and debates on policies and practices. Journals are published frequently, sometimes every week or two, and commonly every quarter, so there is always new information available for the profession. Within the body of each research article is a brief snapshot of the methods used. This is the key to how reliable the data are, for other practitioners in their own context, and with their own patients. Understanding the research methods that have been used is as essential for the reader as for the authors of the articles. Readers need, at a minimum, a working understanding so that they can evaluate the meaning of the results.

Choosing the journal is an important part of deciding how to write your research paper. Most journals have similar, but subtly different requirements of authors. For instance, some require the paper to be sequenced in the classic introduction, methods, results and discussion format. Others do not. Referencing requirements vary between the Vancouver/biomedical referencing systems, and the Harvard or Chicago type social sciences referencing systems. (These referencing systems are explained later in this chapter.)

Information for authors is usually on the cover or inside the cover of the first journal edition of each year. You could photocopy a few journals' author requirements or style guides, and make a file for them, so they are handy as you decide how to prepare your articles for submission.

Here are three examples, one from the *New England Journal of Medicine*, which adopts a medical sciences style of writing and referencing, consistent with the biomedical journal format; one from *Nursing Research*, which leaves style up to the author but asks for a psychological form of referencing; and one from *Medical Teacher*, which adopts the social sciences format.

The *New England Journal of Medicine* requests one original manuscript, no longer than 3000 words, and two hard copies, in triple-spaced typing. 'A covering letter signed by all authors should identify the person (with the address and tele-phone number) responsible for negotiations concerning the manuscript; the letter should make it clear that the final manuscript has been seen and approved by all authors and that they have taken due care to ensure the integrity of the work.' The *NEJM* follows the Uniform requirements format, and requires an abstract of 250 words on a separate page, key words in accordance with the Index Medicus, and references in the biomedical style.[9]

Under the Uniform requirements for manuscripts submitted to biomedical journals, the following format applies for the Introduction, Methods, Results and Discussion sections of the research paper.[10] The Introduction includes the purpose of the article, and a summary of the rationale for the study or observation. The Methods section includes detail on the selection of subjects and their important characteristics, the methods of study or observation, including detail on apparatus and procedures 'in sufficient detail to allow other workers to reproduce the results'. Established methods are referenced, the ethics guidelines followed and the responsible committee for considering the ethics of the research are noted, and the statistics applied to the data are described. The Results section is for the presentation of results in a logical sequence of text, tables and illustrations. The Discussion section is for discussion of new and important aspects of the study, and any implications of those findings. The findings and their limitations are noted, and the findings are related to other studies. An Acknowledgment section allows other people to be noted who have contributed intellectually or technically to the project. A References section contains consecutively numbered citations, in order of reference in the manuscript, and the style is as Index Medicus, which is the Van-couver or biomedical style.

The journal *Nursing Research* asks for manuscript submission to be preceded by an e-mail to the Editor, describing the article. The journal asks for four paper copies and a disk copy of a manuscript when submitted, limited to 14–16 typed pages. The style requested is that in the *Publication Manual of the American Psy-chological Association*, 4th edition, which generally uses the Introduction, Method, Results, Discussion format, and Harvard referencing.[11]

The journal *Medical Teacher* asks contributors to submit four copies of the manuscript, which is double spaced and with designated margin widths. Footnotes are avoided, and Harvard referencing is used. The manuscripts should have an abstract, and a list of 'practice points' at the end of the article.[12] Those points are aimed at clinicians and teachers.

There are different requirements for different types of journal submissions, and the word limits for each are detailed in the author information sections of each journal. A letter to the editor for instance, is one opportunity for you to comment on other writings in a particular journal, or a contemporary professional issue, and perhaps make comment about your own research, in a short article format. Letters to the editor are usually no more than 500 to 1000 words in length.

Brief research reports, of perhaps 1000 or so words, are included in many journals as a way of encouraging the most-up-to-date research to be reported sooner rather than later, and as a way of providing space for information which may not warrant space as a longer article.

Long research articles usually take more time to prepare, and usually take more time to go through the critical process of peer review before acceptance for publication. It is common for a few months to elapse between submission of a research article and completion of peer review.

There will frequently be editorial type articles on specific health issues in journals as well. So, your journal writing need not be limited to the classic research report of your data.

A word of caution though: you are only allowed to submit your piece to one journal at a time. Once submitted, you cannot promise another journal exclusive publication of the piece, and so by copyright restriction, it is not possible to offer the same or slightly varied articles to different journals. Sending your article to a journal means that you are offering them to be the first forum to make your piece publicly available. You will be under a media embargo until the date of publication once the article is accepted.

Your journal choice will be guided by how relevant it is to your own profession, how much interest your research is likely to be to its readership, and whether it is peer reviewed and indexed in a recognised citation index, such as Medline or the Social Sciences Citation Index. Indexing of the journal will mean that the paper will be well regarded academically, as the journal is peer reviewed to an acceptable international standard.

The following steps are normal in journal submission:

- *Submission*: Your piece is submitted to a journal, with a cover letter. The cover letter should include your undertaking that it is not under consideration with another journal, and should give a reason about why it would be of interest to the readership of the journal. The proper address is detailed in the instructions to authors for each journal.
- *Editor acknowledgment*: You will normally receive a postcard or letter (or e-mail) acknowledging receipt of your article from the journal's editorial office, usually within a couple of weeks of it being received. If you send it overseas, allow time for the mail before you start worrying! If you want to be sure of receipt, send it registered mail.
- *Rejection or editorial consideration*: The editor and editorial teams cull the majority of articles that they receive, depending on whether they conform to the journal requirements, as in the author instructions, and whether they appear to be relevant to the readership and credible. You will receive either a polite rejection letter at this stage, or a letter to say that the piece will go to peer review.

If your piece is rejected, consider making some minor changes, and sending it to another journal. Don't lose heart. Every single author has had something rejected. They just usually don't talk about it! In future try to carefully choose an appropriate journal, and try to learn from any comments on your piece.

- *Peer review*: The peer review is a process of critical assessment by two or often three relevant professionals who have significant standing in your field. The review is normally 'blind', that is, the reviewers may not see your name, and you will not know who they are. The peer reviewers can comment on any aspect of your research, from the rationale, to the method and process, to the way you present your results, or analyse and interpret your findings. They send their comments directly to the editor.

  The results of the peer review will determine whether the editor then rejects the article, or sends you a summary of the comments and requests revision, or decides to accept the article as is. The latter is the least common outcome!

  The reviewers' comments should be taken seriously. Making minor revisions will often mean that the article will go on to be accepted. If there are serious differences, you may consider offering the paper elsewhere. Whether you revise at this time, or offer the paper elsewhere, the reviewers' comments are invaluable for you to consider. The comments may prompt you to challenge your assumptions in either the conduct or the presentation of the research. It is part of the writing process in much the same way as your writing group is.

- *Acceptance, galleys and copyright*: Once any revisions are made to the satisfaction of the reviewers and the editor, a typesetting process begins. The journal article is then normally planned to be included in a specific upcoming journal edition, you sign a copyright agreement that the journal can publish your article exclusively, and you are asked to be ready to comment on a 'galley' copy of your piece. Receiving the 'galley' is quite exciting. This is the first time you will see the manuscript looking like it will be published in a journal. Editorial queries about references, wording, spelling and so on will need to be triple-checked at this stage. You may be so close to the article by this stage that you cannot see errors. Your reading group will come in handy to help you check it as well.

References

Referencing is essential when referring to another piece of previously published work, regardless of whether it is fact, process or opinion that you are referring to. The reference gives readers details of who wrote it, in what forum it was published, and enough publication information, such as year and place of publishing, so that readers could find the original source of the information and read it for themselves.

Referencing systems can be found in summary form in the author notes in journals, or in agreed journal requirements like the International Committee of Medical Journal Editors' published requirements, as noted earlier in this chapter. They can be found in full in the style guides, such as the *Chicago Manual of Style*,[13] or books like *Medical Style & Format*.[14] Summaries and comparisons of the styles are given in the Australian Government Publishing Service's *Style Manual for Authors, Editors and Printers*.[15] That style guide favours the social sciences Harvard type style, but does also explain the biomedical style of referencing.

The key features of the Harvard system (Chicago style) and the biomedical (Vancouver) styles are set out in brief below.

The Harvard system is commonly used in government reporting and social sciences. It is also known as the author–date system, because the author's surname and the date (the year) of the referenced work is noted in the text, in parentheses if it is not mentioned in the text: (Surname 2000). At the end of the document, a full reference is given which lists in order:

for a book: Surname, First name (or initial(s), followed by a full stop) Year, Title of book, Publisher, Place of Publishing.

and for an article: Surname, First name (or initial(s), followed by a full stop) Year, 'Title of article', *Journal name*, volume number and month, p. first page – last page.

The Vancouver or biomedical style of referencing is commonly used in medical and health reporting. No brackets are put in the text with author information, but numbers are inserted, usually as superscript at the end of the sentence or after phrase punctuation mark, like this: the number is smaller and raised as in this textbook. Numbers are used in sequence to refer to the full reference at the end of the document, or in the footnotes, where the following information is given:

for a book: 1. Surname Initial. Title of book with optional italics. Place of Publication: Publisher, Year.

for an article: 2. Surname Initial. Title of article. Journal name abbreviated in style of Index Medicus with optional italics Year; volume number: first page – last page.

Notice the different ordering of information in each referencing system, and the different use of punctuation.

Tip: Variations on these styles are commonly requested by publishers of different journals, and their author notes will set out their particular style. The first step is to clarify the style. Then, whichever style is required, use it, and apply it consistently!

Media

When you present a paper at a conference, or a journal publishes your article, a press release may be issued to let the public media know about your work. Press releases are usually prepared by the journal or conference organisers, with an embargo on public release of the information until the piece has been presented or published. The embargo is applied because, in the process of offering your paper, you have promised to allow the journal or conference forum to be the first to publish your work. If a press release is made, you may find that you are contacted by a journalist, and asked to answer some further questions about your research.

It can be useful to ask for a list of anticipated questions before the interview. When the time for the interview arrives, have in your own mind your key findings, your process of research, and a couple of key implications of your research. After the interview, it is also useful to ask to check the copy for accuracy before the journalist's piece is published.

Occasionally, researchers also release their own press statements, through their home hospital or university. Other organisations are more practised at issuing press releases. The format of one ministerial press release, reproduced in part below, shows how the key points are presented in prose form, and are relatively short and simple. Other examples of ministerial press releases can be found in the collection of press releases called the *Ministerial Document Service*.[16]

Generally, press releases are written in prose form, so that journalists can adapt them easily, and there is minimum risk of inaccuracy or misinterpretation. They are simple, short, approximately 500 words long, and contain just a few issues, including the context and the implications of the issue. Consider the following example, with the name and title of the person making the statement at the top (in this case the Minister for Aged Care), the date of release, and a title: 'Young people at high risk of premature hearing loss'.

> Young people need to be aware of the dangers of listening to loud music, especially through headphones, the Minister responsible for Hearing Services, Bronwyn Bishop, warned today.
>
> 'Hearing Awareness Week (23–28 August) provides an excellent opportunity to inform young people that listening to excessively loud music or other loud noises puts them at risk of premature hearing loss,' Mrs Bishop said.

The press release goes on to summarise recent research findings, and to announce government funding for educative processes and hearing services.[17]

If you wish to make a press release, your institution's press officer should be informed, and it should be cleared with your institution, as you are really only acting as an officer of your institution. Your press officer may have templates for media statements which you could see, and you could discuss convenient dates to make the press release. The press or public relations office may even offer to handle it for you. Either way, you will need to be ready to conceptualise your work in a simple and concise style, and synthesise it. This process is very similar to writing a brief abstract which explains your work, and its implications.

Exercise 14.2

As a brief exercise, you could try writing a press release.

This draws on your research skills in collecting, synthesing and summarising information, and then communicating it to others clearly.

Keep your press release brief, no more than 400–500 words.

Summarising the completed research project as a press release is not just a communication and dissemination exercise. It can also crystallise why you embarked on the research in the first place, and highlight what piece of the research puzzle you have helped solve.

The excitement and challenge of being part of research often begins anew after the completion and publication of a research project. There is always another health research quest waiting.

Appendix
Statistics table

Percentage Points of the χ^2-Distribution
The point tabulated is x, where $P(\chi_\nu^2 > x) = p$ and χ_ν^2 has the chi-squared distribution with ν degrees of freedom.

p	.99	.975	.95	.9	.1	.05	.025	.01
ν								
1	0.000	0.000	0.004	0.016	2.706	3.841	5.024	6.635
2	0.020	0.051	0.103	0.211	4.605	5.991	7.378	9.210
3	0.115	0.216	0.352	0.584	6.251	7.815	9.348	11.345
4	0.297	0.484	0.711	1.064	7.779	9.488	11.143	13.277
5	0.554	0.831	1.145	1.610	9.236	11.071	12.833	15.086
6	0.872	1.237	1.635	2.204	10.645	12.592	14.449	16.812
7	1.239	1.690	2.167	2.833	12.017	14.067	16.013	18.475
8	1.646	2.180	2.733	3.490	13.362	15.507	17.535	20.090
9	2.088	2.700	3.325	4.168	14.684	16.919	19.023	21.666
10	2.558	3.247	3.940	4.865	15.987	18.307	20.483	23.209
11	3.053	3.816	4.575	5.578	17.275	19.675	21.920	24.725
12	3.571	4.404	5.226	6.304	18.549	21.026	23.337	26.217
13	4.107	5.009	5.892	7.042	19.812	22.362	24.736	27.688
14	4.660	5.629	6.571	7.790	21.064	23.685	26.119	29.141
15	5.229	6.262	7.261	8.547	22.307	24.996	27.488	30.578
16	5.812	6.908	7.962	9.312	23.542	26.296	28.845	32.000
17	6.408	7.564	8.672	10.085	24.769	27.587	30.191	33.409
18	7.015	8.231	9.390	10.865	25.989	28.869	31.526	34.805
19	7.633	8.907	10.117	11.651	27.204	30.144	32.852	36.191
20	8.260	9.591	10.851	12.443	28.412	31.410	34.170	37.566
21	8.897	10.283	11.591	13.240	29.615	32.671	35.479	38.932
22	9.542	10.982	12.338	14.041	30.813	33.924	36.781	40.289
23	10.196	11.689	13.091	14.848	32.007	35.172	38.076	41.638
24	10.856	12.401	13.848	15.659	33.196	36.415	39.364	42.980
25	11.524	13.120	14.611	16.473	34.382	37.652	40.646	44.314
26	12.198	13.844	15.379	17.292	35.563	38.885	41.923	45.642
27	12.879	14.573	16.151	18.114	36.741	40.113	43.195	46.963
28	13.565	15.308	16.928	18.939	37.916	41.337	44.461	48.278
29	14.256	16.047	17.708	19.768	39.087	42.557	45.722	49.588
30	14.953	16.791	18.493	20.599	40.256	43.773	46.979	50.892
40	22.164	24.433	26.509	29.051	51.805	55.758	59.342	63.691
50	29.707	32.357	34.764	37.689	63.167	67.505	71.420	76.154
60	37.485	40.482	43.188	46.459	74.397	79.082	83.298	88.379
70	45.441	48.758	51.739	55.329	85.527	90.531	95.023	100.425
80	53.541	57.152	60.392	64.278	96.578	101.88	106.628	112.331
90	61.756	65.647	69.126	73.291	107.565	113.145	118.136	124.114
100	70.063	74.222	77.929	82.358	118.498	124.342	129.562	135.808

Notes

Chapter 1: Beginning the quest

1 C.E. Rosenberg, *Explaining epidemics and other studies in the history of medicine*, New York, Cambridge University Press, 1992, p. 114.

2 Ho Peng Yoke, 'China', pp. 191–6, in H. Selin (ed.), *Encyclopaedia of the history of science, technology, and medicine in non-Western cultures*, Dordrecht, Kluwer Academic Publishers, 1997, pp. 193, 195.

3 R. Porter, *The greatest benefit to mankind: A medical history of humanity from antiquity to the present*, London, Harper Collins, 1997, p. 136.

4 E. Temkin and C.L. Temkin, *Ancient medicine: Selected papers of Ludwig Edelstein*, Baltimore, Johns Hopkins University Press, 1987, pp. 225, 236.

5 Preamble to the Constitution of the World Health Organisation, in *World Health Organisation: Basic documents*, 26th edn, World Health Organisation, Geneva, 1976, p. 1.

6 For instance, Australian Medical Association (AMA), *Code of Ethics*, Canberra, 1996, Principle 1.1.2.

7 New Zealand Medical Association, *Code of Ethics*, Auckland, Principle 16.

8 AMA, *Code of Ethics*, Principle 1.4.1.

9 Australian Nursing Council, *Code of Ethics*, Value Statement 3, Explanatory Statement 4, Canberra, 1993.

10 C.A. Berglund and P.M. McNeill, 'Guidelines for research practice in Australia: NHMRC statement & professional codes', *Community Health Studies*, vol. 13, no. 2, 1989, pp. 121–9.

11 British Medical Association, *Core Values for the Medical Profession in the 21st Century*, 1995.

12 B. Russell, 'Science and ethics', chapter 1, pp. 19–27, in J. Rachels (ed.), *Ethical theory 1: The question of objectivity*, Oxford, Oxford University Press, 1998, p. 27.

13 M. Charlesworth, 'Where do research ideas come from?', *Transactions of the Menzies Foundation*, vol. 7, 1984, pp. 9–11, p. 10.

14 D. Saltman, '"Disease model" challenged', chapter 15, pp. 220–37, in P. Baume (ed.), *The Tasks of Medicine: An Ideology of Care*, Sydney, MacLennan and Petty, 1998, p. 225.

15 K. Montgomery Hunter, *Doctors' Stories*, Princeton University Press, Princeton, 1991, pp. 72–3, p. 75.

16 H. Brody, *Stories of Sickness*, Yale University Press, New Haven, 1987, p. 17.

17 K. Montgomery Hunter, *Doctors' Stories*, , p.30.

18 A. Hudson Jones, 'Literature and medicine: Narrative ethics', *Lancet*, vol. 349, 1997, pp. 1243–6.

19 M. Little, 'Cartesian thinking in health and medicine', chapter 6, pp. 75–95, in P. Baume (ed.), *The Tasks of Medicine: An Ideology of Care*, Sydney, MacLennan and Petty, 1998, pp. 78, 81, 83, 86.

20 Little, 'Cartesian thinking in health and medicine', p. 86.

21 W.C. Salmon, 'The importance of scientific understanding', chapter 5, pp. 79–91, in W.C. Salmon, *Causality and Explanation*, Oxford, Oxford University Press, 1998, p. 83.

22 J. Morse, 'What's wrong with random selection?', *Qualitative Health Research*, vol. 8, no. 6, 1998, pp. 733–5.

23 D.L. Morgan, 'Practical strategies for combining qualitative and quantitative methods: applications to health research', *Qualitative Health Research*, vol. 8, no. 3, 1998, pp. 362–76.

24 C. Pope and N. Mays. 'Reaching the parts other methods cannot reach: an introduction to qualitative methods in health and health services research', *British Medical Journal*, vol. 311, 1995, pp. 42–5, at p. 44.

25 M.B. Van der Weyden, 'Databases and evidence-based medicine in general practice: We have built it, but will they come?', *Medical Journal of Australia*, vol. 170, 1999, pp. 52–3.

Chapter 2: Using research in practice

1 D.P. Kernick, 'Lies, damned lies, and evidence-based medicine', *Lancet*, vol. 351, 13 June 1998, p. 1824.

2 Chronowski, G, M.D.chronom 1@ix,netcom.com; viewed 26 October 1999.

3 Kernick, 'Lies, damned lies, and evidence-based medicine', p. 1824.

4 Kernick, 'Lies, damned lies, and evidence-based medicine', p. 1824.

5 National Health and Medical Research Council, *A Guide to the Development, Implementation and Evaluation of Clinical Practice Guidelines*, Canberra, AGPS, 1999.

6 A.J. Brettle, A.F. Long, M.J. Grant, and J. Greenhalgh, 'Searching for information on outcomes: Do you need to be comprehensive?', *Quality in Health Care*, vol. 7, 1998, pp. 163–7.

7 Brettle et al., 'Searching for information on outcomes, p. 166.

8 P. Wright, C. Jensen, and J.C. Wyatt, 'How to limit clinical errors in interpretation of data', *Lancet*, vol. 352, 7 Nov. 1998, pp. 1539–43, p. 1539.

9 Wright et al., 'How to limit clinical errors in interpretation of data', p. 1542.

10 J. Lau, J.P.A. Ioannidis, and C.H. Schmid, 'Summing up evidence: One answer is not enough', *Lancet*, vol. 351, 10 Jan. 1998, pp. 123–7, p. 123.

11 Lau et al., 'Summing up evidence', p. 126.

12 P.G. Shekelle, J.P. Kahan, S.J. Bernstein, L.L. Leape, C.J.Kamberg, and R.E. Park, 'The reproducibility of a method to identify the overuse and underuse of medical procedures', *New England Journal of Medicine*, vol. 338, no. 26, 25 June 1998, pp. 1888–95.

13 A. Kitson, G.Harvey, and B. McCormack, 'Enabling the implementation of evidence-based practice: A conceptual framework', *Quality in Health Care*, vol. 7, 1998, pp. 149–58, p. 149.

14 Kitson et al., 'Enabling the implementation of evidence-based practice, p. 158.

15 K.J. O'Flynn, and M. Irving, 'On the need for evidence-based surgery', *Evidence-based Medicine*, vol. 4, no. 1, Jan./Feb., 1999, pp. 6–7, p. 6.

16 O'Flynn and Irving, 'On the need for evidence-based surgery', p. 7.

17 Editorial, *Medical Journal of Australia*, vol. 169, 5 Oct. 1998, p. 348.

18 M.J. Solomon, and R.S. McLeod, 'Surgery and the randomised controlled trial: Past, present and future', *Medical Journal of Australia*, vol. 169, 5 Oct. 1998, p. 380.

19 M.B. Van Der Weyden (ed.), 'Databases and evidence-based medicine in general practice: We have built it, but will they come', *Medical Journal of Australia*, vol. 170, 18 Jan. 1999, p. 52.

20 J.M. Young, and J.E. Ward, 'General practitioners' use of evidence databases', *Medical Journal of Australia*, vol. 170, 18 Jan. 1999, pp. 56–8.

21 Van Der Weyden, 'Databases and evidence-based medicine in general practice', p. 52.

22 Commonwealth of Australia, *National Statement on Ethical Conduct in Research Involving Humans*, Canberra, AGPS, 1999.

23 *National Statement on Ethical Conduct in Research Involving Humans*, Section 12.

24 *National Statement on Ethical Conduct in Research Involving Humans*, pp. 35, 36.

25 R.O. Day, D.R. Chalmers, K.M. Williams, and T.J. Campbell, 'The death of a healthy volunteer in a human research project: Implications for Australian clinical research', *Medical Journal of Australia*, vol. 168, 1998, pp. 449–51, p. 449.

26 S.N. Bolsin, 'Professional misconduct: The Bristol case', *Medical Journal of Australia*, vol. 169, 1998, pp. 369–72, p. 369.

27 Kernick, 'Lies, damned lies, and evidence-based medicine', p. 1824.

28 The author would like to gratefully acknowledge the valuable assistance, encouragement, and support given to me in the writing of this chapter by the following colleagues and friends: Dr Catherine Berglund, Dr Steven Jurd, Dr Peter the Schaefer, Dr Olav Nielssen, Dr Marilyn McMurchie, Dr Sam Milliken, Dr Trevor Morris, Dr Margot Whitford, Dr Bruce Edelman, Dr Jeremy Bunker, Ann Long, Lena Low, Ms Alexandra Howard, Mr Bill LaGanza, Mr Dieter Steinbusch, The GP HIV Study Group, and the staff at the Australasian Society for HIV Medicine Inc.

Chapter 3: Great expectations

1 G. Osborne and W.F. Mandle, *New History, Studying Australia Today*, Sydney, Allen & Unwin, 1982.

2 A.S. Lyons and J. Petrucelli, *Medicine, An Illustrated History*, New York, Abradale Press, 1978, p. 77.

3 J.F. Nunn, *Ancient Egyptian Medicine*, London, British Museum Press, 1996, p. 24.

4 Nunn, *Ancient Egyptian Medicine*, p. 54.

5 Nunn, *Ancient Egyptian Medicine*, p. 50.

6 Lyons and Petrucelli, *Medicine, An Illustrated History*, p. 90.

7 W. Osler, *The Evolution of Modern Medicine*, Yale, Yale University Press, 1921, p. 16.

8 S. Smith, 'The history and development of forensic medicine', *British Medical Journal*, vol. 1, 24 March 1951, pp. 599–607, pp. 599, 600.

9 Nunn, *Ancient Egyptian Medicine*, pp. 52–4.

10 Nunn, *Ancient Egyptian Medicine*, pp. 43, 54.

11 Nunn, *Ancient Egyptian Medicine*, pp. 43–4.

12 Lyons and Petrucelli, *Medicine, An Illustrated History*, p. 170.

13 Lyons and Petrucelli, *Medicine, An Illustrated History*, p. 192.

14 C. Singer, *A Short History of Anatomy from the Greeks to Harvey (The Evolution of Anatomy)*, New York, Dover Publishing, 1957, p. 10.

15 Lyons and Petrucelli, *Medicine, An Illustrated History*, p. 210.

16 Lyons and Petrucelli, *Medicine, An Illustrated History*, p. 210.

17 R. Porter, *The Cambridge Illustrated History of Medicine*, Cambridge, Cambridge University Press, 1996, p. 92.

18 *Historical Atlas of the World*, Hammond, NJ, 1984, p. H-5.

19 Singer, *A Short History of Anatomy*, p. 38.

20 Singer, *A Short History of Anatomy*, p. 35.

21 Lyons and Petrucelli, *Medicine, An Illustrated History*, p. 251.

22 W.G.H. Duckworth, *Some Notes on Galen's Anatomy*, given as The Linacre Lecture, 6 May 1948, Cambridge, W Heffer & Sons Ltd, 1948, p. 38.

23 Singer, *A Short History of Anatomy*, pp. 52–62.

24 Galen, 'Anatomical Procedures', Book 6, Chapter 11, translated by O. Temkin and W.L. Straus Jnr, 'Galen's dissection of the liver and of the muscles moving the forearm', *Bulletin of the History of Medicine*, vol. 19, 1946, pp. 170–1.

25 R.K. Spiro, 'A backward glance at the study of post-mortem anatomy, Part 1', *International Surgery*, vol. 56, 1971, pp. 27–40, p. 31.

26 B.E. McKnight, *Sung Tz'u: His yuan chi lu* (The washing away of wrongs), Centre for Chinese Studies, University of Michigan, 1981, p. 4.

27 McKnight, *Sung Tz'u: His yuan chi lu*, p. 5.

28 McKnight, *Sung Tz'u: His yuan chi lu*.

29 From E.H. Hume, *The Chinese Way in Medicine*, Baltimore, 1940; and F.W. Kiel, 'Forensic science in China', *Journal of Forensic Science*, vol. 15, 1970, pp. 203–4; as quoted in Y.V. O'Neill and G.R. Chan, 'A Chinese coroner's manual and the evolution of anatomy', *Journal of the History of Medicine and Allied Sciences*, vol. 31, 1976, pp. 3–17, p. 6.

30 As quoted in McKnight, *Sung Tz'u: His yuan chi lu*, pp. 81, 86.

31 E.H. Ackerknecht, *A Short History of Medicine*, Baltimore, Johns Hopkins University Press, 1982, p. 82.

32 Porter, *The Cambridge Illustrated History of Medicine*, p. 73.

33 C.D. O'Malley, *Andreas Vesalius of Brussels 1514–1564*, Berkeley, University of California, 1964, p. 11.

34 A. Castiglioni, *A History of Medicine*, translated by E.B. Krumbhaar, 2nd edn, New York, McClelland & Stewart, 1958, pp. 323–39.

35 Ackerknecht, *A Short History of Medicine*, p. 88.

36 F. Garrison, *History of Medicine*, 4th edn, Philadelphia and London, WB Saunders & Co, 1929, p. 172.

37 K.F. Russell, 'Anatomy and the barber-surgeons', *Medical Journal of Australia*, vol. 1, 1973, pp. 1109–15, p. 1110.

38 Singer, *A Short History of Anatomy*, pp. 71–2.

39 Singer, *A Short History of Anatomy*, p. 71.

40 Singer, *A Short History of Anatomy*, p. 73.

41 R.H. Meade, *An Introduction to the History of General Surgery*, Philadelphia, WB Saunders Co., 1968.

42 R.K. Spiro, 'A backward glance at the study of post-mortem anatomy, Part 1', *International Surgery*, vol. 56, 1971, pp. 27–40, p. 34.

43 Garrison, *History of Medicine*, pp. 196–7, 238.

44 Smith, 'The history and development of forensic medicine', p. 602.

45 R. Palmer, 'Medicine at the papal court in the 16th century', ch. 2 in V. Nutton (ed.), *Medicine at the Courts of Europe 1500–1837*, London, Routledge, 1990, p. 67.

46 Gee and Mason, *The Courts and the Doctor*, Oxford, Oxford University Press, 1990, p. 20.

47 D. Miller, '"After death the doctor", reflections on the Coroners Act and forensic pathology', *Australian Journal of Forensic Sciences*, vol. 3, no. 1, September 1970, pp. 9–14, p. 12.

48 T.R. Forbes, *Surgeons at the Bailey*, New Haven, Yale University Press, 1985, pp. 11–12.

49 From Ambroise Pare, *Reports in Court*, 1575, trans. Th. Johnson, Pub. Th. Cotes and R Yound, London, 1634; as quoted in T.R Forbes TR, *Surgeons at the Bailey*, p. 38.

50 Palmer, 'Medicine at the Papal Court in the 16th century', p. 67.

51 Gee and Mason, *The Courts and the Doctor*, p. 20.

52 Garrison, *History of Medicine*, pp. 196–7, 238.

53 E.R. Long. *A History of Pathology*, New York, Dover Publishers, 1965, p. 30.

54 L. Clendening, *Source Book of Medical History*, New York, Dover Publishers, 1942; O. Saphir, *Autopsy Diagnosis and Technique*, 4th edn, New York, Hoeber-Harber, 1958; Spiro, 'A backward glance at the study of post-mortem anatomy, Part 1', pp. 27–40, p. 35.

55 Garrison, *History of Medicine*, pp. 196–7, 209–10.

56 Saphir, *Autopsy Diagnosis and Technique*, p. 4.

57 R. Major, *Classic Descriptions of Disease*, Oxford, Blackwell Scientific Publications, 1945, pp. 587–8.

58 Porter, *The Cambridge Illustrated History of Medicine*, pp. 312–13.

59 Garrison, *History of Medicine*, pp. 432–3, 569–72.

60 M. Foucault, *The Birth of the Clinic*, trans. A.M. Sheridan Smith, London, Tavistock Publishers, 1973; C. Jones and R. Porter, *Reassessing Foucault*, London, Routledge, 1994.

61 T. Kuhn, *The Essential Tension*, Chicago, University of Chicago Press, 1977.

62 D. Armstrong, *Political Anatomy of the Body, Medical Knowledge in Britain in the 20th Century*, Cambridge, Cambridge University Press, 1983, p. 2.

63 Osborne and Mandle, *New History, Studying Australia Today*.

64 *Medical Journal of Australia*, vol. 161, 1994.

65 For example, H. Attwood, R.W. Home, 'Patients, practitioners and techniques', *2nd National Conference on Medicine and Health in Australia*, Medical History Unit and Department of History and Philosophy of Science, University of Melbourne, 1985.

66 Ackerknecht, *A Short History of Medicine*.

67 Surgeon Redfern to Governor Macquarie 1814. Redfern's Report. HRA, ser 1,8; 274; E. Ford, *The Life and Work of William Redfern*, Australian Medical Publishing Company, Sydney, 1953; A.R. Jones, 'William Redfern (1775? –1833) mutineer to colonial surgeon in New South Wales. Part 1 & 2'. *Journal of Medical Biography*, 1999; R.N. Prescott, Emancipist and Autocrat. The life of Doctor William Redfern and his Relationship with Governor Macquarie, Australian National University. Thesis 1970; M.H. Ellis, *Lachlan Macquarie: His Life, Adventures and Times*, Sydney, Angus & Robertson, 4th edn (rev.), 1965.

68 Acknowledgments: As must all students of Australian medical history, I pay tribute to Brenda Heagney, Librarian of the Royal Australasian College of Physicians. I am grateful, too, to Donna Mendrawi at the same library and to Arthur Easton in the Mitchell section of the State Library of NSW.

Chapter 4: Who needs to plan?

1 S. Hulley and S. Cummings (eds), *Designing Clinical Research*, Baltimore, Williams & Wilkins, 1988, p. vii.

2 Hulley and Cummings, *Designing Clinical Research*.

3 World Health Organization, *Health Research Methodology: A Guide for Training in Research Methods*, Manila, WHO Regional Office for the Western Pacific, 1992.

4 M. Maclure, 'The case-crossover design: A method for studying transient effects on the risk of acute events', *American Journal of Epidemiology*, vol. 133, 1991, pp. 144–53.

5 KJ. Rothman and S. Greenland, *Modern Epidemiology*, Philadelphia, Lippincott-Raven, 1998.

6 A. Bowling, *Research Methods in Health*, Buckingham, Open University Press, 1997.

7 R. Jones, 'Why do qualitative research?', *British Medical Journal*, vol. 311, 1995, p. 2.

8 C. Pope and N. Mays, 'Reaching the parts the methods cannot reach: an introduction to qualitative methods in health and health services research', *British Medical Journal*, vol. 311, 1995, pp. 42–5.

9 Pope and Mays, 'Reaching the parts the methods cannot reach'.

10 Pope and Mays, 'Reaching the parts the methods cannot reach'.

11 P. Norton, E. Dunn, and J. Bain et al., 'Guidelines for the dissemination of new information discovered by researchers', pp. 87–94, in E. Dunn, P. Norton, M. Stewart, F. Tudiver,

and M. Bass (eds), *Disseminating Research/Changing Practice*, Thousand Oaks, CA, Sage, 1994.

Chapter 5: Numbers and more

1   P. Levy and S. Lemeshow, *Sampling of Populations: Methods and Application*, New York, John Wiley & Sons, 1991.

2   S.K. Lwanga and S. Lemeshow, *Sample Size Determination in Health Studies:A Practical Manual*, Geneva, World Health Organization, 1991.

3   Center for Disease Control (CDC), 'Pneumocystic Pneumonia—Los Angeles', *Morbidity and Mortality Weekly*, vol. 30, no. 21, 1981, pp. 250–2.

4   CDC, 'Kaposi's Sarcoma and Pneumocystic Pneumonia—New York City and California', *Morbidity and Mortality Weekly*, vol. 30, no. 25, 1981, pp. 305–8.

5   Australian Bureau of Statistics (ABS), *Catalogue of Publications and Products*, Cat. No. 1101.0, Canberra, ABS, 1999.

6   Australian Institute of Health and Welfare, *Australia's Heath 1998: The Sixth Biennial Health Report of the Australian Institute of Health and Welfare*, AIHW Cat. No. AUS10, Canberra, Australian Institute of Health and Welfare, 1998.

7   D. Rowntree, *Statistics without Tears: A Primer for Non-mathematicians*, London, Penguin Books, 1991.

8   P. Armitage and G. Berry, *Statistical Methods in MedicalResearch*, Oxford, Blackwell Scientific Publications, 1994.

9   ABS, *Estimated Resident Population by Age and Sex: States and Territories of Australia*, Cat. No. 3201.0, Canberra, ABS, 1998.

10 G. Keller and B.Warrack, *Essentials of Business Statistics*, Belmont, CA, Duxbury Press, 1994.

Chapter 6: How is our health?

1   V. Beral, D. Bull, R. Doll, T. Key, R. Peto, and G. Reeves, 'Breast cancer and hormone replacement therapy: Collaborative reanalysis of data from 51 epidemiological studies of 52,705 women with breast cancer and 108,411 women without breast cancer', *Lancet*, vol. 350, 1997, pp. 1047–59.

2   International Agency for Research on Cancer, *IARC Monographs on the Evaluation of Carcinogenic Risks to Humans*, vol. 59: *Hepatitis viruses*, Lyon, International Agency for Research on Cancer, 1994.

3   Centers for Disease Control and Prevention, 'Kaposi's sarcoma and PCP among homosexual men-New York City and California', *Morbidity and Mortality Weekly Report*, vol. 30, 1981, pp. 305–8.

4   L.J. Kinlen, 'Immunosuppression and cancer', pp. 237–53, in H. Vainio, P.N. Magee, D.B. McGregor, and A.J. McMichael (eds), *Mechanisms of Carcinogenesis in Risk Identification*, Lyon, International Agency for Research on Cancer, 1992.

5   M. Burnet, 'Immunological factors in the process of carcinogenesis', *British Medical Bulletin*, vol. 20, 1964, pp. 154–7.

6   Centers for Disease Control and Prevention, '1993 revised classification system for HIV infection and expanded surveillance case definition for AIDS among adolescents and adults', *Morbidity and Mortality Weekly Report*, vol. 41, 1992, pp. 1–18.

7   I. dos Santos Silva, *Cancer Epidemiology: Principles and Methods*, Lyon, International Agency for Research on Cancer, 1999.

8   World Health Organization, *Manual of the International Statistical Classification of Diseases, Injuries, and Causes of Death*, 9th rev., Geneva, WHO, 1977.

9 Centers for Disease Control and Prevention, 'Kaposi's sarcoma and PCP among homosexual men—New York City and California'.

10 National Centre in HIV Epidemiology and Clinical Research, *HIV/AIDS, Hepatitis C and Sexually Transmissible Infections: Annual Surveillance Report 1999*, National Centre in HIV Epidemiology and Clinical Research, Sydney, 1999.

11 dos Santos Silva, *Cancer Epidemiology*.

12 R.J. Biggar, J. Horm, J.J. Goedert, and M. Melbye, 'Cancer in a group at risk of AIDS through 1984', *American Journal of Epidemiology*, vol. 126, 1987, pp. 578–86; R.J. Biggar, W. Burnett, J. Mikl, and P. Nasca, 'Cancer among New York men at risk of acquired immunodeficiency syndrome', *International Journal of Cancer*, vol. 43, 1989, pp. 979–85; C.S. Rabkin and F. Yellin, 'Cancer incidence in a population with a high prevalence of infection with human immunodeficiency virus type 1', *Journal of the National Cancer Institute*, vol. 86, 1995, pp. 1711–16.

13 R.J. Biggar, 'Cancer in acquired immunodeficiency syndrome: an epidemiological assessment', *Seminars in Oncology*, vol. 17, 1990, pp. 251–60.

14 M.S. Coates and B.K. Armstrong, *Cancer in New South Wales: Incidence and Mortality 1995*, Sydney, NSW Cancer Council Sydney, 1998.

15 V. Beral, T.A. Peterman, R.L. Berkelman, and H.W. Jaffe, 'Kaposi's sarcoma among persons with AIDS: a sexually transmitted infection?', *Lancet*, vol. 335, 1990, pp. 123–8.

16 V. Beral, T. Peterman, R. Berkelman, and H. Jaffe, 'AIDS-associated non-Hodgkin's lymphoma', *Lancet*, 337, 1991, pp. 805–9.

17 C. Ateenyi-Agaba, 'Conjunctival squamous cell carcinoma associated with HIV infection in Kampala, Uganda (letter)', *Lancet*, vol. 345, 1995, pp. 695–6.

18 J.J. Goedert, T.R. Cote, P. Virgo, P.M. Scoppa, D.W. Kingma, M.H. Gail, E.S. Jaffe, and R.J. Biggar for the AIDS-Cancer Match study group, 'Spectrum of AIDS-associated malignant disorders', *Lancet*, vol. 358, 1998, pp. 1833–9.

19 C.P. Archibald, M.T. Schechter, T.N. Le, K.J.P. Craib, J.S.G. Montaner, and M.V. O'Shaughnessy, 'Evidence for a sexually transmitted cofactor for AIDS-related Kaposi's sarcoma in a cohort of homosexual men', *Epidemiology*, vol. 3, 1992, pp. 203–9; H.K. Armenian, D.R. Hoover, S. Rubb, S. Metz, R. Kaslow, B. Visscher, J. Chmiel, L. Kingsley, and A. Saah, 'Composite risk score for Kaposi's sarcoma based on a case-control and longitudinal study in the Multicenter AIDS cohort study population', *American Journal of Epidemiology*, vol. 138, 1993, pp. 256–65; A. Grulich, O. Hendry, K. Luo, N. Bodsworth, D. Cooper, and J. Kaldor, 'Risk of Kaposi's sarcoma and oro-anal sexual contact', *American Journal of Epidemiology*, 1997; vol. 145, pp. 673–9.

20 Y. Chang, E. Cesarman, M.S. Pessin, F. Lee, J. Culpepper, D.M. Knowles, and P.S. Moore, 'Identification of Herpesvirus-like DNA sequences in AIDS-associated Kaposi's Sarcoma', *Science*, vol. 266, 1994, pp. 1865–9.

21 D. Whitby, M.R. Howard, M. Tenant-Flowers, M.S. Brink, A. Copas, C. Boschoff, T. Hatzioannou, F.E.A. Suggett, D.M. Aldam, A.S. Denton, R.F. Miller, I.V.D. Weller, R.A. Weiss, R.S. Tedder, and T.F. Schulz, 'Detection of Kaposi's sarcoma associated herpesvirus in peripheral blood of HIV-infected individuals and progression to Kaposi's sarcoma', *Lancet*, vol. 346, 1995, pp. 799–802.

22 J.N. Martin, D.E. Ganem, D.H. Osmond, K.A. Page-Shafer, D. Macrae, and D.H. Kedes, 'Sexual transmission and the natural history of human herpesvirus 8 infection', *New England Journal of Medicine*, vol. 338, 1998, pp. 948–54; A.E. Grulich, S. Olsen, O. Hendry, K. Luo, P. Cunningham, D.A. Cooper, S.J. Gao, Y. Chang, P.S. Moore, and J.M. Kaldor, 'Kaposi's sarcoma associated herpesvirus: a sexually transmissible infection?', *Journal of AIDS & Human Retrovirology*, vol. 20, 1999, pp. 387–93.

23 N.A. Hessol, M.H. Katz, J.Y. Liu, S.P. Buchbinder, C.J. Rubino, and S.D. Holmberg, 'Increased incidence of Hodgkin disease in homosexual men with HIV infection', *Annals of Internal Medicine*, vol. 117, 1992, pp. 309–11; M.V. Ragni, S.H. Belle, R.A. Jaffe, J. Locker, S.L. Duerstein, D.C. Bass, J.E. Addiego, L.M. Aledort, L.E. Barron, D.B. Brettler, G.R. Buchanan, J.C. Gill, B.M. Ewenstein, D. Green, M.W. Hilgartner, W.K. Hoots, T. Kisker, E.W. Lovrien, C.J. Rutherford, N.L. Sanders, K.J. Smith, S.P. Stabler, S. Swindells, G.C. White, and L.A. Kingsley for the hemohpilia malignancy study group, 'AIDS associated NHL as primary and secondary AIDS diagnoses in hemophiliacs', *Journal of AIDS and Human Retrovirology*, vol. 13, 1996, pp.78–86; D.W. Lyter, J. Bryant, R. Thackeray, C.R. Rinaldo, and L.A. Kingsley, 'Incidence of HIV-related and nonrelated malignancies in a large cohort of homosexual men', *Journal of Clinical Oncology*, vol. 13, 1995, pp. 2540–6.

24 S. Franceschi, L. Dal Maso, S. Arniani, P. Crosignani, M. Vercelli, L. Simonata, F. Falcini, R. Zanetti, A. Barchielli, D. Serraino, and G. Rezza for the Cancer and AIDS Registry Linkage Study, 'Risk of cancer other than Kaposi's sarcoma and non-Hodgkin's lymphoma in persons with AIDS in Italy', *British Journal of Cancer*, vol. 78, 1998, pp. 966–70; J.J. Goedert and T.R. Coté, 'Conjunctival malignant disease with AIDS in USA', *Lancet*, vol. 346, 1995, pp. 257–8; A. Grulich, X. Wan, M. Law, M. Coates, and J. Kaldor, 'Cancer incidence rates in people with AIDS in NSW, Australia', *AIDS*, vol. 13, 1999, pp. 839–43.

25 J.L. Jones, D.L. Hanson, M.S. Dworkin, J.W. Ward, and H.W. Jaffe, and the Adult/adolescent Spectrum of HIV Disease Project Group, 'Effect of anti-retroviral therapy on recent trends in selected cancers among HIV-infected persons', *Journal of AIDS*, vol. 21, 1999, pp. S11–S17.

26 D.F. Martin, B.D. Kupperman, R.A. Wolitz, A.G. Palestine, M.S. Hong Li, and C.A. Robinsons, Roche Ganciclovir Study Group, 'Oral ganciclovir for patients with cytomegalovirus retinitus treated with a ganciclovir implant', *New England Journal of Medicine*, vol. 340, no. 14, 1999, pp. 1063–70.

Chapter 7: Meaningful categories

1 A. Agresti, *An Introduction to Categorical Data Analysis*, New York, Wiley, 1996.

2 E.B. Andersen, *Introduction to the Statistical Analysis of Categorical Data*, New York, Springer-Verlag, 1997.

3 C. Canaris and S. Jurd, 'The diagnosis of alcohol-related brain damage: a retrospective study in alcoholics undergoing in-patient rehabilitation', *Drug and Alcohol Review*, vol. 10, 1991, pp. 85–8.

4 SMS (School of Mathematics and Statistics), *DMS Tables*, Sydney, University of Sydney, 1991.

5 C. Plato, D. Rucknagel, and H. Gershowitz, 'Studies of the distribution of glucose-6-phosphate dehydorgenase deficiency, thalassemia, and other genetic traits in the coastal and mountain villages of Cyprus', *American Journal of Human Genetics*, vol. 16, 1964, pp. 267–83.

6 W.G. Cochran, 'Some methods of strengthening the common c^2', *Biometrics*, vol. 10, 1954, pp. 417–51.

7 B. Rosner, *Fundamentals of Biostatistics*, 3rd edn, Boston, PWS-KENT, 1990.

8 J.E. Higgins and G.G. Koch, 'Variable selection and generalized chi-square analysis of categorical data applied to a large cross-sectional occupational health survey', *International Statistical Review*, vol. 45, 1977, pp. 51–62 (as cited in Andrews and Herzberg).

9 D.P. Byar, C. Blackard and the VACURG, 'Comparisons of placebo, pyridoxine, and topical thiotepa in preventing recurrence of stage 1 bladder cancer,' *Urology*, vol. 10, 1977, pp. 556–61.

10 D. Andrews and A. Herzberg, *Data*, New York, Springer-Verlag 1985.

11 T.C. Beard, D.R. Woodward, P.J. Ball, H. Hornsby, R.J. von Witt and T. Dwyer, 'The Hobart Salt Study 1995', *Medical Journal of Australia*, vol. 166, no. 8, 1997, pp. 404–7.

12 Rosner, *Fundamentals of Biostatistics*.

13 S. Johnson and R. Johnson, 'Tonsillectomy history in Hodgkin's disease', *New England Journal of Medicine*, vol. 287, 1972, pp. 1122–5.

14 Q. McNemar, 'Note on the sampling error of the difference between correlated proportions or percentages', *Psychometrika*, vol. 12, 1947, pp. 153–7.

15 Canaris and Jurd, 'The diagnosis of alcohol-related brain damage'.

16 Rosner, *Fundamentals of Biostatistics*.

17 H.O. Lancaster, *Quantitative Methods in Biological and Medical Sciences: A Historical Essay*, New York, Springer-Verlag, 1994.

18 J.C. Prichard, *A Treatise on Insanity and Other Disorders Affecting the Mind*, 1835/1995.

19 C.C. Clogg and E.S. Shihadeh, *Statistical Models for Ordinal Variables*, Thousand Oaks, CA, Sage Publications, 1994; W.J. Conover, *Practical Nonparametric Statistics*, 2nd edn, New York, Wiley, 1980; M. Ishii-Kuntz, *Ordinal Log-linear Models*, Thousand Oaks, CA, Sage Publications, 1994; V.E. Johnson and J.H. Albert, *Ordinal Data Modeling*, New York, Springer, 1999; P. Sprent, *Applied Nonparametric Statistical Methods*, 2nd edn, London, Chapman & Hall, 1993; T.D. Wickens, *Multiway Contingency Tables Analysis for the Social Sciences*, Hillsdale, NJ, Lawrence Erlbaum, 1989; R.R. Wilcox, *New Statistical Procedures for the Social Sciences: Modern Solutions To Basic Problems*, Hillsdale, NJ, Lawrence Erlbaum, 1987.

Chapter 8: So, how is the treatment going?

1 I. McDowell I and C. Newell, *Measuring Health: A Guide to Rating Scales and Questionnaires*, New York, Oxford University Press, 1996; D. Streiner and G. Norman, *Health Measurement Scales: A Practical Guide to their Development and Use*, New York, Oxford University Press, 1996; and H. MacBeth, *Health Outcomes: Biological, Social and Economic Perspectives*, New York, Oxford University Press, 1996.

2 J.C. Linder, 'Outcomes measurement: Compliance tool or strategic initiative?', *Health Care Management Review*, vol. 16, no. 4 , 1991, pp. 21–33, p. 25.

3 R. Batalden, E. Nelson and J. Roberts, 'Linking outcomes measurement to continual improvement: The serial 'V' way of thinking about improving clinical care', *Joint Commission Journal of Quality Improvement*, vol. 20, no. 4, 1994, pp. 167–80.

4 L. Bero and D. Rennie, 'The Cochrane Collaboration: Preparing, maintaining and disseminating systematic reviews of the effects of health care', *Journal of the American Medical Association*, vol. 274, no. 24, 1995, pp. 1935–8; W. Silverman, 'Effectiveness, efficiency ... and subjective choice', *Perspectives in Biology and Medicine*, vol. 38, no. 3, 1995, pp. 480–95.

5 J. Hayward, 'Promoting clinical effectiveness: A welcome initiative, but both clinical and health policy need to be based on evidence', *British Medical Journal*, vol. 312, no. 7045, 1996, pp. 1491–2.

6 E.H. Walters and J.A.E. Walters, 'Many reports of RCTs give insufficient data for Cochrane reviewers', *British Medical Journal*, vol. 319, no. 7204, 1999, pp. 257.

7 Australian Institute of Health and Welfare, *Australia's Health, 1998*, Canberra, AGPS, 1998.

8 Australian Institute of Health and Welfare, *Australia's Children: Their Health and Wellbeing 1998*, Canberra, AGPS, 1998.

9 D.M. Gels and J.R. Banks, 'The effects of drug therapy on long-term outcome of childhood asthma: A possible preview of the international guidelines', *Pediatrics*, vol. 102, no. 2, 1998, p. 451.

10 Gels and Banks, 'The effects of drug therapy on long-term outcome of childhood asthma'.

11 G. Rose, L. Arlian, D. Bernstein, A. Grant, M. Lopez, J. Metzger, S. Wasserman, and T.A.E. Plattsmills, 'Evaluation of household dust mite exposure and levels of specific IGE and IGG antibodies in asthmatic patients enrolled in a trial of immunotherapy', *Journal of Allergy & Clinical Immunology*, vol. 97, no. 5, 1996, pp. 1071–8.

12 H. Reddel, C. Jenkins, and A. Woolcott, 'Diurnal variability time to change asthma guidelines', *British Medical Journal*, vol. 319, no. 7201, 1999, pp. 45–7.

13 Gels and Banks, 'The effects of drug therapy on long-term outcome of childhood asthma'.

14 Reddel, Jenkins, and Woolcott, 'Diurnal variability time to change asthma guidelines'.

15 J.F. Fries and P.W. Spitz, 'The hierarchy of patient outcomes', in B. Spilker (ed.), *Quality of Life Assessment in Clinical Trials*, New York, Raven Press, 1990, pp. 25–36, p. 25.

16 A. Leplege and S. Hunt, 'The problem of quality of life in medicine', *Journal of the American Medical Association*, vol. 278, no. 1, 1997, pp. 47–50; T. Gill and A. Feinstein, 'A critical appraisal of the quality of quality-of-life measures', *Journal of the American Medical Association*, vol. 272, no. 8, 1994, pp. 619–26; D. Berwick, 'Harvesting knowledge for improvement', *Journal of the American Medical Association*, vol. 275, no. 11, 1996, pp. 877–8, p. 877.

17 Leplege and Hunt, 'The problem of quality of life in medicine', p. 47.

18 A. Giuffrida, H. Gravelle, and M. Roland, 'Measuring quality of care with routine data: avoiding confusion between performance indicators and health outcomes', *British Medical Journal*, vol. 319, no. 7202, 1999, pp. 94–8; M.C. Gulliford, 'Evaluating prognostic factors: Implications for measurement of health care outcome', *Journal of Epidemiology & Community Health*, vol. 46, no. 4, 1992, pp. 323–6; L. Aharony, and S. Strasser, 'Patient satisfaction: What we know about it and what we still need to explore', *Medical Care Review*, vol. 50, no. 1, 1993, pp 49–79.

19 Gulliford, 'Evaluating prognostic factors'.

20 Gill and Feinstein, 'A critical appraisal of the quality of quality-of-life measures'.

21 G. Guyatt and D. Cook, 'Health status, quality of life and the individual', *Journal of the American Medical Association*, vol. 272, no. 8, 1994, pp. 630–1; M. Testa and D. Simonson, 'Current concepts: Assessment of quality-of-life outcomes', *New England Journal of Medicine*, vol. 334, no.13, 1996, pp. 835–40.

22 C. Lefant, N. Khaltaev, A.L. Sheffer, M Bartal, J. Bousquet, Y.Z. Chen, A.G. Chuchalin, T.J.H. Clark, R. Dahl, L.M. Fabbri, S.T. Holgate, P. Mahapatra, S. Makino, C.K.Naspitz, M.R. Partridge, R. Pauwels, V. Spicak, W.C. Tan, K.B. Weiss, A.J. Woolcock, M.N. Xabamokoena, and N.S. Zhong, 'Global strategy for asthma—management and prevention. NHLBI/WHO workshop report', *Revue Française d'Allergologie et d'Immunologie Clinique*, vol. 36, no. 6, 1996, pp. 563 ff.

23 McDowell and Newell, *Measuring Health*.

24 Australian Institute of Health and Welfare, *Australia's Children*.

25 Australian Institute of Health and Welfare, *Australia's Children*.

26 D.C. Goodman, P. Lozano, T.A. Stukel, C.H. Chang, and J. Hecht, 'Has asthma medication use in children become more frequent, more appropriate or both?', *Pediatrics*, vol. 104 , no. 2, 1999, pp. 187–94.

27 R. MacFaul, E.J. Glass, and S. Jones, 'Appropriateness of paediatric admission', *Archives of Disease in Childhood*, vol. 71, no. 1, 1994, pp. 50–8.

28 Reddel, Jenkins, and Woolcott, 'Diurnal variability time to change asthma guidelines'.

29 Gels and Banks, 'The effects of drug therapy on long-term outcome of childhood asthma'.

30 Department of Housing and Community Services, 'Enough to make you sick: How income and environment affect health', *National Health Strategy Research Paper No. 1*, Canberra, Australian Government Printers, 1992.

31 Gels and Banks, 'The effects of drug therapy on long-term outcome of childhood asthma'.

32 B. Jalaludin, T. Chey, M. Holmwood, J. Chipps, R. Hanson, S. Corbett, and S. Leeder, 'Admission rates as an indicator of the prevalence of severe asthma in the community', *Australian and New Zealand Journal of Public Health*, vol. 22, no. 2, 1998, pp. 214–15.

33 T. Voigt, M. Bailey, and M. Abramson, 'Air Pollution in the Latrobe Valley and its impact upon respiratory morbidity', *Australian and New Zealand Journal of Public Health*, vol. 22, no. 5, 1998, pp. 556.

34 Jalaludin, Chey, Holmwood, Chipps, Hanson, Corbett, and Leeder, 'Admission rates as an indicator of the prevalence of severe asthma in the community'.

35 L.H. Plotnick and F.M. Ducharme, 'Should inhaled anticholinergies be added to beta$_2$ agonists for treating acute childhood and adolescent asthma?: A systematic review', *British Medical Journal*, vol. 317, no. 7164, 1998, pp. 971–7.

36 Gels and Banks, 'The effects of drug therapy on long-term outcome of childhood asthma'.

37 International Study of Asthma and Allergies in Childhood Steering Committee, 'Worldwide variation in prevalence of symptoms of asthma, allergic rhinoconjunctivits, and atopic eczema: ISAAC', *Lancet*, vol. 351, no. 9111, 1998, pp. 1225–32.

38 Jalaludin, Chey, Holmwood, Chipps, Hanson, Corbett, and Leeder, 'Admission rates as an indicator of the prevalence of severe asthma in the community'.

39 Berwick, 'Harvesting knowledge for improvement'.

40 P. Trye, R. Jackson, R.L. Yee, and R. Beaglehole, 'Trends in the use of blood pressure lowering medications in Auckland, and associated costs, 1982–94', *New Zealand Medical Journal*, vol. 109, no. 1026, 1996, pp. 270–2.

41 P. Pinna Pintor, R. Torta, S. Bartolozzi, R. Borio, E. Caruzzo, A. Cicolin, M. Giammaria, F. Mariana, G. Ravarino, F. Triumbari, O. Alfieri, and L. Ravizza, 'Clinical outcome and emotional behaviour status after isolated coronary surgery', *Quality of Life Research*, vol. 1, 1992, pp. 177–85; D. Booth, R. Deupree, H. Hultgren, A. De Maria, S. Scott, and R. Luch , 'Quality of life after bypass surgery for unstable angina; 5-year follow-up results of Veterans Affairs Cooperative Study', *Circulation*, vol. 83, 1991, pp. 87–95.

42 E. Lindal, 'Post-operative depression and coronary bypass surgery', *International Disability Studies*, vol. 12, 1990, pp. 704.

43 P.J. Shaw, 'The incidence and nature of neurological morbidity following cardiac surgery: a review', *Perfusion*, vol. 4, no. 2, 1989, pp. 83–92.

Chapter 9: Not everything can be reduced to numbers

1 National Health and Medical Research Council (NHMRC), *Ethical Aspects of Qualitative Methods in Health Research*, Canberra, National Health and Medical Research Council, 1995.

2 M. LeCompte and J. Preissle, *Ethnography and Qualitative Design in Educational Research*, 2nd edn, San Diego, CA, Academic Press Inc., 1993, p. 42.

3 P. Maguire, *Doing Participatory Research: A Feminist Perspective*, Amherst, Center for International Education, University of Massachusetts, 1987.

4 T. Kuhn, *The Structure Of Scientific Revolutions*, Chicago, University of Chicago Press, 1970.

5 N. Denzin and Y. Lincoln (eds), *Handbook of Qualitative Research*, Thousand Oaks, CA, Sage Publications, 1994.

6 E.G. Guba and Y.S. Lincoln, 'Competing paradigms in qualitative research', in Denzin and Lincoln (eds), *Handbook of Qualitative Research*, pp. 105–17.

7 M.B. Miles and A.M. Huberman, *Qualitative Data Analysis: A Sourcebook of New Methods*, Newbury Park, CA, Sage Publications, 1984, p. 37.

8 National Health and Medical Research Council (NHMRC), *Ethical Aspects of Qualitative Methods in Health Research*, Canberra, National Health and Medical Research Council, 1995.

9 R. Stake, 'Case studies', in Denzin and Lincoln (eds), *Handbook of Qualitative Research*, pp. 236–47.

10 LeCompte and Preissle, *Ethnography and Qualitative Design in Educational Research*.

11 M.Q. Patton, *Qualitative Evaluation and Research Methods*, 2nd edn, Newbury Park, CA, Sage Publications, 1990.

12 A. Strauss and J. Corbin, *Basics of Qualitative Research: Grounded Theory Procedures and Techniques*, Newbury Park, CA, Sage Publications, 1994.

13 See for example, S. Quine, 'Sampling in non-numerical research', in C. Kerr, R. Taylor, and G. Heard (eds), *Handbook of Public Health Methods*, Sydney, McGraw-Hill, 1998, pp. 539–42.

14 M. Ely, *Doing Qualitative Research: Circles within Circles*, London, Falmer Press, 1991.

15 Denzin and Lincoln (eds), *Handbook of Qualitative Research*.

16 N.K. Denzin, *The Research Act*, 2nd edn, New York, McGraw-Hill, 1978.

17 Y.S. Lincoln and E.G. Guba , *Naturalistic Inquiry*, Beverly Hills, CA, Sage Publications, 1985; E.G. Guba and Y.S. Lincoln, *Fourth Generation Evaluation*, Newbury Park, CA, Sage Publications, 1989.

18 Guba and Lincoln, *Fourth Generation Evaluation*.

19 J. Morse, '"Perfectly healthy, but dead": The myth of inter-rater reliability', *Qualitative Health Research*, vol. 7, no. 4, 1997, pp. 445–7.

20 C. Grbich, *Qualitative Research in Health: An Introduction*, St Leonards, NSW, Allen & Unwin, 1999.

21 Grbich, *Qualitative Research in Health*.

22 Patton, *Qualitative Evaluation and Research Methods*.

23 D.W. Stewart and P.N. Shamdasani, *Focus Groups: Theory and practice*, Newbury Park, CA, Sage Publications, 1990.

24 Patton, *Qualitative Evaluation and Research Methods*.

25 Stewart and Shamdasani, *Focus Groups*.

26 Strauss and Corbin, *Basics of Qualitative Research*.

27 S. Chapman, D. Lupton, *The Fight for Public Health: Principles and Practice of Media Advocacy*, London, BMJ Publishing Group, 1994.

28 D. Lupton, 'Discourse analysis: A new method for understanding the ideologies of health and illness', *Australian Journal of Public Health*, vol. 16, 1992, pp. 145–50.

29 M. Lewis, 'Historical analysis', in Kerr, Taylor, and Heard (eds), *Handbook of Public Health Methods*, pp. 516–21.

30 As in J.P. Spradley, *Participant Observation*, New York, Holt, Rinehart and Winston, 1980.

31 Grbich, *Qualitative Research in Health*.

32 Denzin and Lincoln (eds), *Handbook of Qualitative Research*.

33 LeCompte and Preissle, *Ethnography and Qualitative Design in Educational Research*.

34 Miles and Huberman, *Qualitative Data Analysis*.

35 A.M. Huberman and M.B. Miles, 'Data management and analysis methods', in Denzin and Lincoln (eds), *Handbook of Qualitative Research*, pp. 428–44.

36 Miles and Huberman, *Qualitative Data Analysis*, p. 21.

37   Miles and Huberman, *Qualitative Data Analysis*, p. 21.

38   V.J. Janesick, 'The dance of qualitative research design: Metaphor, methodolatry, and meaning', in Denzin and Lincoln (eds), *Handbook of Qualitative Research*, pp. 209–19.

39   QSR, 1999, 'Announcing NUD*IST Vivo', NUD*IST Newsletter, http://www.qsr.com.au.

40   P.L. Munhall, *Qualitative Research Proposals and Reports: A Guide*, New York, National League for Nursing Press, 1994.

41   Southern Community Health Research Unit (SCHRU), *Planning Health Communities: A Guide to Doing Community Needs Assessment*, Bedford Park, SA, Flinders Medical Centre, 1991.

42   M. Torres, 'South American women's perceptions and experience of menopause', unpublished Master of Public Health project report, University of New South Wales, 1999.

43   S.R. Woolfenden, J. Ritchie, R. Hanson, and V. Nossar, 'Parental use of a paediatric emergency department as an ambulatory care service', *Australian & New Zealand Journal of Public Health*, vol. 24, no. 2, 2000, pp. 204–6.

44   L. Ashton, 'The role of prevention in the practice of rural community nurses', unpublished Master of Public Health project report, University of New South Wales, 1999.

45   F. Trede, 'The role of knowledge and artistry in clinical expertise: A pilot study with rheumology physiotherapists', *Focus on Health Professional Education: A Multidisciplinary Journal*, vol. 2, no. 1, 2000, pp. 48–57.

46   M. Eisenbruch, 'Children with failure to thrive, epilepsy and STI/AIDS: Indigenous taxonomies, attributions and ritual treatments', *Clinical Child Psychology and Psychiatry*, vol. 3, no. 4, 1998, pp. 505–18.

47   R. Stake, 'Case studies', in Denzin and Lincoln (eds), *Handbook of Qualitative Research*, p. 236.

48   K. Kavanagh, 'Performing Miracles? The role and the reality of practice for nurse discharge planners', unpublished Master of Health Personnel Education project report, University of New South Wales, 1996.

49   J.E. Ritchie, 'There's something different in what's happening to us: Participatory action research in a work setting', *Promotion and Education*, vol. 3, no.4, 1997, pp. 16–20.

50   F. Baum, *The New Public Health: An Australian Perspective*, Melbourne, Oxford University Press, 1998.

51   Ritchie, 'There's something different in what's happening to us'.

52   J.E. Ritchie, 'Promoting the health and quality of life of residents of retirement villages', unpublished research report, NSW Ageing and Disability Department, 1999.

53   D.L. Sackett, W.S. Richardson, W. Rosenberg, and R.B. Haynes, *Evidence-based Medicine*, Edinburgh, Churchill Livingstone, 1996.

54   K. Cox, *Doctor and patient—Exploring Clinical Thinking*, Sydney, University of New South Wales Press, 1998, p. 114.

55   J. Ritchie, 'Using qualitative research to enhance the evidence-based practice of health care providers', *Australian Journal of Physiotherapy*, vol. 45, 1999, pp. 251–6.

56   Ritchie, 'Using qualitative research to enhance the evidence-based practice of health care providers', p. 255.

Chapter 10: Quality and quantity

1   A. Strauss and J. Corbin, *Basics of Qualitative Research: Grounded Theory Procedures and Techniques*, Newbury Park, CA, Sage Publications Inc., 1990.

2   Y. Wadsworth, *Everyday Evaluation on the Run*, Melbourne, Action Research Issues Association (Inc.), 1991.

3   S. Labovitz and R. Hagedorn, *Introduction to Social Research*, New York, McGraw-Hill, 1971, p. 65.

4   R.P. Gephart, *Ethnostatistics*, vol. 12, Qualitative Foundations for Quantitative Research, Qualitative Research Methods. Newbury Park, CA, Sage Publications Inc., 1988.

5   D.C. Saltman, I.W. Webster, and G.A. Therin, 'Older persons' definitions of good health: implications for general practitioners', *Medical Journal of Australia*. 1989; vol. 150, no. 8, pp. 426, 428.

6   G.A. Colditz, 'The Nurses Health Study: A cohort of US women followed since 1976', *Journal of the American Medical Women's Association*, vol. 50, no. 2, pp.40–4.

7   D. Saltman, B. Veale, and G. Bloom, 'Developing a mental health resource for consumers', *Australian Journal of Primary Health—Interchange*, vol. 3, no. 4, 1997, pp. 40–8.

8   T.A. Welborn (ed.), *The Busselton study: mapping population health (cardiovascular and respiratory disease risk factors in Busselton, Australia*, North Sydney, Australian Medical Publishing Co., 1998.

9   H. Hemingway, M. Stafford, S. Stansfeld, M. Shipley, and M. Marmot, 'Is the SF-36 a valid measure of change in population health? Results from the Whitehall II Study', *British Medical Journal*, vol. 315, no. 7118, 1997, pp.1273–9.

10 K. Messing, 'Women's occupational health: a critical review and discussion of current issues', *Women and Health*, 1997 vol. 25, no. 4, pp. 39–68.

11 J. Sechzer, A. Griffin, and S.M. Pfafflin (eds), 'Forging a women's health research agenda: Policy issues for the 1990s', *Annals of the New York Academy of Sciences*, vol. 736, 1994, pp. 21–48.

12 S. Leeder (ed.), *Transactions of Menzies Foundation: A handbook for researchers*, vol. 7, pp. 33–44, Melbourne, Menzies Foundation, 1984.

13 T. Richards and L. Richards, NUD*IST, Bundoora, Vic., Replee Pty Ltd, 1990.

14 M. Hammersley and P. Atkinson, *Ethnograpy—Ethnography: Principles in practice*, 2nd edn, New York, Routlege, 1995.

15 SPSS Inc., *SPSS Reference Guide*, Chicago, SPSS Inc., 1990.

16 StataCorp. Stata Statistical Software: Release 6.0. College Station, TX, Stata Corporation, 1999.

17 Z.R. Wolf and M.M. Heinzer, 'Substruction: illustrating the connections from research question to analysis,' *Journal of Professional Nursing*, vol. 15, no. 1, 1999, pp. 33–7.

Chapter 11: Assistants and mentors

1   J.H. Abrahamson, *Survey Methods in Community Medicine*, Edinburgh, Churchill Livingston, 1990, p. 30.

2   National Health and Medical Research Council (NHMRC), *National Statement on Ethical Conduct in Research Involving Humans*, Canberra, NHMRC, 1999.

3   Norusis MJ/SPSS Inc., *SPSS for Windows: Base System Users' Guide*, Release 6.0. SPSS, 1993.

4   SAS Institute Inc., *Introducing the SAS system*, Version 6, 1st edn, Cary, NC, SAS Institute, 1991.

5   T. Richards, L. Richards, J. McGalliard, and B. Sharrock, *NUDIST 2.3 User Manual*, Eltham, Vic., Replee, 1992.

6   P. Hawe, D. Degeling, and J. Hall, *Evaluating Health Promotion*, Artarmon, NSW, MacLennan & Petty, 1994, pp. 148–9.

7   R. Bhopal, J. Rankin, E. McColl, L. Thomas, E. Kaner, R. Stacy, P. Pearson, B. Vernon, and H. Rodgers, 'The vexed question of authorship—Views of researchers in a British medical faculty', *British Medical Journal*, vol. 314, no. 7086, 1997, pp. 1009–12.

8   International Committee of Medical Journal Editors, 'Guidelines on authorship: International Committee of Medical Journal Editors', *Medical Journal of Australia*, vol. 143, no. 11, 1985, pp. 520–1.

9 B. Moore (ed.), *The Australian Concise Oxford Dictionary*, 3rd edn, Melbourne, Oxford University Press, 1998.

10 K. Tyler, 'Mentoring programs link employees and experienced execs', *HRMagazine*, vol. 43, no. 5, April, 1998, pp. 98–103.

11 M. Messmer, 'Power/knowledge and psychosocial dynamics in mentoring', *Management and Learning*, vol. 30, March 1999, pp. 7–24

12 S. Bochner, 'Mentoring in higher education: Issues to be addressed in developing a mentoring program', *ERA/AARE Joint Conference Papers*, Nov. 1996; J.R. Baird, 'Mentoring for professional development of tertiary educators', *Australian Teacher Education Association Annual Conference Papers*, July, 1994.

13 S. Johnston and C. McCormack, 'Developing research potential through a structured mentoring program: Issues arising', *Higher Education*, vol. 33, no. 3, 1997, pp. 251–64.

14 D. Roesler, 'Teach your people well', *Financial Executive*, vol. 13, no. 2, March/April 1997, pp. 43–5.

15 M. McDougall and R. Beattie, 'Peer into the future', *People in Management*, vol. 4, no. 9, April 1998, p. 56.

16 McDougall and Beattie, 'Peer into the future'.

17 J.B. Ritchie, 'Ray Miles as a teacher and mentor', *Journal of Management Inquiry*, vol. 7, no. 4, December 1998, pp. 307–8.

18 Roesler, 'Teach your people well'.

19 Ritchie, 'Ray Miles as a teacher and mentor'.

20 C. Bridges-Webb, H. Britt, D.A. Miles, S. Neary, J. Charles, and V. Traynor, 'Morbidity and treatment in general practice in Australia', *Australian Family Physician*, vol. 22, no. 3, 1993, pp. 336–9, 342–6.

21 D. Pond, C. Berglund, V. Traynor, D. Gietzelt, P. McNeill, E. Comino, and M. Harris, *Ethical Issues in General Practice: GPs' and Consumers' Perspectives*, Final report to the General Practice Evaluation Program (GPEP), Canberra, 1997.

Chapter 12: Ethics as part of research

1 National Health and Medical Research Council, *National Statement on Ethical Conduct in Research Involving Humans*, Canberra, Commonwealth of Australia, 28 June 1999. Page references noted in this chapter are to this NHMRC document.

2 C. Berglund and S. Dodds, 'Ethical concepts and issues in research involving humans', Section 2, in P. Komesaroff, S. Dodds, P.M. McNeill, and L. Skene (eds), *Ethical Issues in Research: Operations Manual for Human Research Ethics Committees in Australia*, Canberra, Australian Health Ethics Committee, in press, p. 2-2.

3 You may like to read further about the history of the Belmont principles in the original Belmont Report: United States Department of Health, Education, and Welfare, *Ethical Principles and Guidelines for the Protection of Human Subjects of Research*, DHEW Publication No. OS 78-0012, Washington, DC, United States Department of Health, Education, and Welfare, 1978.

4 C.A. Berglund, *Ethics for Health Care*, Melbourne, Oxford University Press, 1998, p. 160.

5 Berglund and Dodds, 'Ethical concepts and issues in research involving humans', p. 2-3.

6 Berglund, *Ethics for Health Care*, p. 13.

7 A. Campbell, M Charlesworth, G. Gillett, and G. Jones, 'Theories of medical ethics', ch. 1, *Medical Ethics*, 2nd edn, Oxford, Oxford University Press, 1997, pp. 2–9.

8 T.L. Beauchamp and J.F. Childress, *Principles of Biomedical Ethics*, 4th edn, New York, Oxford University Press, 1994.

9 Berglund, *Ethics for Health Care*, pp. 7–8.

10 R.J. Levine, *Ethics and Regulation of Clinical Research*, 2nd edn, Baltimore-Munich, Urban & Schwarzenberg, 1986; R.H. Nicholson, *Medical Research with Children: Ethics, Law and Practice*, Oxford, Oxford University Press, 1986; A.M. Capron, 'Human experimentation: Basic issues', in W.T. Reich (ed,), *Encyclopedia of Bioethics*, New York, The Free Press, 1978, pp. 692–9.

11 C.A. Berglund, 'Children in medical research: Australian ethical standards', *Child: care, health and development*, vol. 21 no. 2, 1995, pp. 149–59.

12 NHMRC, *General Guidelines for Medical Practitioners on Providing Information to Patients*, Canberra, NHMRC, June 1993.

13 NHMRC, *General Guidelines for Medical Practitioners on Providing Information to Patients*.

14 P. Baume, *A question of Balance: Report on the Future of Drug Evaluation in Australia*, commissioned by the Minister for Aged, Family, and Health Services, the Hon. Peter Staples, AGPS, Canberra, 1991.

15 K.R. Mitchell, I.H. Kerridge, and T.J. Lovat, *Bioethics and Clinical Ethics FOR Health Care Professionals*, 2nd edn, Wentworth Falls, Social Sciences Press, 1996.

16 NHMRC, *General Guidelines for Medical Practitioners on Providing Information to Patients*.

17 P. Finucane, C. Myser, and S. Ticehurst, "Is she fit to sign doctor?' - Practical ethical issues in assessing the competence of elderly patients', *Medical Journal of Australia*, vol. 159, 1993, pp. 400–3.

18 Berglund and Dodds, 'Ethical concepts and issues in research involving humans', p. 2-9.

19 Berglund, *Ethics for Health Care*, p. 83.

20 NHMRC, *Aspects of Privacy in Medical Research*, Canberra, NHMRC, 1995.

21 Such as: Office of the Privacy Commissioner, *National Principles for the Fair Handling of Personal Information*, Sydney, Human Rights and Equal Opportunity Commission, January 1999; NSW Health Department, *Discussion Paper: Ethical Management of Health Information*, Sydney, December 1999.

22 Berglund and Dodds, 'Ethical concepts and issues in research involving humans', p. 2-5. A discussion paper by the NHMRC may be useful in regards to a committee's considerations of justice: NHMRC, *Discussion Paper on Ethics and Resource Allocation in Health Care*, Canberra, AGPS, 1990.

23 Berglund, *Ethics for Health Care*, pp. 158–9.

Chapter 13: Disciplines and boundaries

1 National Health and Medical Research Council, *National Statement on Ethical Conduct in Research Involving Humans*, Canberra, NHMRC, 28 June 1999.

2 P. Komesaroff, S. Dodds, P.M. McNeill, and L. Skene (eds), *Ethical Issues in Research: Operations Manual for Human Research Ethics Committees in Australia*, Canberra, Australian Health Ethics Committee, in press.

3 J. Devereux and N. Cuffe, *A Guide to Legal Research in the Solomon Islands*, Brisbane, Queensland Law Reform Commission and Griffith University, 1995.

4 R. Balkin and J. Davis, *The Law of Torts*, Sydney, Butterworths, 1996.

5 D. Gardiner and F. McGlone, *An Introduction to the Law of Torts*, Sydney, Butterworths, 1996.

6 R.G. Kenny, *An Introduction to Criminal Law in Queensland and Western Australia*, 5th edn, Sydney, Butterworths, 1999.

7 C. Enright, *Studying Law*, 5th edn, Sydney, Federation Press, 1995, p. 166.

8 Enright, *Studying Law*, p. 166.

9   G. Morris, C. Cook, R. Creyke, and R. Geddes, *Laying Down the Law: The Foundations of Legal Reasoning, Research and Writing in Australia and New Zealand*, 4th edn, Sydney, Butterworths, 1996.

10 R.B. Vermeesch and K.E. Lindgren, *Business Law in Australia*, 9th edn, Sydney, 1999, p. 506.

11 On copyright generally see Vermeesch and Lindgren, *Business Law in Australia*.

12 *Copyright Act 1968* (Cwlth), s. 35(2).

13 *Copyright Act 1968* (Cwlth), s. 35(6).

14 [1972] 1 All ER 1023.

15 Kenny, *An Introduction to Criminal Law in Queensland and Western Australia*, p. 143.

16 Kenny, *An Introduction to Criminal Law in Queensland and Western Australia*, pp.140, 141.

17 Kenny, *An Introduction to Criminal Law in Queensland and Western Australia*, pp.141, 142.

18 J. Fitzgerald, 'A background to the ethical and legal issues in maintaining confidentiality when conducting research into illegal behaviours', in *Ethical and Legal issues when Conducting Research into Illegal Behaviours*, University of Melbourne, 8 August 1995.

19 See generally, Fitzgerald, 'A background to the ethical and legal issues in maintaining confidentiality when conducting research into illegal behaviours'.

Chapter 14: Writing and publishing

1   L.J. Cuba, *A Short Guide to Writing about Social Science*, Glenview, Ill.: Scott, Foresman and Co., 1988, p. 31.

2   D.O. McCarthy and B.J. Bowers, 'Implementation of writing-to-learn in a program of nursing', *Nurse Educator*, vol. 19, no. 3, 1994, pp. 32–5.

3   P.C. Broussard and M.G. Oberleitner, 'Writing and thinking: A process to critical understanding', *Journal of Nursing Education*, vol. 36, no. 7, 1997, pp. 334–6, p. 336.

4   Broussard and Oberleitner, 'Writing and thinking', p. 335.

5   S.P. MacDonald, *Professional Academic Writing in the Humanities and Social Sciences*, Carbondale and Edwardsville, Southern Illinois University Press, 1994, pp. 21–2.

6   H.S. Becker, Tricks of the Trade: How to think about your research while you're doing it, Chicago, University of Chicago Press, 1998, pp. 9, 79.

7   Becker, Tricks of the trade, p. 96.

8   International Committee of Medical Journal Editors, 'Uniform requirements for manuscripts submitted to biomedical journals', *New England Journal of Medicine*, vol. 336, no. 4, 1997, pp. 309–315, p. 311.

9   New England Journal of Medicine, 'Information for authors', *New England Journal of Medicine*, vol. 340, no. 18, 1999, p. 1435.

10 International Committee of Medical Journal Editors, 'Uniform requirements for manuscripts submitted to biomedical journals'.

11 'Information for authors', *Nursing Research*, vol. 48, no. 1, 1999, back page unnumbered.

12 'Notes for contributors', *Medical Teacher*, vol. 21, no. 4, 1999, back page inside back cover unnumbered.

13 Chicago Manual of Style: The Essential Guide for Writers, Editors and Publishers, 14th edn, Chicago and London, The University of Chicago Press, 1993.

14 E.J. Huth., Medical Style & Format: An International Manual For Authors, Editors, and Publishers, Philadelphia, ISI Press, 1987.

15 Australian Government Publishing Service, *Style Manual for Authors, Editors and Printers*, 5th edn, Canberra, AGPS, 1996.

16 Ministerial Document Service: Daily Collation of Ministers' and Opposition Leaders' Statements, Canberra, Ausinfo, Department of Finance and Administration.

17 Bishop, Bronwyn MP, Minister for Aged Care, Member for Mackellar. Media Release BB62/99, 23 Aug. 1999. 'Young people at high risk of premature hearing loss', *Ministerial Document Service* 1999–2000, no. 16, p. 417.

Bibliography

J.H. Abrahamson, *Survey Methods in Community Medicine*, Edinburgh, Churchill Livingston, 1990.

E.H. Ackerknecht, *A Short History of Medicine*, Baltimore, MD, Johns Hopkins University Press, 1982.

A. Agresti, *An Introduction to Categorical Data Analysis*, New York, Wiley, 1996.

A.L. Aharony and S. Strasser, 'Patient satisfaction: What we know about it and what we still need to explore', *Medical Care Review*, vol. 50, no. 1, 1993, pp. 49–79.

E.B. Andersen, *Introduction to the Statistical Analysis of Categorical Data*, New York, Springer-Verlag, 1997.

D. Andrews and A. Herzberg, *Data*, New York, Springer-Verlag 1985.

H.K. Armenian, D.R. Hoover, S. Rubb, S. Metz, R. Kaslow, B. Visscher, J. Chmiel, L. Kingsley, and A. Saah, 'Composite risk score for Kaposi's sarcoma based on a case-control and longitudinal study in the Multicenter AIDS cohort study population', *American Journal of Epidemiology*, vol. 138, 1993, pp. 256–65.

P. Armitage and G. Berry, *Statistical Methods in MedicalResearch*, Oxford, Blackwell Scientific Publications, 1994.

D. Armstrong, *Political Anatomy of the Body, Medical Knowledge in Britain in the 20th Century*, Cambridge, Cambridge University Press, 1983.

L. Ashton, The role of prevention in the practice of rural community nurses, unpublished master of Public Health project report, University of New South Wales, 1999.

C. Ateenyi-Agaba, 'Conjunctival squamous cell carcinoma associated with HIV infection in Kampala, Uganda (letter)', *Lancet*, vol. 345, 1995, pp. 695–6.

H. Attwood and R.W. Home, Patients, practitioners and techniques; *2nd National Conference on Medicine and Health in Australia*, Medical History Unit and Department of History and Philosophy of Science, University of Melbourne, 1985.

Australian Bureau of Statistics (ABS), *Estimated Resident Population by Age and Sex: States and Territories of Australia*, catalogue no. 3201. 0, Canberra, ABS, 1998.

Australian Bureau of Statistics (ABS), *Catalogue of Publications and Products*, catalogue no. 1101. 0, Canberra, ABS, 1999.

The Australian Concise Oxford Dictionary, 3rd edn, ed. B. Moore, Melbourne, Oxford University Press, 1998.

Australian Government Publishing Service, *Style Manual for Authors, Editors and Printers*, 5th edn, Canberra, AGPS, 1996.

Australian Institute of Health and Welfare, *Australia's Health, 1998*, Canberra, AGPS, 1998.

Australian Institute of Health and Welfare, *Australia's Children, Their Health and Wellbeing 1998*, Canberra, AGPS, 1998.

Australian Institute of Health and Welfare, *Australia's Heath 1998: The Sixth Biennial Health Report of the Australian Institute of Health and Welfare*, AIHW catalogue no. AUS10, Canberra, Australian Institute of Health and Welfare, 1998.

Australian Medical Association, *Code of Ethics*, Canberra, 1996.

Australian Nursing Council, *Code of Ethics*, Canberra, 1993.

J.R. Baird, 'Mentoring for professional development of tertiary educators', *Australian Teacher Education Association Annual Conference Papers,* July, 1994.

R. Balkin and J. Davis, *The Law of Torts,* Sydney, Butterworths, 1996.

M. Bass, *Disseminating Research/Changing Practice,* Thousand Oaks, CA, Sage, 1994.

R. Batalden, E. Nelson, and J. Roberts, 'Linking outcomes measurement to continual improvement: The serial "V" way of thinking about improving clinical care', *Joint Commission Journal of Quality Improvement,* vol. 20, no. 4, 1994, pp. 167–80.

F. Baum, *The New Public Health: An Australian Perspective,* Melbourne, Oxford University Press, 1998.

P. Baume, *A Question of Balance: Report on the Future of Drug Evaluation in Australia,* commissioned by the Minister for Aged, Family, and Health Services, the Hon. Peter Staples, Canberra, AGPS, 1991.

P. Baume (ed.), *The Tasks of Medicine: An Ideology of Care,* Sydney, MacLennan & Petty, 1998.

T.C. Beard, D.R. Woodward, P.J. Ball, H. Hornsby, R.J. von Witt and T. Dwyer, 'The Hobart Salt Study 1995' *Medical Journal of Australia,* vol. 166, no. 8, 1997, pp. 404–7.

T.L. Beauchamp and J.F. Childress, *Principles of Biomedical Ethics,* 4th edn, New York, Oxford University Press, 1994.

H.S. Becker, *Tricks of the Trade: How to think about your research while you're doing it,* Chicago, University of Chicago Press, 1998.

V. Beral, T.A. Peterman, R.L. Berkelman, and H.W. Jaffe, 'Kaposi's sarcoma among persons with AIDS: A sexually transmitted infection?', *Lancet,* vol. 335, 1990, pp. 123–8.

V. Beral, T. Peterman, R. Berkelman, and H. Jaffe, 'AIDS-associated non-Hodgkin's lymphoma', *Lancet,* vol. 337, 1991, pp. 805–9.

R.J. Biggar, 'Cancer in acquired immunodeficiency syndrome: An epidemiological assessment', *Seminars in Oncology,* vol. 17, 1990, pp. 251–60.

R.J. Biggar for the AIDS-Cancer Match study group, 'Spectrum of AIDS-associated malignant disorders', *Lancet,* vol. 358, 1998, pp. 1833–9.

V. Beral, D. Bull, R. Doll, T. Key, R. Peto, and G. Reeves, 'Breast cancer and hormone replacement therapy: Collaborative reanalysis of data from 51 epidemiological studies of 52,705 women with breast cancer and 108,411 women without breast cancer', *Lancet,* vol. 350, 1997, pp. 1047–59.

R.J. Biggar, W. Burnett, J. Mikl, and P. Nasca, 'Cancer among New York men at risk of acquired immunodeficiency syndrome', *International Journal of Cancer,* vol. 43, 1989, pp. 979–85.

R.J. Biggar, J. Horm, J.J. Goedert, and M. Melbye, 'Cancer in a group at risk of AIDS through 1984', *American Journal of Epidemiology,* vol. 126, 1987, pp. 578–86.

M. Burnet, 'Immunological factors in the process of carcinogenesis', *British Medical Bulletin,* vol. 20, 1964, pp. 154–7.

C.A. Berglund and P.M. McNeill, 'Guidelines for research practice in Australia: NHMRC Statement & Professional Codes', *Community Health Studies,* vol. 13, no. 2, 1989, pp. 121–9.

C.A. Berglund, 'Children in medical research: Australian ethical standards', *Child: Care, Health and Development,* vol. 21 no. 2, 1995, pp. 149–59.

C.A. Berglund, *Ethics for Health Care,* Melbourne, Oxford University Press, 1998.

L. Bero and D. Rennie, 'The Cochrane Collaboration: preparing, maintaining and disseminating systematic reviews of the effects of health care', *Journal of the American Medical Association*, vol. 274, no. 24, 1995, pp. 1935–8.

D. Berwick, 'Harvesting knowledge for improvement', *Journal of the American Medical Association*, vol. 275, no. 11, 1996, pp. 877–8.

R. Bhopal, J. Rankin, E. McColl, L. Thomas, E. Kaner, R. Stacy, P. Pearson, B. Vernon, and H. Rodgers, 'The vexed question of authorship—views of researchers in a British medical faculty', *British Medical Journal*, vol. 314, no. 7086, 1997, pp. 1009–12.

Bishop, Bronwyn MP, Minister for Aged Care, Member for Mackellar. Media Release BB62/99, 23 Aug. 1999: 'Young people at high risk of premature hearing loss'. *Ministerial Document Service* 1999–2000, no. 16, p. 417.

S. Bochner, 'Mentoring in Higher Education: Issues to be Addressed in Developing a Mentoring Program', *ERA/AARE Joint Conference Papers*, Nov. 1996.

S.N. Bolsin, 'Professional misconduct: the Bristol case', *Medical Journal of Australia*, vol. 169, 1998, pp. 369–72.

D. Booth, D.R. Deupree, H. Hultgren, A. De Maria, S. Scott, and R. Luch, 'Quality of life after bypass surgery for unstable angina; 5-year follow-up results of Veterans Affairs Cooperative Study', *Circulation*, vol. 83, 1991, pp. 87–95.

A. Bowling, *Research Methods in Health*, Buckingham, Open University Press, 1997.

British Medical Association, *Core Values for the Medical Profession in the 21st Century*, 1995.

A.J. Brettle, A.F. Long, M.J. Grant, and J. Greenhalgh, 'Searching for information on outcomes: do you need to be comprehensive?', *Quality in Health Care*, vol. 7, 1998, pp. 163–7.

C. Bridges-Webb, H. Britt, D.A. Miles, S. Neary, J. Charles, and V. Traynor, 'Morbidity and treatment in general practice in Australia', *Australian Family Physician*, vol. 22, no. 3, 1993, pp. 336–9, 342–6.

H. Brody, *Stories of Sickness*, New Haven, CT, Yale University Press, 1987.

P.C. Broussard and M.G. Oberleitner, 'Writing and thinking: A process to critical understanding', *Journal of Nursing Education*, vol. 36, no. 7, 1997, pp. 334–6.

D.P. Byar, C. Blackard and the VACURG, 'Comparisons of placebo, pyridoxine, and topical thiotepa in preventing recurrence of stage 1 bladder cancer,' *Urology*, vol. 10, 1977, pp. 556–61.

A. Campbell, M. Charlesworth, G. Gillett, and G. Jones, *Medical Ethics*, 2nd edn, Oxford, Oxford University Press, 1997.

C. Canaris and S. Jurd, 'The diagnosis of alcohol-related brain damage: a retrospective study in alcoholics undergoing in-patient rehabilitation', *Drug and Alcohol Review*, vol. 10, 1991, pp. 85–8.

A. Castiglioni, *A History of Medicine*, 2nd edn, trans. by E.B. Krumbhaar, New York, McClelland & Stewart, 1958.

Centers for Disease Control, 'Pneumocystic pneumonia—Los Angeles', *Morbidity and Mortality Weekly*, vol. 30, no. 21, 1981, pp. 250–2.

Centers for Disease Control, 'Kaposi's Sarcoma and Pneumocystic Pneumonia – New York City and California', *Morbidity and Mortality Weekly*, vol. 30, no. 25, 1981, pp. 305–8.

Centers for Disease Control and Prevention, '1993 revised classification system for HIV infection and expanded surveillance case definition for AIDS among adolescents and adults', *Morbidity and Mortality Weekly Report*, vol. 41, 1992, pp. 1–18.

Y. Chang, E. Cesarman, M.S. Pessin, F. Lee, J. Culpepper, D.M. Knowles, and P.S. Moore, 'Identification of Herpesvirus-like DNA sequences in AIDS-associated Kaposi's Sarcoma', *Science*, vol. 266, 1994, pp. 1865–9.

S. Chapman and D. Lupton, *The Fight for Public Health: Principles and Practice of Media Advocacy*, London, BMJ Publishing Group, 1994.

M. Charlesworth, 'Where do research ideas come from?', *Transactions of the Menzies Foundation*, vol. 7, 1984, pp. 9–11.

Chicago Manual of Style: The essential guide for writers, editors and publishers, 14th edn, Chicago and London, University of Chicago Press, 1993.

G. Chronowski, MD, chronom 1@ix, netcom. com.

L. Clendening, *Source Book of Medical History*, New York, Dover Publishers, 1942.

C.C. Clogg and E.S. Shihadeh, *Statistical Models for Ordinal Variables*, Thousand Oaks, CA, Sage Publications, 1994.

M.S. Coates and B.K. Armstrong, *Cancer in New South Wales: Incidence and Mortality 1995*, Sydney, NSW Cancer Council Sydney, 1998.

W.G. Cochran, 'Some methods of strengthening the common χ^2', *Biometrics*, vol. 10, 1954, pp. 417–51.

G.A. Colditz, 'The Nurses Health Study: A cohort of US women followed since 1976', *Journal of the American Medical Womens Association*, vol. 50, no. 2, pp. 40–4.

W.J. Conover, *Practical Nonparametric Statistics*, 2nd edn, New York, Wiley, 1980.

K. Cox, *Doctor and Patient—Exploring Clinical Thinking*, Sydney, University of New South Wales Press, 1998.

L.J. Cuba, *A Short Guide to Writing about Social Science*, Glenview, IL: Scott, Foresman and Co., 1988.

R.O. Day, D.R. Chalmers, K.M. Williams, and T.J. Campbell, 'The death of a healthy volunteer in a human research project: implications for Australian clinical research', *Medical Journal of Australia*, vol. 168, 1998, pp. 449–51.

N.K. Denzin, *The Research Act*, 2nd edn, New York, McGraw-Hill, 1978.

N. Denzin and Y. Lincoln (eds), *Handbook of Qualitative Research*, Thousand Oaks, CA, Sage Publications, 1994.

Department of Housing and Community Services, 'Enough to make you sick: How income and environment affect health', *National Health Strategy Research Paper No. 1*, Canberra, AGPS, 1992.

J. Devereux, *Medical Law: Text, Cases and Materials*, Sydney, Cavedish, 1997.

J. Devereux and N. Cuffe, *A Guide to Legal Research in the Solomon Islands*, Brisbane, Queensland Law Reform Commission and Griffith University, 1995.

W.G.H. Duckworth, *Some Notes on Galen's Anatomy*, given as The Linacre Lecture, 6 May 1948, Cambridge, W. Heffer & Sons Ltd, 1948, p. 38.

Editorial, *Medical Journal of Australia*, vol. 169, 5 Oct. 1998, p. 348.

M. Eisenbruch, 'Children with failure to thrive, epilepsy and STI/AIDS: Indigenous taxonomies, attributions and ritual treatments', *Clinical Child Psychology and Psychiatry*, vol. 3, no. 4, 1998, pp. 505–18.

M.H. Ellis, *Lachlan Macquarie: His Life, Adventures and Times*, 4th edn (rev.), Sydney, Angus & Robertson, 1965.

M. Ely, *Doing Qualitative Research: Circles within Circles*, London, Falmer Press, 1991.

C. Enright, *Studying Law*, 5th edn, Sydney, Federation Press, 1995.

P. Finucane, C. Myser, and S. Ticehurst, "Is she fit to sign doctor?'—Practical ethical issues in assessing the competence of elderly patients', *Medical Journal of Australia*, vol. 159, 1993, pp. 400–3.

J. Fitzgerald, 'A background to the ethical and legal issues in maintaining confidentiality when conducting research into illegal behaviours' in *Ethical and Legal issues when Conducting Research into Illegal Behaviours*, University of Melbourne, 8 August 1995.

S. Franceschi, L. Dal Maso, S. Arniani, P. Crosignani, M. Vercelli, L. Simonata, F. Falcini, R. Zanetti, A. Barchielli, D. Serraino, and G. Rezza for the Cancer and AIDS Registry Linkage Study, 'Risk of cancer other than Kaposi's sarcoma and non-Hodgkin's lymphoma in persons with AIDS in Italy', *British Journal of Cancer*, vol. 78, 1998, pp. 966–70.

J.F. Fries and P.W. Spitz, 'The hierarchy of patient outcomes', in B. Spilker (ed.), *Quality of Life Assessment in Clinical Trials*, New York, Raven Press, 1990.

T.R. Forbes, *Surgeons at the Bailey*, New Haven, CT, Yale University Press, 1985.

M. Foucault, *The Birth of the CLINIC*, trans. A.M. Sheridan Smith, London, Tavistock Publishers, 1973.

E. Ford, *The Life and Work of William Redfern*, Australian Medical Publishing Company, Sydney, 1953.

Galen, 'Anatomical Procedures', Book 6, Chapter 11, trans. by O. Temkin and W.L. Straus Jnr, *Galen's Dissection of the Liver and of the Muscles moving the Forearm* (from the Edward Ford Collection, Library of the Royal College of Physicians of Australasia).

D. Gardiner and F. McGlone, *An Introduction to the Law of Torts*, Sydney, Butterworths, 1996.

F. Garrison, *History of Medicine*, 4th edn, Philedelphia and London, WB Saunders & Co., 1929.

Gee & Mason, *The Courts and the Doctor*, Oxford, Oxford University Press, 1990.

D.M. Gels and J.R. Banks, 'The effects of drug therapy on long-term outcome of childhood asthma: A possible preview of the international guidelines', *Pediatrics*, vol. 102, no. 2, 1998, p. 451.

R.P. Gephart, *Ethnostatistics*, vol. 12, Qualitative Foundations for Quantitative Research. Qualitative Research Methods, Newbury Park, CA, Sage Publications Inc., 1988.

T. Gill and A. Feinstein, 'A critical appraisal of the quality of quality-of-life measures', *Journal of the American Medical Association*, vol. 272, no. 8, 1994, pp. 619–26.

A. Giuffrida, H. Gravelle, and M. Roland, 'Measuring quality of care with routine data: avoiding confusion between performance indicators and health outcomes', *British Medical Journal*, vol. 319, no. 7202, 1999, pp. 94–8.

J.J. Goedert and T.R. Coté, 'Conjunctival malignant disease with AIDS in USA', *Lancet*, vol. 346, 1995, pp. 257–8.

J.J. Goedert, T.R. Coté, P.Virgo, P.M. Scoppa, D.W. Kingma, M.H. Gail, E.S. Jaffe, C.P. Archibald, M.T. Schechter, T.N. Le, K.J.P. Craib, J.S.G. Montaner, and M.V. O'Shaughnessy, 'Evidence for a sexually transmitted cofactor for AIDS-related Kaposi's sarcoma in a cohort of homosexual men', *Epidemiology*, vol. 3, 1992, pp. 203–9.

D.C. Goodman, P. Lozano, T.A. Stukel, C.H. Chang, and J. Hecht, 'Has asthma medication use in children become more frequent, more appropriate or both?', *Pediatrics*, vol. 104, no. 2, 1999, pp. 187–94.

C. Grbich, *Qualitative Research in Health: An Introduction*, St Leonards, NSW, Allan & Unwin, 1999.

A. Grulich, O. Hendry, K. Luo, N. Bodsworth, D. Cooper, J. Kaldor, 'Risk of Kaposi's sarcoma and oro-anal sexual contact', *American Journal of Epidemiology*, 1997; vol. 145, pp. 673–679.

A.E. Grulich, S. Olsen, O. Hendry, K. Luo, P. Cunningham, D.A. Cooper, S.J. Gao, Y. Chang, P.S. Moore, and J.M. Kaldor, 'Kaposi's sarcoma associated herpesvirus: a sexually transmissible infection?', *Journal of AIDS & Human Retrovirology*, vol. 20, 1999, pp. 387–393.

A. Grulich, X. Wan, M. Law, M. Coates, and J. Kaldor, 'Cancer incidence rates in people with AIDS in NSW, Australia', *AIDS*, vol. 13, 1999, pp. 839–43.

M.C. Gulliford, 'Evaluating prognostic factors: implications for measurement of health care outcome', *Journal of Epidemiology & Community Health*, vol. 46, no. 4, 1992, pp. 323–6.

E.G. Guba and Y.S. Lincoln, *Fourth generation evaluation*, Newbury Park, CA, Sage Publications, 1989.

E.G. Guba and Y.S. Lincoln, 'Competing paradigms in qualitative research', in N. Denzin and Y. Lincoln (eds), *Handbook of Qualitative Research*, Sage Publications, Thousand Oaks, CA, 1994.

G. Guyatt, D. Cook, 'Health status, quality of life and the individual', *Journal of the American Medical Association*, vol. 272, no. 8, 1994, pp. 630–1.

M. Hammersley and P. Atkinson, *Ethnograph. Ethnography: Principles in Practice*. 2nd edn, New York, Routlege, 1995.

Hammond Publishers, *Historical Atlas of the World*, Hammond, NJ, 1984, p. H-5.

P. Hawe, D. Degeling, and J. Hall, *Evaluating Health Promotion*, Artarmon, NSW, MacLennan & Petty, 1994.

J. Hayward, 'Promoting clinical effectiveness: a welcome initiative, but both clinical and health policy need to be based on evidence', *British Medical Journal*, vol. 312, no. 7045, 1996, pp. 1491–2.

H. Hemingway, M. Stafford, S. Stansfeld, M. Shipley, and M. Marmot, 'Is the SF-36 a valid measure of change in population health? Results from the Whitehall II Study', *British Medical Journal*, vol. 315, no. 7118, 1997, pp. 1273–9.

N.A. Hessol, M.H. Katz, J.Y. Liu, S.P. Buchbinder, C.J. Rubino, and S.D. Holmberg, 'Increased incidence of Hodgkin disease in homosexual men with HIV infection', *Annals of Internal Medicine*, vol. 117, 1992, pp. 309–11.

J.E. Higgins and G.G. Koch, 'Variable selection and generalized chi-square analysis', of categorical data applied to a large cross-sectional occupational health survey', *International Statistical Review*, vol. 45, 1977, pp. 51–62.

A.M. Huberman, and M.B. Miles, 'Data management and analysis methods', in N. Denzin and Y. Lincoln (eds), *Handbook of Qualitative Research*, Thousand Oaks, CA, Sage Publications, 1994.

A. Hudson Jones, 'Literature and medicine: narrative ethics', *Lancet*, vol. 349, 1997, pp. 1243–1246.

S. Hulley, S. Cummings (eds), *Designing Clinical Research*, Baltimore, MD, Williams & Wilkins, 1988.

E.H. Hume, *The Chinese Way in Medicine*, Baltimore, MD, 1940.

E.J. Huth, *Medical Style & Format: An International Manual for Authors, Editors, and Publishers*, Philadelphia, ISI Press, 1987.

'Information for authors', *New England Journal of Medicine*, vol. 340, no. 18, 1999, p. 1435.

'Information for authors', *Nursing Research*, vol. 48, no. 1, 1999, back page unnumbered.

International Agency for Research on Cancer, 'IARC monographs on the evaluation of carcinogenic risks to humans', vol. 59: *Hepatitis viruses*, Lyon, International Agency for Research on Cancer, 1994.

International Committee of Medical Journal Editors, 'Guidelines on authorship: International Committee of Medical Journal Editors', *Medical Journal of Australia*, vol. 143, no. 11, 1985, pp. 520–1.

International Committee of Medical Journal Editors, 'Uniform requirements for manuscripts submitted to biomedical journals', *New England Journal of Medicine*, vol. 336, no. 4, 1997, pp. 309–15.

International Study of Asthma and Allergies in Childhood Steering Committee, 'Worldwide variation in prevalence of symptoms of asthma, allergic rhinoconjunctivits, and atopic eczema: ISAAC', *Lancet*, vol. 351, no. 9111, 1998, pp. 1225–32.

M. Ishii-Kuntz, *Ordinal Log-linear Models*, Thousand Oaks, CA, Sage Publications, 1994.

V.E. Johnson and J.H. Albert, *Ordinal Data Modeling*. New York, Springer, 1999.

B. Jalaludin, T. Chey, Holmwood, J. Chipps, R. Hanson, S. Corbett, and S. Leeder, 'Admission rates as an indicator of the prevalence of severe asthma in the community', *Australian & New Zealand Journal of Public Health*, vol. 22, no. 2, 1998, pp. 214–15.

V.J. Janesick, 'The dance of qualitative research design: Metaphor, methodolatry, and meaning', in N. Denzin and Y. Lincoln (eds), *Handbook of Qualitative Research*, Thousand Oaks, CA, Sage Publications, 1994.

S. Johnson and R. Johnson, 'Tonsillectomy history in Hodgkin's disease', *New England Journal of Medicine*, vol. 287, 1972, pp. 1122–25.

S. Johnston and C. McCormack, 'Developing research potential through a structured mentoring program: Issues arising', *Higher Education*, vol. 33, no. 3, 1997, pp. 251–64.

A.R. Jones, 'William Redfern (1775? –1833) mutineer to colonial surgeon in New South Wales. Part 1 & 2', *Journal of Medical Biography*, 1999.

C. Jones and R. Porter, *Reassessing Foucault*, London, Routledge, 1994.

J. L. Jones, D.L. Hanson, M.S. Dworkin, J.W. Ward, H.W. Jaffe, and the Adult/adolescent Spectrum of HIV Disease Project Group, 'Effect of anti-retroviral therapy on recent trends in selected cancers among HIV-infected persons', *Journal of AIDS*, vol. 21, 1999, pp. S11–S17.

R. Jones, 'Why do qualitative research?', *British Medical Journal*, vol. 311, 1995, p. 2.

K. Kavanagh, Performing miracles? The role and the reality of practice for nurse discharge planners, unpublished Master of Health Personnel Education project report, University of New South Wales, 1996.

G. Keller and B. Warrack, *Essentials of Business Statistics*, Belmont, CA, Duxbury Press, 1994.

R.G. Kenny, *An Introduction to Criminal Law in Queensland and Western Australia*, 5th edn, Sydney, Butterworths, 1999.

D.P. Kernick, 'Lies, damned lies, and evidence-based medicine', *Lancet*, vol. 351, 13 June 1998, p. 1824.

F.W. Kiel, Forensic science in China, *Journal of Forensic Science*, vol. 15, 1970, pp. 203–4.

L.J. Kinlen, 'Immunosuppression and cancer', in H. Vainio, P.N. Magee, D.B. McGregor, and A.J. McMichael (eds), *Mechanisms of Carcinogenesis in Risk Identification*, Lyon, International Agency for Research on Cancer, 1992, pp. 237–53.

A. Kitson, G. Harvey, and B. McCormack, 'Enabling the implementation of evidence-based practice: a conceptual framework', *Quality in Health Care*, 1998, vol. 7, pp. 149–58.

P. Komesaroff, S. Dodds, P.M. McNeill, and L. Skene (eds), *Ethical Issues in Research: Operations Manual for Human Research Ethics Committees in Australia*, Canberra, Australian Health Ethics Committee, in press.

T. Kuhn, *The Structure of Scientific Revolutions*, Chicago, University of Chicago Press, 1970.

T. Kuhn, *The Essential Tension*, Chicago, University of Chicago Press, 1977.

S. Labovitz and R. Hagedorn, *Introduction to Social Research*, New York, McGraw-Hill, 1971.

H.O. Lancaster, *Quantitative Methods in Biological and Medical Sciences : A Historical Essay*, New York, Springer-Verlag, 1994.

J. Lau, J.P.A. Ioannidis, C.H. Schmid, 'Summing up evidence: One answer is not enough', *Lancet*, vol. 351, Jan 10, 1998, pp. 123–7.

M. LeCompte and J. Preissle, *Ethnography and Qualitative Design in Educational Research*, 2nd edn, San Diego, CA, Academic Press Inc., 1993.

S. Leeder (ed.), *Transactions of Menzies Foundation: A Handbook for Researchers*, vol. 7, pp. 33–44. Menzies Foundation, Australia, 1994.

C. Lefant, N. Khaltaev, A.L. Sheffer, M Bartal, J. Bousquet, Y.Z. Chen, A.G. Chuchalin, T.J.H. Clark, R. Dahl, L.M. Fabbri, S.T. Holgate, P. Mahapatra, S. Makino, C.K. Naspitz, M.R. Partridge, R. Pauwels, V. Spicak, W.C. Tan, K.B. Weiss, A.J. Woolcock, M.N. Xabamokoena, and N.S. Zhong, 'Global strategy for asthma—management and prevention. NHLBI/WHO workshop report', *Revue Française d'Allergologie et d'Immunologie Clinique*, vol. 36, no. 6, 1996, p. 563 ff.

A. Leplege and S. Hunt, 'The problem of quality of life in medicine', *Journal of the American Medical Association*, vol. 278, no. 1, 1997, pp. 47–50.

R.J. Levine, *Ethics and Regulation of Clinical Research*, 2nd edn, Baltimore and Munich, Urban & Schwarzenberg, 1986.

P. Levy and S. Lemeshow, *Sampling of Populations: Methods and Application*, New York, John Wiley & Sons, Inc., 1991.

M. Lewis, 'Historical analysis', in C. Kerr, R. Taylor and G. Heard (eds), *Handbook of Public Health Methods*, Sydney, McGraw-Hill, 1998.

Y.S. Lincoln and E.G. Guba, *Naturalistic Inquiry*, Beverly Hills, CA, Sage Publications, 1985.

E. Lindal, 'Post-operative depression and coronary bypass surgery', *International Disability Studies*, vol. 12, 1990, pp. 704.

J.C. Linder, 'Outcomes measurement: Compliance tool or strategic initiative?', *Health Care Management Review*, vol. 16, no. 4, 1991, pp. 21–33.

M. Little, 'Cartesian Thinking in Health and Medicine', in P. Baume (ed.), *The Tasks of Medicine: An Ideology of Care*, Sydney, MacLennan & Petty, 1998, ch. 6, pp. 75–95.

E.R. Long. *A History of Pathology*, New York, Dover Publishers, 1965.

D. Lupton, 'Discourse analysis: A new method for understanding the ideologies of health and illness', *Australian Journal of Public Health*, vol. 16, 1992, pp. 145–50.

S.K. Lwanga and S. Lemeshow, *Sample Size Determination in Health Studies: A Practical Manual*, Geneva, World Health Organization, 1991.

A.S. Lyons and J. Petrucelli, *Medicine, An Illustrated History*, New York, Abradale Press, 1978.

D.W. Lyter, J. Bryant, R. Thackeray, C.R. Rinaldo, and L.A. Kingsley, 'Incidence of HIV-related and nonrelated malignancies in a large cohort of homosexual men', *Journal of Clinical Oncology*, vol. 13, 1995, pp. 2540–6.

H. MacBeth, *Health Outcomes: Biological, Social and Economic Perspectives*, New York, Oxford University Press, 1996.

D.O. McCarthy, B.J. Bowers, 'Implementation of writing-to-learn in a program of nursing', *Nurse Educator*, vol. 19, no. 3, 1994, pp. 32–5.

S.P. MacDonald, *Professional Academic Writing in the Humanities and Social Sciences*, Carbondale and Edwardsville, Southern Illinois University Press, 1994, pp. 21–2.

M. McDougall and R. Beattie, 'Peer into the future', *People in Management*, vol. 4, no. 9, April 1998, p. 56.

I. McDowell and C. Newell, *Measuring Health: A Guide to Rating Scales and Questionnaires*, New York, Oxford University Press, 1996.

R. MacFaul, E.J. Glass, and S. Jones, 'Appropriateness of paediatric admission', *Archives of Disease in Childhood*, vol. 71, no. 1, 1994, pp. 50–8.

M. Maclure, 'The case-crossover design: a method for studying transient effects on the risk of acute events', *American Journal of Epidemiology*, vol. 133, 1991, pp. 144–53.

B.E. McKnight, *Sung Tz'u: His yuan chi lu* (The washing away of wrongs), Centre for Chinese Studies, University of Michigan, 1981.

Q. McNemar, 'Note on the sampling error of the difference between correlated proportions or percentages', *Psychometrika*, vol. 12, 1947, pp. 153–7.

P. Maguire, *Doing Participatory Research: A Feminist Perspective*, Amherst, Mass., Center for International Education, University of Massachusetts, 1987.

R. Major, *Classic Descriptions of Disease*, Oxford, Blackwell Scientific Publications, 1945.

D.F. Martin, B.D. Kupperman, R.A. Wolitz, A.G. Palestine, M.S. Hong Li, C.A. Robinsons, Roche Ganciclovir Study Group, 'Oral ganciclovir for patients with cytomegalovirus retinitus treated with a ganciclovir implant', *New England Journal of Medicine*, vol. 340, no. 14, 1999, pp. 1063–70.

J.N. Martin, D.E. Ganem, D.H. Osmond, K.A. Page-Shafer, D. Macrae, and D.H. Kedes, 'Sexual transmission and the natural history of human herpesvirus 8 infection', *New England Journal of Medicine*, vol. 338, 1998, pp. 948–54.

N. Mays and C. Pope, 'Rigour and qualitative research', *British Medical Journal*, vol. 311, 1995, p. 109–12.

R.H. Meade, *An Introduction to the History of General Surgery*, Philadelphia, WB Saunders Co, 1968.

Medical Teacher, 'Notes for contributors', *Medical Teacher*, vol. 21, no. 4, 1999, back page inside back cover unnumbered.

K. Messing, 'Women's occupational health: a critical review and discussion of current issues', *Women and Health*, vol. 25, no. 4, 1997, pp. 39–68.

M. Messmer, 'Power/knowledge and psychosocial dynamics in mentoring', *Management and Learning*, vol. 30, March 1999, pp. 7–24.

M.B. Miles and A.M. Huberman, *Qualitative Data Analysis: A Sourcebook of New Methods*, Newbury Park, CA, Sage Publications, 1984.

D. Miller, '"After death the doctor", reflections on the Coroners Act and forensic pathology', *Australian Journal of Forensic Sciences*, vol. 3, no. 1, September, 1970, pp. 9–14.

K. R. Mitchell, I.H. Kerridge, and T.J. Lovat, *Bioethics and Clinical Ethics for Health Care Professionals*, 2nd edn, Wentworth Falls, NSW, Social Sciences Press, 1996.

K. Montgomery Hunter, *Doctors' Stories*, Princeton, NJ, Princeton University Press, 1991.

D.L. Morgan, 'Practical strategies for combining qualitative and quantitative methods: Applications to health research', *Qualitative Health Research*, vol. 8, no. 3, 1998, pp. 362–76.

G. Morris, C. Cook, R. Creyke, and R. Geddes, *Laying Down the Law: The Foundations of Legal Reasoning, Research and Writing in Australia and New Zealand*, 4th edn, Sydney, Butterworths, 1996.

J. Morse, '"Perfectly healthy, but dead": The myth of inter-rater reliability', *Qualitative Health Research*, vol. 7, no. 4, 1997, pp. 445–7.

J. Morse, 'What's wrong with random selection?', *Qualitative Health Research*, vol. 8, no. 6, 1998, pp. 733–5.

P.L. Munhall, *Qualitative Research Proposals and Reports: A Guide*, New York, National League for Nursing Press, 1994.

National Centre in HIV Epidemiology and Clinical Research. *HIV/AIDS, Hepatitis C and Sexually Transmissible Infections: Annual Surveillance Report 1999*, Sydney, National Centre in HIV Epidemiology and Clinical Research, 1999.

National Health and Medical Research Council, *Discussion Paper on Ethics and Resource Allocation in Health Care*, Canberra, AGPS, 1990.

National Health and Medical Research Council, *Aspects of Privacy in Medical Research*, Canberra, NHMRC, 1995.

National Health and Medical Research Council, *General Guidelines for Medical Practitioners on Providing Information to Patients*, Canberra, NHMRC, June 1993.

National Health and Medical Research Council, *Ethical Aspects of Qualitative Methods in Health Research: An Information Paper for Institutional Ethics Committees.* Canberra, AGPS, 1995.

National Health and Medical Research Council, *A Guide to the Development, Implementation and Evaluation of Clinical Practice Guidelines*, Canberra, AGPS, 1999.

National Health and Medical Research Council, *National Statement on Ethical Conduct in Research Involving Humans*, Canberra, Commonwealth of Australia, 28 June 1999.

New South Wales Health Department, *Discussion Paper: Ethical Management of Health Information*, Sydney, December 1999.

New Zealand Medical Association, *Code of Ethics*, Auckland.

R.H. Nicholson, *Medical Research with Children: Ethics, Law and Practice*, Oxford, Oxford University Press, 1986.

P. Norton, E. Dunn, J. Bain et al., 'Guidelines for the dissemination of new information discovered by researchers' in E. Dunn, P. Norton, M. Stewart, F. Tudiver, and Norusis MJ/SPSS Inc., *SPSS for Windows: Base System Users' Guide*, Release 6. 0. SPSS, 1993.

J.F. Nunn, *Ancient Egyptian Medicine*, London, British Museum Press, 1996.

Office of the Privacy Commissioner, *National Principles for the Fair Handling of Personal Information*, Sydney, Human Rights and Equal Opportunity Commission, January 1999.

K.J. O'Flynn and M. Irving, 'On the need for evidence-based surgery', *Evidence-based medicine*, vol. 4, no. 1, Jan./Feb. 1999, pp. 6–7.

C.D. O'Malley, *Andreas Vesalius of Brussels 1514–1564*, Berkeley, University of California Press, 1964.

Y.V. O'Neill and G.R. Chan, 'A Chinese coroner's manual and the evolution of anatomy', *Journal of the History of Medicine and Allied Sciences*, vol. 31, 1976, pp. 3–17.

G. Osborne and W.F. Mandle, *New History, Studying Australia Today*, Sydney, Allen & Unwin, 1982.

W. Osler, *The Evolution of Modern Medicine*, New Haven, CT, Yale University Press, 1921.

R. Palmer, 'Medicine at the papal court in the 16th century', in V. Nutton, *Medicine at the courts of Europe 1500–1837*, London, Routledge, 1990, ch. 2.

M.Q. Patton, *Qualitative Evaluation and Research Methods*, 2nd edn, Newbury Park, CA, Sage Publications, 1990.

Ho Peng Yoke, 'China', in H. Selin (ed.), *Encyclopaedia of the History of Science, Technology, and Medicine in Non-Western Cultures*, Dordrecht, Kluwer Academic Publishers, 1997, pp. 191–6.

P. Pinna Pintor, R. Torta, S. Bartolozzi, R. Borio, E. Caruzzo, A. Cicolin, M. Giammaria, F. Mariana, G. Ravarino, F. Triumbari, O. Alfieri, and L. Ravizza, 'Clinical outcome and emotional behaviour status after isolated coronary surgery', *Quality of Life Research*, vol. 1, 1992, pp. 177–85.

C. Plato, D. Rucknagel, and H. Gershowitz, 'Studies of the distribution of glucose-6-phosphate dehydorgenase deficiency, thalassemia, and other genetic traits in the coastal and mountain villages of Cyprus', *American Journal of Human Genetics*, vol. 16, 1964, pp. 267–83.

L. H. Plotnick and F. M. Ducharme, 'Should inhaled anticholinergies be added to beta$_2$ agonists for treating acute childhood and adolescent asthma?: A systematic review', *British Medical Journal*, vol. 317, no. 7164, 1998, pp. 971–7.

D. Pond, C. Berglund, V. Traynor, D. Gietzelt, P. McNeill, E. Comino, and M. Harris, *Ethical Issues in General Practice: GPs' and Consumers' Perspectives*, Final report to the General Practice Evaluation Program (GPEP), Canberra, 1997.

C. Pope and N. Mays, 'Reaching the parts other methods cannot reach: An introduction to qualitative methods in health and health services research', *British Medical Journal*, vol. 311, 1995, pp. 42–5.

R. Porter, *The Cambridge Illustrated History of Medicine*, Cambridge, Cambridge University Press, 1996.

R. Porter, *The greatest benefit to mankind: A medical history of humanity from antiquity to the present*, London, Harper Collins, 1997.

R.N. Prescott, Emancipist and Autocrat. The Life of Doctor William Redfern and his Relationship with Governor Macquarie, thesis, Australian National University, 1970.

J.C. Prichard, *A Treatise on Insanity and Other Disorders Affecting the Mind*, 1835/1995.

S. Quine, 'Sampling in non-numerical research', in C. Kerr, R. Taylor, and G. Heard (eds), *Handbook of Public Health Methods*, Sydney, McGraw-Hill, 1998.

C.S. Rabkin and F. Yellin, 'Cancer incidence in a population with a high prevalence of infection with human immunodeficiency virus type 1', *Journal of the National Cancer Institute*, vol. 86, 1995, pp. 1711–16.

M.V. Ragni, S.H. Belle, R.A. Jaffe, J.Locker, S. L. Duerstein, D.C. Bass, J.E. Addiego, L.M. Aledort, L.E. Barron, D.B. Brettler, G.R. Buchanan, J.C. Gill, B.M. Ewenstein, D.Green, M.W. Hilgartner, W.K. Hoots, T.Kisker, E.W. Lovrien, C.J. Rutehrford, N.L. Sanders, K.J. Smith, S.P. Stabler, S. Swindells, G.C. White, and L.A. Kingsley for the hemohpilia malignancy study group, 'AIDS associated NHL as primary and secondary AIDS diagnoses in hemophiliacs', *Journal of AIDS and Human Retrovirology*, vol. 13, 1996, pp. 78–86.

H. Reddel, C. Jenkins, and A. Woolcott, 'Diurnal Variability time to change asthma guidelines', *British Medical Journal*, vol. 319, no. 7201, 1999, pp. 45–7.

W.T. Reich (ed.). *Encyclopedia of Bioethics*, New York, The Free Press, 1978.

T. Richards and L. Richards, *NUD*IST*, Bundoora, Vic., Replee Pty Ltd, 1990.

T. Richards, L. Richards, J. McGalliard, and B. Sharrock, *NUDIST 2. 3 User Manual*, Eltham, Vic., Replee, 1992.

J.B. Ritchie, 'Ray Miles as a teacher and mentor', *Journal of Management Inquiry*, vol. 7, no. 4, Dec. 1998, pp. 307–8.

J. Ritchie, 'Using qualitative research to enhance the evidence-based practice of health care providers', *Australian Journal of Physiotherapy*, vol. 45, 1999, pp. 251–6.

J.E. Ritchie, 'There's something different in what's happening to us: Participatory action research in a work setting', *Promotion and Education*, vol. 3, no. 4, 1997, pp. 16–20.

J.E. Ritchie, Promoting the health and quality of life of residents of retirement villages, unpublished research report, NSW Ageing and Disability Department, 1999.

D. Roesler, 'Teach your people well', *Financial Executive*, 1997, vol. 13, no. 2, March/April, pp. 43–5.

G. Rose, L. Arlian, D. Bernstein, A. Grant, M. Lopez, J. Metzger, S. Wasserman, and T.A.E. Plattsmills, 'Evaluation of household dust mite exposure and levels of specific IGE and IGG antibodies in asthmatic patients enrolled in a trial of immunotherapy', *Journal of Allergy & Clinical Immunology*, vol. 97, no. 5, 1996, pp. 1071–8.

C.E. Rosenberg, *Explaining Epidemics and Other Studies in the History of Medicine*, New York, Cambridge University Press, 1992.

B. Rosner, *Fundamentals of Biostatistics*, 3rd edn, Boston, PWS-KENT, 1990.

K.J. Rothman and S. Greenland, *Modern Epidemiology*, Philadelphia, Lippincott-Raven, 1998.

D. Rowntree, *Statistics without Tears: A Primer for Non-mathematicians*, London, Penguin Books, 1991.

B. Russell, 'Science and ethics', in J. Rachels (ed.), *Ethical Theory 1: The Question of Objectivity*, Oxford, Oxford University Press, 1998, ch. 1, pp. 19–27.

K.F. Russell, 'Anatomy and the barber-surgeons', *Medical Journal of Australia*, vol. 1, 1973, pp. 1109–15.

D.L. Sackett, W.S. Richardson, W. Rosenberg, and R.B. Haynes, *Evidence-based Medicine*, Edinburgh, Churchill Livingstone, 1996.

W.C. Salmon, 'The importance of scientific understanding', *Causality and Explanation*, Oxford, Oxford University Press, 1998, ch. 5, pp. 79–91.

D. Saltman, '"Disease model" challenged', in P. Baume (ed.), *The Tasks of Medicine: An Ideology of Care*, Sydney, MacLennan & Petty, 1998, ch. 15, pp. 220–37.

D. Saltman, B. Veale, and G. Bloom, 'Developing a mental health resource for consumers', *Australian Journal of Primary Health – Interchange*, vol. 3, no. 4, 1997, pp. 40–8.

D.C. Saltman, I.W. Webster, and G.A. Therin, 'Older persons' definitions of good health: Implications for general practitioners', *Medical Journal of Australia*. 1989; vol. 150, no. 8, pp. 426, 428.

I. dos Santos Silva, *Cancer Epidemiology: Principles and Methods*, Lyon, International Agency for Research on Cancer, 1999.

O. Saphir, *Autopsy Diagnosis and Technique*, 4th edn, New York, Hoeber-Harber, USA, 1958.

School of Mathematics and Statistics, *DMS Tables*, Sydney, University of Sydney, 1991.

SAS Institute Inc., *Introducing the SAS system*, Version 6, 1ˢᵗ edn, Cary, NC: SAS Institute, 1991.

J. Sechzer, A. Griffin, and S.M. Pfafflin (eds), 'Forging a women's health research agenda: Policy issues for the 1990s', *Annals of the New York Academy of Sciences*, vol. 736, 1994, pp. 21–48.

P.J. Shaw, 'The incidence and nature of neurological morbidity following cardiac surgery: A review', *Perfusion*, vol. 4, no. 2, 1989, pp. 83–92.

P.G. Shekelle, J.P. Kahan, S.J. Bernstein, L.L. Leape, C.J. Kamberg, R.E. Park, 'The reproducibility of a method to identify the overuse and underuse of medical procedures', *The New England Journal of Medicine*, vol. 338, no. 26, 25 June 1998, pp. 1888–95.

W. Silverman, 'Effectiveness, efficiency . and subjective choice', *Perspectives in Biology and Medicine*, vol. 38, no. 3, 1995, pp. 480–95.

C. Singer, *A Short History of Anatomy from the Greeks to Harvey (The evolution of anatomy)*, New York, Dover Publishing, 1957.

S. Smith, 'The history and development of forensic medicine', *British Medical Journal*, vol. 1, 24 March 1951, pp. 599–607.

M.J. Solomon and R.S. McLeod, 'Surgery and the randomised controlled trial: Past, present and future', *Medical Journal of Australia*, vol. 169, 5 Oct. 1998, p. 380.

R.K. Spiro, 'A backward glance at the study of post-mortem anatomy, Part 1', *International Surgery*, vol. 56, 1971, pp. 27–40.

J.P. Spradley, *Participant Observation*, New York, Holt, Rinehart and Winston, 1980.

P. Sprent, *Applied Nonparametric Statistical Methods*, 2ⁿᵈ edn, London, Chapman & Hall, 1993.

R. Stake, 'Case studies', in N. Denzin and Y. Lincoln (eds), *Handbook of Qualitative Research*, Thousand Oaks, CA, Sage Publications, 1994.

D.W. Stewart and P.N. Shamdasani, *Focus Groups: Theory and Practice*, Newbury Park, CA, Sage Publications, 1990.

Southern Community Health Research Unit (SCHRU), *Planning Health Communities: A Guide to Doing Community Needs Assessment*, Bedford Park, SA, Flinders Medical Centre, 1991.

SPSS Inc., *SPSS Reference Guide*, Chicago, SPSS Inc., 1990.

StataCorp., *Stata Statistical Software: Release 6.0*, College Station, TX: Stata Corporation. 1999.

A. Strauss and J. Corbin, *Basics of Qualitative Research: Grounded Theory Procedures and Techniques*, Newbury Park, CA, Sage Publications, 1994.

D. Streiner and G. Norman, *Health Measurement Scales: A Practical Guide to their Development and Use*, New York, Oxford University Press, 1996.

Surgeon Redfern to Governor Macquarie 1814. Redfern's Report. HRA, ser 1, 8; 274.

E. Temkin and C.L. Temkin, *Ancient Medicine: Selected Papers of Ludwig Edelstein*, Baltimore, MD, Johns Hopkins University Press, 1987.

M. Testa and D. Simonson, 'Current concepts: Assessment of quality-of-life outcomes', *New England Journal of Medicine*, vol. 334, no. 13, 1996, pp. 835–40.

M. Torres, South American women's perceptions and experience of menopause, unpublished Master of Public Health project report, University of New South Wales, 1999.

F. Trede, 'The role of knowledge and artistry in clinical expertise: A pilot study with rheumology physiotherapists', *Focus on Health Professional Education: A multidisciplinary journal*, vol. 2, no. 1, 2000, pp. 48–57.

P. Trye, R. Jackson, R. L. Yee, and R. Beaglehole, 'Trends in the use of blood pressure lowering medications in Auckland, and associated costs, 1982–94', *New Zealand Medical Journal*, vol. 109, no. 1026, 1996, pp. 270–2.

K. Tyler, 'Mentoring programs link employees and experienced execs', *HRMagazine*, vol. 43, no. 5, April 1998, pp. 98–103.

United States Department of Health, Education, and Welfare, *Ethical Principles and Guidelines for the Protection of Human Subjects of Research*, DHEW Publication No. OS 78-0012, The Belmont Report, Washington DC, United States Department of Health, Education, and Welfare, 1978.

M.B. Van der Weyden, 'Databases and evidence-based medicine in general practice: We have built it, but will they come?', *Medical Journal of Australia*, vol. 170, 1999, pp. 52–3.

R.B. Vermeesch and K.E. Lindgren, *Business Law in Australia*, 9th edn, Sydney, 1999.

T. Voigt, M. Bailey, and M. Abramson, 'Air Pollution in the Latrobe Valley and its impact upon respiratory morbidity', *Australian and New Zealand Journal of Public Health*, vol. 22, no. 5, 1998, p. 556.

Y. Wadsworth, *Everyday Evaluation on the Run*, Melbourne Action Research Issues Association (Incorporated), 1991.

E.H. Walters and J.A.E. Walters, 'Many reports of RCTs give insufficient data for Cochrane reviewers', *British Medical Journal*, vol. 319, no. 7204, 1999, p. 257.

T.A. Welborn (ed.), *The Busselton Study: Mapping Population Health (Cardiovascular and Respiratory Disease Risk Factors In Busselton, Australia)*, Australian Medical Publishing Co., 1998.

D. Whitby, M.R. Howard, M. Tenant-Flowers, M.S. Brink, A. Copas, C. Boschoff, T. Hatzioannou, F.E.A. Suggett, D.M. Aldam, A.S. Denton, R.F. Miller, I.V.D. Weller, R.A. Weiss, R.S. Tedder, and T.F. Schulz, 'Detection of Kaposi's sarcoma associated herpesvirus in peripheral blood of HIV-infected individuals and progression to Kaposi's sarcoma', *Lancet*, vol. 346, 1995, pp. 799–802.

T.D. Wickens, *Multiway Contingency Tables Analysis for the Social Sciences*, Hillsdale, NJ, Lawrence Erlbaum, 1989.

R.R. Wilcox, *New Statistical Procedures for the Social Sciences: Modern Solutions to Basic Problems*, Hillsdale, NJ, Lawrence Erlbaum, 1987.

Z.R. Wolf and M.M. Heinzer, 'Substruction: Illustrating the connections from research question to analysis,' *Journal of Professional Nursing*, vol. 15, no. 1, 1999, pp. 33–7.

S.R. Woolfenden, J. Ritchie, R. Hanson, and V. Nossar, 'Parental use of a paediatric emergency department as an ambulatory care service', *Australian & New Zealand Journal of Public Health*, vol. 24, no. 2, 2000, pp. 204–6.

World Health Organization, *Basic Documents*, 26th edn, World Health Organization, Geneva, 1976.

World Health Organization, *Manual of the International Statistical Classification of Diseases, Injuries, and Causes of Death*, 9th revision, Geneva, World Health Organization, 1977.

World Health Organization. *Health Research Methodology: A Guide for Training in Research Methods*, Manilla, WHO Regional Office for the Western Pacific, 1992.

P. Wright, C. Jensen, and J.C. Wyatt, 'How to limit clinical errors in interpretation of data', *Lancet*, vol. 352, 7 Nov. 1998, pp. 1539–43.

J.M. Young and J.E. Ward, 'General practitioners' use of evidence databases', *Medical Journal of Australia*, vol. 170, 1999, pp. 56–8.

Index

Entries in **bold** indicate major entries.